Obstetric Triage and Emergency Care Protocols

Diane J. Angelini, EdD, CNM, NEA-BC, FACNM, FAAN, is the Director of Midwifery at Women & Infants Hospital and Clinical Professor, Department of Obstetrics and Gynecology at the Alpert Medical School of Brown University. Dr. Angelini was founding director of the nurse-midwifery graduate education programs at the University of Southern California and the University of Rhode Island. She is an advanced practice nurse executive, board certified. Her publications include 18 peer-reviewed journal articles, 13 nonpeer-reviewed publications, including two book chapters, and two books, *Case Studies in Perinatal Nursing* and *Perinatal Nursing*. She is the senior editor and founding coeditor of the *Journal of Perinatal and Neonatal Nursing*, associate editor of *Journal Watch Women's Health*, and past editorial consultant and current peer reviewer for the *Journal of Midwifery and Women's Health*. She is a fellow of the American Academy of Nursing, a fellow of the American College of Nurse Midwives, and, by invitation, a member of the International Academy of Nursing Editors. She is a national presenter and consultant in obstetric triage.

Donna LaFontaine, MD, SANE, is the former Director of the Division of Obstetrics and Gynecological Emergency Medicine at Women & Infants Hospital and Clinical Associate Professor in the Department of Obstetrics and Gynecology at the Alpert Medical School of Brown University. Her publishing credits include three journal articles and one book chapter. Dr. LaFontaine serves on several hospital committees including emergency preparedness, pain management, obstetrics and gynecology, and guidelines committee, all at Women & Infants Hospital. She is a certified sexual assault forensic examiner and has been directing the sexual assault program at Women & Infants Hospital since 2004. Dr. LaFontaine has received over 20 teaching awards throughout her 24-year career as a physician.

Obstetric Triage and Emergency Care Protocols

Editors

Diane J. Angelini, EdD, CNM, NEA-BC, FACNM, FAAN

Donna LaFontaine, MD, SANE

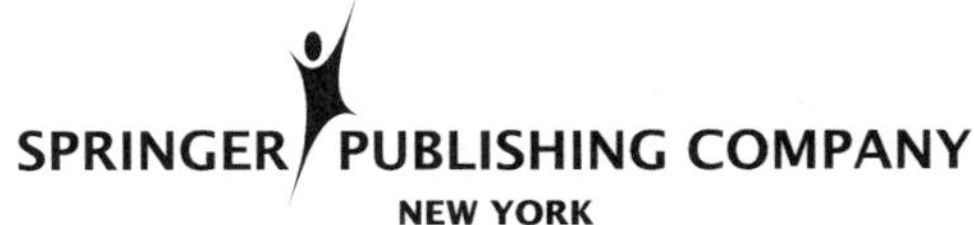

Springer Publishing Company, LLC
11 West 42nd Street
New York, NY 10036
www.springerpub.com

Acquisitions Editor: Margaret Zuccharini
Composition: Newgen Imaging

ISBN: 978-0-8261-0890-6
E-book ISBN: 978-0-8261-0891-3
12 13 14 15 / 5 4 3 2 1

Library of Congress Cataloging-in-Publication Data
Obstetric triage and emergency care protocols / Diane J. Angelini, Donna LaFontaine, editors.
p. ; cm.
Includes bibliographical references and index.
ISBN 978-0-8261-0890-6 — ISBN 978-0-8261-0891-3 (e-ISBN)
I. Angelini, Diane J., 1948- II. LaFontaine, Donna.
[DNLM: 1. Pregnancy Complications. 2. Emergency Medical Services—methods.
3. Triage--methods. WQ 240]
LC classification not assigned
618.2'025—dc23 2012017006

Printed in the United States of America by Bang Printing.

To my husband, David.

D. J. A

To all my patients—I hope I have taught them as much as they have taught me. And to John, Trini, and Jack—my work would be meaningless without their love and support.

D. L.

Contents

Contributors

Brenna L. Anderson, MD, MS
Chief of the Reproductive Infectious Disease Consultative Service
Women & Infants Hospital
Associate Professor
Obstetrics and Gynecology
Alpert Medical School of Brown University
Providence, Rhode Island

Diane J. Angelini, EdD, CNM, NEA-BC, FACNM, FAAN
Director of Midwifery
Women & Infants Hospital
Clinical Professor
Department of Obstetrics and Gynecology
Alpert Medical School of Brown University
Providence, Rhode Island

Karen Archabald, MD
Maternal Fetal Medicine Fellow
Department of Obstetrics and Gynecology
Yale School of Medicine
New Haven, Connecticut

Courtney Clark Bilodeau, MD
Attending Physician
Obstetric Medicine and Women's Primary Care
Women's Medicine Collaborative, Lifespan
Providence, Rhode Island

Robert J. Blaskiewicz, MD
Professor
Department of Obstetrics, Gynecology and Women's Health
St. Louis University School of Medicine
Director
General Division of Obstetrics
Director
Medical Student Education
St. Louis, Missouri

Chelsy Caren, MD, FACOG
Attending Obstetrician–Gynecologist
Division of Obstetrics and Gynecological Emergency Medicine
Women & Infants Hospital
Clinical Assistant Professor
Alpert Medical School of Brown University
Providence, Rhode Island

Rebecca Christophersen, MSN, PHMNP-BC
Psychiatric Mental Health Nurse Practitioner
Postpartum Depression Day Hospital
Women & Infants Hospital
Providence, Rhode Island

Agatha S. Critchfield, MD
Fellow
Maternal Fetal Medicine
Department of Obstetrics and Gynecology
Tufts Medical Center
Boston, Massachusetts

Luu Cortes Doan, MD, MPH
Resident
Obstetrics and Gynecology
Women & Infants Hospital
Alpert Medical School of Brown University
Providence, Rhode Island

David A. Edmonson, MD, FACS
Attending Physician
Breast Health Center
Women & Infants Hospital
Clinical Assistant Professor
Obstetrics and Gynecology
Alpert Medical School of Brown University
Providence, Rhode Island

Alex Friedman, MD
Fellow
Maternal Fetal Medicine
Department of Obstetrics and Gynecology
University of Pennsylvania School of Medicine
Philadelphia, Pennsylvania

Catherine Friedman, MD
Assistant Professor Clinical
Department of Psychiatry and Human Behavior
Alpert Medical School of Brown University
Providence, Rhode Island

Robyn A. Gray, DO, FACOG
Attending Obstetrician–Gynecologist
Division of Obstetrics and Gynecological Emergency Medicine
Clinical Assistant Professor
Department of Obstetrics and Gynecology
Alpert Medical School of Brown University
Providence, Rhode Island

Asha J. Heard, MD
Fellow
Maternal Fetal Medicine
Department of Obstetrics and Gynecology
Tufts Medical Center
Boston, Massachusetts

Elisabeth D. Howard, PhD, CNM
Midwife
Academic Midwifery Section
Women & Infants Hospital
Clinical Assistant Professor
Department of Obstetrics and Gynecology
Warren Alpert Medical School of Brown University
Providence, Rhode Island

Margaret Howard, PhD
Director
Postpartum Depression Day Hospital
Women & Infants Hospital
Clinical Associate Professor
Department of Psychiatry and Human Behavior
Department of Obstetric Medicine
Alpert Medical School of Brown University
Providence, Rhode Island

Linda A. Hunter, EdD, CNM
Midwife
Academic Midwifery Section
Women & Infants Hospital
Clinical Assistant Professor
Department of Obstetrics and Gynecology
Alpert Medical School of Brown University
Providence, Rhode Island

Moune Jabre Raughley, MD, MA, FACOG
Attending Obstetrician–Gynecologist
Division of Obstetrics and Gynecological Emergency Medicine
Women & Infants Hospital
Assistant Clinical Professor
Obstetrics and Gynecology
Alpert Medical School of Brown University
Providence, Rhode Island

Dotti C. James, PhD, RNC-OB, C-EFM
Director
Clinical Education
Talent Development and Optimization
Mercy, East Community
St. Louis, Missouri

Julie M. Johnson, MD
Maternal Fetal Medicine Specialist
Clinical Assistant Professor
Obstetrics and Gynecology
Alpert Medical School of Brown University
Providence, Rhode Island

Donna LaFontaine, MD, SANE
Attending Obstetrician–Gynecologist
Division of Obstetrics and Gynecological Emergency Medicine
Women & Infants Hospital
Clinical Associate Professor
Department of Obstetrics and Gynecology
Alpert Medical School of Brown University
Providence, Rhode Island

Lucia Larson, MD
Associate Professor
Medicine and Obstetrics and Gynecology
Alpert Medical School of Brown University
Providence, Rhode Island.
Division Director
Obstetric Medicine
Women's Medicine Collaborative, Lifespan
Providence, Rhode Island

Jan M. Kriebs, MSN, CNM, FACNM
Assistant Professor
Director
Midwifery Division
University of Maryland School of Medicine
Baltimore, Maryland

Mary Ann Maher, MSN, RNC-OB, C-EFM
Advanced Nurse Clinician
Labor and Delivery
Women's Evaluation Unit
Mercy Hospital
St. Louis, Missouri

Edie McConaughey, MS, CNM
Midwife
Academic Midwifery Section
Women & Infants Hospital
Senior Clinical Teaching Associate
Department of Obstetrics and Gynecology
Alpert Medical School of Brown University
Providence, Rhode Island

Mollie A. McDonnold, MD
Fellow
Maternal Fetal Medicine
University of Texas Medical Branch
Galveston, Texas

Alyson J. McGregor, MD, MA, FACEP
Attending Physician
Rhode Island Hospital Emergency Department
Assistant Professor
Emergency Medicine
Alpert Medical School of Brown University
Providence, Rhode Island

Srilakshmi Mitta, MD
Assistant Professor
Clinical Medicine
Department of Medicine
Division of Clinical Practice
Department of Obstetrics and Gynecology
Columbia University Medical Center
New York, New York

Martha Pizzarello, MD, FACOG
Attending Obstetrician–Gynecologist
Division of Obstetrics and Gynecological Emergency Medicine
Women & Infants Hospital
Assistant Clinical Professor
Alpert Brown School of Medicine
Providence, Rhode Island

Karen Rosene-Montella, MD
Senior Vice President
Women's Services and Clinical Integration, Lifespan
Vice Chair
Medicine for Quality and Outcomes
Professor
Medicine and Obstetrics and Gynecology
Alpert Medical School
Brown University
Providence, Rhode Island

Janet Singer, MSN, CNM
Midwife
Academic Midwifery Section
Women & Infants Hospital
Senior Clinical Teaching Associate
Department of Obstetrics and Gynecology
Alpert Medical School of Brown University
Providence, Rhode Island

Amy L. Snyder, MD, FACOG
Attending Obstetrician–Gynecologist
Division of Obstetrics and Gynecological Emergency Medicine
Women & Infants Hospital
Assistant Clinical Professor
Obstetrics and Gynecology
Alpert Medical School of Brown University
Providence, Rhode Island

Linda Steinhardt, MS, CNM, FNP-C
Midwife
Academic Midwifery Section
Women & Infants Hospital
Senior Clinical Teaching Associate
Department of Obstetrics and Gynecology
Alpert Medical School of Brown University
Providence, Rhode Island

Roxanne A. Vrees, MD, FACOG
Interim Director
Division of Obstetrics and Gynecological Emergency Medicine
Women & Infants Hospital
Associate Residency Program Director
Obstetrics and Gynecology
Women & Infants Hospital
Clinical Assistant Professor
Obstetrics and Gynecology
Alpert Medical School of Brown University
Providence, Rhode Island

Emily White, MD, MPH, FACOG
Attending Obstetrician–Gynecologist
Division of Obstetrics and Gynecological Emergency Medicine
Women & Infants Hospital
Assistant Clinical Professor
Obstetrics and Gynecology
Alpert Medical School of Brown University
Providence, Rhode Island

Preface

The idea for writing *Obstetric Triage and Emergency Care Protocols* has been long in coming, finally seeing its way through to completion. Working in obstetric triage units and obstetric emergency settings has formed a good part of the professional careers of the editors. We felt the time was right for a book on obstetric triage since many large hospitals have now developed such a unit or are beginning to expand obstetric emergency services. The use of a handbook/e-book to guide the clinician in the obstetric triage setting seemed appropriately timed.

As noted in Chapter 1, obstetric triage has developed into a specialty area/unit within obstetrics with multifunctional aspects. In some institutions, the obstetric triage setting is primarily a screening area for laboring women; while in other settings, it serves multiple functions including labor evaluation, assessment of obstetric emergencies, and management of obstetric conditions post viability.

We developed the use of narrative protocols as the primary format for this book. These guidelines are partitioned both by timing in pregnancy and by topic to provide a quick read and guide for the learner. The book is robust in imaging and rich in tables, figures, and exhibits to enhance learning and quick assessment. A standard format is primarily used across most chapters. Quick and easy access to topically focused guidelines is tailored to the obstetric triage and obstetric emergency setting. The two introductory chapters provide the framework, background, and legal considerations encompassing obstetric triage. Management of obstetric conditions in early pregnancy, often at the threshold of viability, is the second section followed by clinical management of obstetric and medical conditions presenting at greater than viability including fetal evaluation, labor management, and common obstetric and medical complications. Other conditions, seen throughout pregnancy, such as surgical emergencies, infections, and biohazardous exposure are included. Lastly, postpartum complications commonly seen in obstetric triage or an emergency setting are presented.

The primary audience for this handbook/e-book encompasses all advanced health care practitioners who work in an obstetric triage or obstetric emergency setting. This would include all levels of residents, both obstetric and those in emergency services, obstetricians, emergency department physicians, family practice physicians, midwives, nurse practitioners, physician assistants, and radiologists. Learners in all these subspecialties will find this book helpful. It is our hope that this book, in its narrative format, will provide a quick read, timely access by topic and gestational age, up-to-date imaging, and evidence-based clinical management.

Diane J. Angelini
Donna LaFontaine

Acknowledgments

We would like to thank the following people who assisted in bringing this book to completion:

Dena Bassett for her administrative support and detail-oriented work in getting every chapter in order prior to submission to the publisher.

Dr. Liz Lazarus who supplied us with multiple images to support each chapter in this book, and without whose assistance we could not have completed this work.

We also want to thank Dotty Calvano and Dr. Raymond Powrie who facilitated obtaining the authorization to utilize images and forms from Women & Infants Hospital.

Others who helped us are Nancy Ross, Librarian at Women & Infants Hospital, Dr. Rebecca Allen, Dr. Julie Johnson, and other reviewers who assisted in reviewing manuscripts and advising on content.

I: INTRODUCTION

Overview of Obstetric Triage and Potential Pitfalls

1

Diane J. Angelini

The concept of triage as applied to obstetrics has come of age since the 1980s and early 1990s. Obstetric (OB) triage units were created for various reasons, some of which include increased patient volume in obstetrics, more effective utilization and productivity of staff and resources, need for heightened assessment of fetal and maternal surveillance, and assessment of labor. A review of the draft core competencies for the new Society of OB/GYN Hospitalists now includes OB triage content (Jancin, 2011). Clearly, OB triage has become one of the most critical perinatal services to emerge in the last two decades in OB care within the United States (Angelini, 2006).

FUNCTIONS OF OB TRIAGE UNITS

Two of the most common reasons for development of OB triage units have been (a) decompression of labor and birthing settings, which have become burdened by numerous OB evaluations (many of these women do not go on to deliver); and (b) evaluation of all labor complaints in a setting outside of labor/delivery, thus freeing up critical bed capacity within labor and delivery proper.

The increased demand to evaluate urgent and emergent pregnancy complaints outside the office setting has added to the need for a functioning unit in which all pregnancy complaints, including labor, can be fully evaluated. Many pregnant women present to OB triage in prodromal, latent, or false labor. However, laboring women can be more effectively evaluated in a setting without utilizing a labor bed. This improves patient flow in labor and delivery, decreases turnover costs, and increases bed capacity to better accommodate women in more active labor. In addition, many OB triage units with large OB volume function as a holding unit until inpatient labor beds become available.

The OB triage unit often improves utilization of both personnel and bed capacity. It manages OB volume as a "gatekeeper," evaluating complaints, prioritizing care, and improving inpatient utilization. OB triage can help to limit diversions from labor and delivery at a time of high census, as well. Multiple functions of OB triage units are noted in Exhibit 1.1.

Most OB triage units are located within close proximity to labor and birthing units (Angelini, 1999). However, there has been wide diversity

EXHIBIT 1.1

Multiple Functions of OB Triage Units

- Labor assessment and evaluation
- Decompression of labor and delivery
- Use as a holding unit (when labor and delivery is at capacity)
- Fetal evaluation and assessment
- Evaluation of medical and OB complaints (often after office/clinic hours)
- Initial stabilization of OB complications
- Evaluation of OB referrals/transfers
- Triaging of OB telephone calls
- Selected OB procedures
- Source of OB care when normal source of medical care is inaccessible or unavailable

as to where OB triage units are located; whether they are placed in close proximity to labor and delivery or whether they are remote from the labor and delivery setting. Often, pregnant women with OB complaints at less than viability (23–24 weeks) are evaluated in a main emergency department. Pregnancies greater than viability are mostly evaluated in OB triage units within close proximity to labor and delivery (Angelini, 1999). Staffing for OB units can include attending OB/GYN physicians, nurse midwives, nurse practitioners, and OB residents, among others. Access to direct imaging, laboratory services, fetal evaluation, consultations, and immediate care by an OB provider makes OB triage units highly valuable in delivering high reliability perinatal care. OB triage is also a setting where women with nonemergent OB and medical conditions present when their normal source of medical care is inaccessible or unavailable (Matteson, Weitzen, LaFontaine, & Phipps, 2008).

OB TRIAGE, ACTIVE LABOR, AND EMTALA

Labor and birthing units, and consequently OB triage units, meet several criteria for the Emergency Medical Treatment and Active Labor Act (EMTALA), which is part of the Federal Omnibus Bill under the direction of the Centers for Medicare and Medicaid (Glass, Rebstock, & Handberg, 2004). EMTALA is the federal law governing emergency medical treatment and active labor (EMTALA, 2011). Pregnant women seek care when they have an urgent pregnancy problem, often without a previously scheduled appointment; typically more than one-third of all laboring visits or OB visits are unscheduled (Caliendo, Millbauer, Moore, & Kitchen, 2004). EMTALA defines an emergency medical condition as one that manifests itself in acute symptoms of sufficient severity such that the absence of immediate medical attention could reasonably be expected to result in or pose a threat to the health and safety of a pregnant woman or unborn child. EMTALA also mandates that all pregnant women presenting to an emergency department, labor, or triage setting have a medical screening examination (MSE).

EMTALA mandates that (a) medical treatment be provided so that no material deterioration of the pregnancy condition is likely to result from or occur during transfer from a facility or (b) that the woman has delivered the child and the placenta. With EMTALA, routinely keeping patients waiting so long that they leave against medical advice (AMA) can also be a violation of the federal law. The EMTALA enforcement process is governed by the Department of Health and Human Services (DHHS), Centers for Medicare and Medicaid, which has the authority to pull facility and provider status. In addition, the office of the Inspector General has the authority to execute facility and practitioner fines (Glass et al., 2004).

CATEGORIES OF RISK IN OB TRIAGE

Major categories of risk in OB triage involve patient safety concerns. These include, but are not limited to, assessment in a timely manner, appropriate and complete evaluation and documentation, discharge from OB triage without evidence of fetal well-being, recognizing active labor and discharging the pregnant woman in false labor, delay in timely response from consultants, and the use of clinical handoffs.

Assessment in a Timely Manner

In an OB triage unit, pregnant women who are contracting need to be assessed ahead of other women who present with less emergent OB complaints. The fact that pregnant women are contracting and could be in active labor places them within the purview of EMTALA. Any pregnant woman at greater than viability with complaints of uterine contractions, needs quick and emergent assessment. However, patient care policies around this issue should be flexible and not overly specific. Strict guidelines can often open the door to liability if not met for every patient encounter. However, it is critical to avoid treatment delays. It may become necessary to move up the chain of command/communication when disagreements or differences in clinical opinion occur to prevent any treatment delays.

It is crucial to determine what the parameters for fetal assessment are in each specific OB setting. However, in most cases, if there is a combined OB and GYN unit, pregnant women would be assessed ahead of non-pregnant women or ahead of those women with less emergent problems. Pregnant women with decreased fetal movement and with active bleeding are two examples of the need for emergent screening. It is critical to place pregnant women with a viable pregnancy on a fetal monitor and obtain a baseline fetal heart rate tracing. If the fetal tracing is nonreactive or a non-Category 1 tracing, further fetal testing measures will need to be implemented, and intrauterine resuscitative measures initiated. Notification to the provider of fetal/maternal status needs to occur promptly, and patient care expedited. OB triage personnel have the responsibility to initiate intrauterine resuscitative measures, notify the provider in a timely fashion of nonreactive fetal status, initiate an action plan, and ensure a safe transfer of care to the intrapartum provider responsible for the longer term management plan.

Appropriate and Complete Evaluation and Documentation

Pregnant women often present to OB triage with the following generalized symptoms: abdominal pain, vomiting, diarrhea, nausea, epigastric pain, and dizziness. It is usually risky to address such complaints via the telephone alone. Differential diagnoses will always include both pregnant and nonpregnant possibilities. Use of imaging techniques such as ultrasound, computed tomography, and magnetic resonance imaging, as well as consultations and extensive laboratory data, may be necessary to complete a full and adequate maternal and fetal evaluation and workup.

Access to timely laboratory and imaging results is crucial in the OB triage setting so as to not discharge a pregnant woman who might still have an impending, emergent problem. For example, appendicitis and cholecystitis, often evaluated in the triage setting, are the two most common reasons for non-OB surgical intervention in pregnancy and can be associated with significant maternal/fetal morbidity (Gilo, Amini, & Landy, 2009). Full documentation of all negative findings and counseling of the pregnant patient are necessary. In addition, there is no downside to extended observation when clinical findings are unclear or symptomatology is rapidly changing.

Discharge From OB Triage Without Evidence of Fetal Well-Being

Assessing the fetal heart rate tracing, or following up on changes within the fetal monitor strip while a woman is in triage, becomes part of the overall assessment even though a pregnant woman may be evaluated in OB triage for a different pregnancy complaint. Two commonly seen OB triage liability issues regarding fetal status are as follows: failure to adequately assess the fetal heart rate tracing and failure to respond to a non-Category 1 fetal tracing. Discharge from the OB triage unit must include documentation of fetal well-being.

Recognizing Active Labor and Discharging the Pregnant Woman in False Labor

Evaluating and assessing active labor are part of the EMTALA law. Consequently, it triggers an emergency medical condition that needs to be assessed by a qualified medical provider (QMP). EMTALA regulations (Angelini & Mahlmeister, 2005) state that a woman who presents having contractions is only deemed stable when (a) the infant and placenta are delivered, (b) labor contractions are gone, or (c) it is certified that the woman is in false labor. EMTALA requires an MSE to determine labor, especially if transfer is necessary.

The Technical Advisory Group (TAG) of the Centers for Medicaid and Medicare make recommendations for any changes to the EMTALA law. Effective October 1, 2006, a certified nurse midwife or other qualified medical person, acting within the scope of his/her practice, can certify that a pregnant woman is in false labor. Prior to this time, the Centers for Medicare and Medicaid stated that only a physician could certify false labor.

The EMTALA rules state that a woman experiencing contractions is in true labor, unless it is certified that the woman is in false labor. When a QMP makes a diagnosis that a woman is in false labor, the QMP is required to certify that diagnosis before the woman can be discharged. Nurses acting in this role need to ensure that they are credentialed by their institutions (hospital bylaws), and that it is within their scope of practice to perform this function within the state nurse practice act or state rules and regulations governing nursing practice. Telephone consultation with the medical provider may be necessary prior to patient discharge depending on who is the designated qualified medical person.

Delay in Timely Response From Consultants

EMTALA mandates lists of consultants who are on-call. These must be available at all times or be readily available electronically. Some reasons for delay in response from consultants include the following: not relaying a sense of urgency to the consultant, miscommunication issues between parties, or unclear consultative relationships. It is important to document when the consultant called back or the number of times it took to receive a response. Record keeping is an essential component of EMTALA. Both on-call lists and patient logs must be available upon request.

Use of Clinical Handoffs

Handoffs are one of the biggest concerns for patient safety in the OB triage setting (Kitch et al., 2008; Solet, Norvell, Rutan, & Frankel, 2005). Handoffs need to be practiced repetitively to reduce errors. Checklists and computerized charting help to avoid errors during handoff situations. Clinical handoffs commonly occur at change of shift, with change in provider status, change in the level of provider, change in patient status, and during a team update or debriefing.

In 2008, the Joint Commission called for a standardized approach to handoffs through communication with an opportunity to ask and respond to questions (Joint Commission Perspectives in Patient Safety, 2006). One recommended technique using the concept of Situation, Background, Assessment, Recommendation (SBAR) utilizes a framework for communication among members of the health care team regarding a patient's condition (Bello, Quinn, & Horrell, 2011; Freitag & Carroll, 2011).

Patient handoffs involve the transfer of rights, duties, and obligations from one person or team to another. It is best performed if it involves face-to-face communication. There have been reports of patient harm during handoffs and an increase in handoff errors with trainees. The use of the electronic medical record has been helpful to minimize problematic handoffs (Kitch et al., 2008). Errors in judgment, teamwork breakdowns, lack of technical competence, and communication errors (Ong & Coiera, 2011) have been reported during handoffs (Kitch et al., 2008), especially with trainees (Singh, Thomas, Peterson, & Studdert, 2007) and potentially during resident signouts (Angelini, Stevens, MacDonald, Wiener, & Wieczorek, 2009; Arora, Kao, Lovinger, Seiden, & Meltzer, 2007). Potential errors with clinical patient handoffs are noted in Exhibit 1.2.

EXHIBIT 1.2

Errors During Clinical Patient Handoffs in OB Triage

- Errors in judgment
- Teamwork breakdowns
- Medication errors
- Lack of technical competence
- Lack of supervision with handoff difficulties
- Increased errors with trainees
- Misdiagnosis and decision making
- Lack of adequate monitoring of the patient or situation
- Miscommunication and communication breakdowns during intra-hospital transfers
- Lack of communication of critical information

Source: Adapted from Kitch et al. (2008), Singh et al. (2007), Arora et al. (2007), and Ong & Coiera (2011).

OTHER SAFETY-RELATED ISSUES IN OB TRIAGE

Other patient-related safety issues in OB triage involve excessive waiting times, crowding, and delays in early recognition of significant clinical events. There is often a myriad of patient complaints at the triage desk, which makes the task of effective triage challenging. The first person to assess the pregnant woman is the gatekeeper and this is the starting place for information. Utilizing a guided script may be useful for providers and caregivers and may ensure the appropriate assessment of symptoms. Is the woman contracting or not? Is there fetal movement or not? Knowing the key questions to ask helps to expedite the assessment process at the point of care avoiding placing a potentially at-risk or high-risk patient in the waiting room.

At this critical point, it may be useful to have a more experienced medical or nursing provider at the triage desk or entry. Using standardized screening guidelines or checklists (for questions, laboratory tests, etc.) can improve reliability of care and safety for patients at the point of service. Timely access to clinical databases, both online and hard copy records as well as provider on-call lists, improves what can be accomplished at the starting point in the triage process.

Crowding is an issue commonly noted in OB triage settings. Ironically, many OB triage units were initially developed to decompress the crowding associated with labor/delivery units. However, triage units can themselves become overwhelmed and overcrowded. Having a surge policy to deal with crowding is critical, especially when a clinical crisis arises, as was seen with the H1N1 virus. An alert to patient crowding is necessary so that contingency plans can be implemented. Use of fast track rooms and observation/holding rooms is helpful. Deciding which pregnant women can/should be seen and others with less emergent problems kept waiting is important. Diversion, if implemented, will trigger strict EMTALA guidelines. If the institution is a tertiary level OB/neonatal unit, and if it is a catchment area for rural facilities with minimal OB services, most units will rarely be placed on diversion status. Overcrowding, in general, cannot affect decision making or timing of care. If pregnant women are regularly kept waiting as a routine, this could trigger an EMTALA violation. Minimization of any waiting time would be a long-term goal for an OB triage unit.

When labor units or inpatient antepartum units are at capacity, OB triage can easily back up and experience overcrowding. Alerts to the potential for emergency births and the impact on all patients in labor who are awaiting care, need careful consideration.

Early recognition of events occurring in the waiting area or early in the screening process can avoid missteps and treatment delays later on. Deciding if the pregnancy is viable or not, often 24 weeks or greater, and what resuscitative parameters are necessary, can be helpful. Is there a need for more targeted fetal monitoring and assessment, and is the patient stable or not, will all affect timing of care and early treatment decisions. Making an accurate and early assessment will avoid going down the wrong clinical pathway later on.

Risk Reduction Strategies in OB Triage

All care providers need to be knowledgeable about the standard of care in the OB triage setting and familiar with the EMTALA law as it applies to pregnant women who are contracting, in active labor, or undergoing transfer. Knowledge and familiarity with best practices, guidelines, and hospital policies are imperative. Clinical management is always driven by best evidence. Use of computerized databases at the point of care is useful in this regard. The ability to access medical records in the electronic medical record system or having a hard copy is key. Ease of access to consultants and knowing where the consultant or on-call lists are posted adds to efficiency of service. Having access to an OB generalist/internist as well as specialists can be helpful when medical, surgical, and OB emergencies arise.

Evaluating patient status and disposition minimally every 4 hours and having a plan for any ongoing observation are critical. Communicating this plan among all care providers, especially if working in large teams, is necessary to decrease patient errors and improve safety.

Establishing thresholds for care, especially if telephone triage is part of the OB triage unit, can be useful. Use a chain of command/communication policy to resolve disputes and have an escalation policy available. Be mindful of transfer of care to another service or institution and the appropriate documentation and level of personnel needed for safe transport. Begin to assess the number of handoffs that occur and develop ways to decrease these numbers. Audits of sentinel events, use of debriefings (Arafeh, Hansen, & Nichols, 2010), mock sessions and drills, team training, simulation, and identification of near misses are all good quality measures and strategies. Missed opportunities and good catches should be reviewed and become part of a standardized quality improvement program for OB triage (Mahlmeister, 2006).

Staff competency and competency maintenance need to be documented and available if requested by review agencies. Numerous documentation issues also need to be addressed in triage. These include the need for complete notes as well as transfer notes, medication reconciliation, review and rereview of fetal tracings as necessary, procedures, laboratory findings, discussion with consultants, timing of calls, negative/positive findings, and written/oral discharge instructions.

PROPOSED FUTURE STANDARDS AND QUALITY ISSUES FOR OB TRIAGE UNITS

Call backs for at-risk pregnant women who departed OB triage without being seen and those who left against medical advice can be developed as part of a quality improvement program. Direct patient surveys sent to women post clinical care are always a useful tool. Evaluation of length of stay (LOS) as well as time to provider and admission-to-transfer time can also be tracked and compared with national benchmarks. Assessment of the average number of handoffs, outcomes during handoffs, and addressing ongoing issues are a good starting place for quality monitoring in OB triage. A review of readmits and rerepresentations, as with laboring women or those with recurring abdominal pain, may be warranted.

Some common standards for evaluation of care in an OB triage unit include evaluation of the following: women discharged without evidence of fetal well-being or discharged in active labor, delays in initiating fetal assessment or incorrectly managing fetal tracings, and timeliness of emergency drug initiation (i.e., with hypertension/preeclampsia). Developing a quality improvement plan, utilizing some of the above standards, can pave the way toward improved patient safety in OB triage settings.

REFERENCES

Angelini, D. (1999). The utilization of nurse midwives as providers of obstetric triage services. *Journal of Nurse Midwifery, 44*(5), 431–438.

Angelini, D. (2006). Obstetric triage: State of the practice. *Journal of Perinatal and Neonatal Nursing, 20*(1), 74–75.

Angelini, D. J., & Mahlmeister, L. (2005). Liability in triage: Management of EMTALA regulations and common obstetric risks. *Journal of Midwifery and Women's Health, 50*(6), 472–478.

Angelini, D., Stevens, E., MacDonald, A., Wiener, S., & Wieczorek, B. (2009). Obstetric triage: Models and trends in resident education by midwives. *Journal of Midwifery and Women's Health, 54*(4), 294–300.

Arafeh, J. M., Hansen, S. S., & Nichols, A. (2010). Debriefing in simulation-based learning: Facilitating a reflective discussion. *Journal of Perinatal and Neonatal Nursing, 24*(4), 302–309.

Arora, V., Kao, J., Lovinger, D., Seiden, S. C., & Meltzer, D. (2007). Medication discrepancies in resident sign-outs and their potential to harm. *Journal of General Internal Medicine, 22*(12), 1751–1755.

Bello, J., Quinn, P., & Horrell, L. (2011). Maintaining patient safety through innovation: an electic SBAR communication tool. *Computer Informatics Nursing, 29*(9), 481–483.

Caliendo, C., Millbauer, L., Moore, B., & Kitchen, E. (2004). Obstetric triage and EMTALA. *AWHONN Lifelines, 8*(5), 442–448.

EMTALA. (2011). Regulations and guidance. Retrieved from http://www.cms.gov

Freitag, M., & Carroll, V. S. (2011). Handoff communication using failure modes and effects analysis to improve the transition in care process. *Quality Management in Health Care, 20*(2), 103–109.

Gilo, N. B., Amini, D., & Landy, H. J. (2009) Appendicitis and cholecystitis in pregnancy. *Clinic in Obstetrics and Gynecology, 52*(4), 586–596.

Glass, D. L., Rebstock, J., & Handberg, E. (2004). Emergency Treatment and Labor Act (EMTALA). Avoiding the pitfalls. *Journal of Perinatal and Neonatal Nursing, 18*(2), 103–114.

Jancin, B. (2011). OB/GYN hospitalists hold inaugural meeting. *Ob Gyn News, 46*(11), p. 1, 7.

Joint Commission Perspectives in Patient Safety. (2006). Improving handoff communications: Meeting national patient safety. Goal, Z.E. *Joint Commission Resources, 6*(8), 9–15.

Kitch, B., Cooper, J., Zapol, W., Marder, J., Karson, A., Hutter, M., & Campbell, E. G. (2008). Handoffs causing patient harm: A survey of medical and surgical house staff. *Joint Commission Journal on Quality and Patient Safety, 34(10)*, 563–570.

Mahlmeister, L. (2006) Best practices in perinatal care: Reporting "near misses" and "good catches" as a risk reduction strategy. *Journal of Perinatal and Neonatal Nursing, 20*(3), 197–199.

Matteson, K. A., Weitzen, S. H., LaFontaine, D., Phipps, M. G. (2008). Accessing care: Use of a specialized women's emergency care facility for non-emergent problems. *Journal of Women's Health, 17*(2), 269–277.

Ong, M. S., & Coiera, E. (2011). A systematic review of failures in handoffs communication during intrahospital transfers. *Joint Commission Journal on Quality and Patient Safety, 37*, (6), 274–284.

Singh, H., Thomas, E. J., Peterson, L. A., & Studdert, D. M. (2007). Medical errors involving trainees: A study of closed malpractice claims from 5 insurers. *Archives of Internal Medicine, 167*(19), 2030–2036.

Solet, D., Norvell, J., Rutan, G., Frankel, R. (2005). Lost in translation: Challenges and opportunities in physician-to-physician communication during patient handoffs. *Academic Medicine, 80*(12), 1094–1099.

Legal Considerations in Obstetric Triage: EMTALA and HIPAA

2

Jan M. Kriebs

A pregnant woman presenting to obstetric triage may have a pregnancy-related problem, a medical condition complicating pregnancy, an injury, or simply be anticipating the birth of a healthy child. Legal requirements for emergency and labor care are addressed specifically by the Emergency Medical Treatment and Active Labor Act (EMTALA) of 1986 and the Health Information Portability and Accountability Act (HIPAA) of 1996. Documentation and follow-up care, as essential components of the triage process, are discussed in the context of legal liability.

EMERGENCY MEDICAL TREATMENT AND ACTIVE LABOR ACT (EMTALA)

The requirements placed on institutions by EMTALA are possibly the most critical legal concerns specific to obstetric triage. The law was passed to ensure public access to emergency services including labor and birth care. It prevents discrimination based on financial status, that is, whether one has insurance or the ability to self pay. The guarantee of care extends only to hospitals that accept Medicare; however, virtually all nonmilitary hospitals in the United States fall under the statute.

The law applies to every person seeking emergency care. The ability to pay for care does not eliminate a hospital's duty to meet the EMTALA standards (Cohen, 2007). Even if an insurance plan requires that care be received in certain hospitals, other facilities cannot turn someone away on that basis. In practice, any claim of discriminatory care (e.g., based on race, religion, lifestyle choices) may be considered under EMTALA.

The burden of EMTALA falls on the hospital, not the provider (Dowdy, Friend, & Rangel, 1996). This becomes an issue when community providers cover emergency services in rotation or when providers who are not physicians are the primary caregivers in the emergency department. It is the facility's task to maintain adequate staffing within the limits of the hospital's ability to provide care and to ensure that staff members understand the requirements of EMTALA. The civil penalty to a hospital for a single negligent violation is $50,000 ($25,000 for hospitals with fewer than 100 beds). In addition, any provider who violates EMTALA may also be subject to a civil penalty of $50,000. As Bitterman (2002) points out, the Centers for Medicare and Medicaid Services do not care whether harm has come to a woman, but whether the rules concerning care and transfer have been broken. Repeated violations can lead to the hospital's or provider's exclusion from Medicare and Medicaid participation.

The federal EMTALA law does not take the place of state liability tort laws. A diagnosis rendered in good faith may be in error, leading to an adverse outcome and legal liability for poor care. Failure to diagnose or treat is a medical malpractice issue. So, for example, the misdiagnosis of an ectopic pregnancy as a spontaneous abortion will generate a liability claim, but in general, not an EMTALA claim. Care that is not adequate to find the cause of emergent symptoms does not fall under EMTALA, unless it can be shown that the individual was not screened in the same way as any other patient (Hughes, 2008).

EMTALA defines an emergency as any "condition manifesting itself by acute symptoms of sufficient severity (including severe pain) such that the absence of immediate medical attention could reasonably be expected to result in placing the individual's health (or the health of an unborn child) in serious jeopardy, serious impairment to bodily functions, or serious dysfunction of bodily organs, or with respect to a pregnant woman who is having contractions that there is inadequate time to effect a safe transfer to another hospital before delivery, or that transfer may pose a threat to the health or safety of the woman or the unborn child" (EMTALA, 1986).

The essential components of the law include medical evaluation and transfer of care. Any person presenting to an emergency department (ED; or an obstetric triage unit if that is where pregnant women are evaluated) must receive a medical screening examination (MSE) that goes beyond the initial triage (EMTALA, 1986). The woman must then be treated for the emergency condition, including stabilization prior to transport. Nonemergent conditions are not covered under EMTALA solely because someone has been presented to an ED or obstetric suite. In practice, however, many facilities provide initial treatment for routine conditions.

Medical Screening Examination (MSE)

An MSE is different from triage, which determines in what order or how rapidly an individual must be seen. Although triage initiates care, it does not complete the hospital's duty under EMTALA. The MSE is provided by an appropriate licensed provider and should be similar in all women based on initial complaint. It includes the appropriate tests or procedures to identify conditions suspected based on history and physical examination. This requirement speaks to the benefit of standardizing guidelines for common conditions. Clinical judgment always plays a role in patient evaluation. The rationale for providing care that is different from the norm must be documented. Excluding tests out of a cost or time concern may expose the hospital to an EMTALA claim.

Only in cases of labor are other health care practitioners (certified nurse-midwives) specifically mentioned as appropriate providers of a MSE. When a nonphysician provider is assigned to perform the MSE, then the job description and credentialing documents must clearly reflect the facility's approval of this role. Whether or when a physician should review triage decisions made by another provider is also part of the institution's protocols.

Emergency Treatment

Following the MSE, a hospital is required to ensure that appropriate care is provided to all outpatients in the emergency unit. There is no national standard for care required by EMTALA. The level of care provided varies depending on the availability of services (Cohen, 2007). For example, a hospital that does not offer obstetric care will transfer the woman who presents with possible preterm labor. Another hospital with obstetric practitioners available will evaluate the same woman, treat, and discharge her home.

Treatment includes the provision of appropriate tests and procedures. It also includes follow-up care mandated by the emergency condition. However, if a woman refuses further care or refuses transport, then the EMTALA criteria for discharge have been met. Necessary documentation includes what treatment was recommended and refused, and that risks and benefits of both treatment and no treatment were explained. Just as with anyone leaving "against medical advice" or AMA, having the woman sign a refusal of treatment is best practice.

Transport

Reasons to transfer include need for a higher level of care, lack of capacity at the transferring hospital, and/or patient request for transport (see Exhibit 2.1 for specific transport criteria). Just as a woman can refuse a transfer and decline further treatment, a woman has the right to request transfer away from a facility prior to stabilizing treatment. This regulation is found at 42 CFR 489.24(e)(1)(ii)(A) (EMTALA.com, 2011).

Under EMTALA, transports must be "appropriate"; the medical benefits have to outweigh the risks. For example, the woman must be stable for transport (e.g., not in active labor) or the danger of remaining in the original location must be greater than the risk of giving birth in an ambulance. The decision that transport is necessary rests with the referring physician, not the receiving physician. As long as the receiving hospital can provide the needed services and has the space to do so, it is obligated under the law to accept transfers. The complete available records from the transporting hospital are to travel with the

EXHIBIT 2.1

Requirements for Transport Under EMTALA

- Medical screening examination (MSE)
- Stabilization within the abilities of transferring facility
- Need for services not available at transferring facility or medical benefits of transport outweigh risks or patient/responsible person requests transfer
- Contact with receiving hospital to approve/accept transport
- Written certification by physician of need
- Records sent with the patient
- Appropriate method of transport used

Source: EMTALA (1986).

EXHIBIT 2.2

EMTALA Transfer Form

Women & Infants Hospital
EMTALA Physician Assessment and Certification

Patient Condition

1. _____ The patient has been stabilized such that within reasonable medical probability, no material deterioration of the patient's condition or the condition of the unborn child(ren) is likely to result from transfer.
2. _____ The patient's condition has not stabilized.
3. _____ The patient is in labor.

Transfer Requirements

1. _____ The receiving facility, ______________________________, has available space and qualified personnel for treatment as acknowledged by: ____ __________________________.
2. _____ The receiving facility has agreed to accept transfer and to provide appropriate medical treatment as acknowledged by: ________ ____ __________.
3. _____ Appropriate medical records of the examination and treatment of the patient are provided at the time of transfer.
4. _____ The patient will be transferred by qualified personnel and transportation equipment as required, including the use of necessary and medically appropriate life support measures.

Provider Certification

I have examined the patient and explained the following risks and benefits of being transferred/refusing transfer to the patient:
____
____
____

Based on these reasonable risks and benefits to the patient and/or newborn child(ren), and based upon the information available at the time of the patient's examination, I certify that the medical benefits reasonably to be expected from the provision of appropriate medical treatment at another medical facility outweigh the increased risks, if any to the individual's medical condition from effecting the transfer.

____
Signature of physician or other qualified medical person **Date**

____
Title ____

Source: Courtesy of Women & Infants Hospital, Providence, Rhode Island.

woman. As long as the emergency condition persists, EMTALA dictates the procedures required. Financial concerns cannot overrule the need for transfer.

Transfer, particularly of an unstable patient, requires documentation of the patient's condition, transfer requirements, and certification that the provider has counseled the woman appropriately. See Exhibit 2.2 for an example of an EMTALA transfer form.

Labor and Birth

Labor is a special case under EMTALA, with a definition that runs counter to both the original title of the act and standard obstetric practice. As defined by EMTALA, labor means the process of childbirth beginning with the latent or early phase of labor and continuing through the delivery of the placenta. A woman experiencing contractions is in true labor unless a physician, certified nurse midwife, or other qualified medical person acting within the scope of practice as defined in hospital medical staff bylaws and state law, certifies that, after a reasonable time of observation, the woman is in false labor (EMTALA, 1986).

No reference is made to any other specific condition in the law. In the case of childbirth, care to stabilize or resolve (i.e., deliver) the pregnancy is required. Although latent labor is not "false" in a medical sense, a difficulty in interpreting EMTALA arises because the language used in the law is not the same as that used by health care practitioners. Because the law defines labor as the onset of contractions and refers to latent labor, the individual providing the MSE must be able to justify the decision to discharge. A woman with two prior cesarean sections and preterm contractions may need to be admitted as unstable for discharge (or transported to a facility with more appropriate obstetric services), whereas a primigravida at term with the same pelvic examination might not. The normal variation in labor progress and a host of contributing factors—parity, prior surgeries, contraction pattern, fetal well-being—make it imperative that the discharge note clearly states the rationale for deciding that a woman is not in active labor.

Record Keeping and Patient Follow-Up

After the emergency is resolved, information needs to flow back to a woman's primary provider. The "long, fragile feedback loops" that come into play whenever multiple institutions or providers are involved in care can lead to failures in diagnosis and timely treatment of complications (Gandhi & Lee, 2010). New or altered medications, referrals, pending results all can be lost when communication is not ensured. One study found that as many as 41% of discharged patients had pending tests and that neither the ordering provider nor the primary care provider were aware of significant findings (Roy et al., 2005). About 30 times as many outpatient visits as hospital discharges occur each year, and errors in diagnosis, often discovered after discharge, are the primary cause of paid liability claims in outpatient care (Bishop, Ryan, & Casalino, 2011).

EMTALA and Risk Reduction

Facilities can reduce the risk of an EMTALA violation by having the policies and documents in place that reinforce the requirements. Among the recommendations of Glass, Rebstock, & Handberg (2004) are: having a multidisciplinary educational curriculum for all affected areas (ED, obstetric triage); reviewing policies/protocols to ensure that performance of the MSE is performed by appropriately trained personnel; using templates for transfer documentation; and maintaining transfer and discharge records. In addition, obstetric triage settings need firm policies and protocols for communication to both patient and provider and tracking logs for pending test results at transfer or discharge. Finally, the development of guidelines for evaluation of common obstetric events can help ensure that the same level of care is offered for each woman.

HEALTH INFORMATION PORTABILITY AND ACCOUNTABILITY ACT (HIPAA)

While EMTALA is emergency specific, the Health Insurance Portability and Accountability Act (HIPAA), applies to all clinical encounters. The Act sets a balance between protection of privacy and provision of quality care (HIPAA, 1996). The Act includes both the Privacy Rule, discussed here, and the Security Rule, which addresses confidentiality of electronic health records. Given the variety of settings in which obstetric triage may occur, and the likelihood that information from a triage visit will be transmitted to others for continued care, the requirements of HIPAA often affect the process.

HIPAA requires that patient privacy be maintained. As Annas (2003) has pointed out, HIPAA is a complex way to apply basic privacy doctrine to modern health care and ensure that only the necessary minimum of information is released to accomplish any purpose. Examples of times when HIPAA can be violated inadvertently include elevator conversations, signing in at reception, or telephone scheduling. Speaking softly or not at all in public areas, keeping records out of casual view, not shouting out information, moving the "whiteboard" with identifying information out of sight are all obvious ways to provide privacy. But triage areas are more likely than most settings to offer minimal protection against overheard discussions. It is important to be conscious of possible listeners when asking the woman or family sensitive questions.

Disclosure of Health Information

Protected health information (PHI) covered under HIPAA includes both medical and financial records; psychiatric records have separate requirements from general medical care. In the context of emergent care, the ability to obtain records from prior providers and to relay information back to the appropriate primary site directly affects the quality of care. HIPAA specifically permits this exchange of information without written consent to facilitate quality care, such as with specialist consultation or care of a woman arriving at a clinical site different from the location of her usual care (Department of Health and Human Services [DHHS], 2011). However, some facilities may require written consent before they will release records. The decision to require formal consent, but not the choice whether to provide records, is the prerogative of the facility or provider.

There are times when PHI can be disclosed with informal consent or when the woman's consent is not required. Informal consent occurs when a family member, friend, or other individual is present during a conversation, and the patient declines an offer of privacy or does not ask for privacy. When a woman goes to cesarean section emergently and a family member is in the waiting room, the provider can safely give information without violating HIPAA. However, the "friend" who calls to ask if someone has arrived has a limited right to knowledge about the woman, and staff must be careful to limit phone information to that published in the hospital directory (DHHS 2011). Informal consent to disclosure also covers activities such as a woman requesting that a brother pick up a prescription. By sending him to the pharmacy, she consented to the disclosure of information. Professional judgment is the deciding factor about what information to release in these cases. Individual facilities may decide to have more stringent requirements, such as written consent for disclosure of information to family members.

Electronic Media and HIPAA

Communications between providers, or between a provider and a friend or colleague from another setting, can also lead to serious HIPAA violations. Even if e-mail messages are used within an institution as a common method of relaying information about care, consideration must be given to the security of the system and to the specific content of the message. It is the institution's responsibility to set standards to which individuals are required to adhere. For example, using a home e-mail address to send updates to practice partners is inherently less safe than using a hospital system limited to staff. Staying within the facility's firewall does not guarantee confidentiality but lessens the chance of accidentally releasing PHI. Using attachments to send information, password protection, and encrypting documents are ways to decrease the risk of unintended violations of HIPAA (DHHS, 2011).

The proliferation of social media, blogs, electronic discussion lists, and other general access communication forums have led to increased risks of an unconsidered release of PHI. Contributing factors to violations of patient privacy summarized by Cronquist and Spector (2011) include beliefs that a posting or communication is private, that deleted comments cannot be retrieved, that limited disclosure to an intended recipient is harmless, or that the use of nonspecific identifiers is adequate to maintain confidentiality; failure to refrain from sharing information other than for a health care related need; and the ease of posting combined with the commonplace sharing of personal information on social media.

In fact, virtually any posting or e-mail can be forwarded, copied and resent, retrieved by a webmaster, and used as evidence of publication of PHI. Investigations by a state licensing board, workplace discipline/firing, a federal HIPAA investigation, or a liability suit sound like extreme responses to a casual online comment or photo posting, but may be the legitimate response to an electronic disclosure (Hader & Brown, 2010).

Care of the Adolescent

The care of adolescent women raises confidentiality issues that go beyond the scope of HIPAA. Adolescent women's right to confidentiality is governed by a complex of state and federal laws, Title X, Medicaid, HIPAA, and court cases. HIPAA generally defers to state requirements for parental disclosure, consent to care, access to medical records, and the like (Annas, 2003; English & Ford, 2004). Parents are able to access their minor child's records with three exceptions, which are: the minor has given consent for care, and parental consent is not required by state law; the minor's care is obtained at the direction of the court or someone appointed by the court; or the parent has agreed to a confidential relationship between the child and provider within the limits of that agreement (DHHS, 2011).

Reproductive health care is often considered a special case, again with differing requirements by jurisdiction. Both adolescents and their parents may be unclear on the issues of confidentiality. Minor consent laws are based on either status (e.g., pregnancy) or specific area of care (e.g., mental health; Berlin & Bravender, 2009). Each individual should be aware of jurisdictional requirements relating to adolescent care. Accessing confidential care is difficult enough for teens—knowing what can be promised can prevent later conflicts and loss of trust.

REFERENCES

Annas, G. J. (2003). HIPAA regulations—A new era of medical record privacy? *New England Journal of Medicine, 348*(*15*), 1486–1490.

Berlin, E. D., & Bravender, T. (2009). Confidentiality, consent and caring fro the adolescent patient. *Current Opinions in Pediatrics, 21*(*4*), 450–456.

Bishop, T. F., Ryan, A. M., & Casalino, L. P. (2011). Paid malpractice claims for adverse events in inpatient and outpatient settings. *Journal of American Medical Association, 305*(*23*), 2427–2431.

Bitterman, R. A. (2002). Explaining the EMTALA paradox. *Annals of Internal Medicine, 40*, 470–475.

Cohen, B. (2007). Disentangling EMTALA from medical malpractice: Revising EMTALA's screening standard to differentiate between ordinary negligence and discriminatory denials of care. *Tulane Law Review, 82*, 645–692.

Cronquist, R., & Spector, N. (2011). Nurses and social media: Regulatory concerns and guidelines. *Journal of Nursing Regulation, 2*(3), 37–40.

Department of Health and Human Services (DHHS). (2011). Health Information Privacy. Retrieved from http://www.hhs.gov/ocr/privacy/ (accessed on November 29, 2011).

Dowdy, A. K., Friend, G. N., & Rangel, J. L. (1996). The anatomy of EMTALA: A litigator's guide. *St. Mary's Law Journal, 27*(*3*), 464–511.

Emergency Medical Treatment and Active Labor Act (EMTALA), P.L 89–97. U.S. Code. Title 42, § 1395dd (1986). Retrieved from http://www.law.cornell.edu/uscode/42/1395dd.html (accessed on November 29, 2011).

EMTALA.com. (2011). Frequently asked questions. Retrieved from http://www.emtala.com/index.html (accessed on November 29, 2011).

English, A., & Ford, C. A. (2004). The HIPAA privacy rule and adolescents: Legal questions and clinical challenges. *Perspectives on Sexual and Reproductive Health, 36*(2), 80–86.

Gandhi, T. K. & Lee, T. H. (2011). Patient safety beyond the hospital. *New England Journal of Medicine, 363*(*11*), 1001–1003.

Glass, D. L., Rebstock, J., & Handberg, E. (2004). Emergency treatment and labor act (EMTALA): Avoiding the pitfalls. *Journal of Perinatal & Neonatal Nursing, 18*(2), 103–114.

Hader, A. L. & Brown, E. D. (2010). Patient privacy and social media. *AANA Journal, 78*(*4*), 270–245.

Health Insurance Portability and Accountability Act (HIPAA), P.L. 104–191 (1996). Retrieved from http://www.hhs.gov/ocr/privacy/hipaa/administrative/statute/hipaastatutepdf.pdf (accessed on November 29, 2011).

Hughes, L. M. (Ed.). (2008). Health care access. *Georgetown Journal of Gender and the Law, IX*, 1183–1220.

Roy, C. L., Poon, E. G., Karson, A. S., Ladak-Merchant, Z., Johnson, R. E., Maviglia, S. M., & Gandhi, T. K. (2005). Patient safety concerns arising from test results that return after hospital discharge. *Annals of Internal Medicine, 143*(2), 121–128.

II: MANAGEMENT OF OBSTETRIC CONDITIONS IN EARLY PREGNANCY (LESS THAN VIABILITY)

Management of Ectopic Pregnancy

3

Roxanne A. Vrees

Ectopic pregnancy, frequently referred to as tubal pregnancy, is a potentially life-threatening condition in which a fertilized ovum implants and develops outside of the endometrial cavity. Overall trends in ectopic pregnancies have remained fairly stable since the 1990s. In the United States, ectopic pregnancies account for 2% of all first trimester pregnancies (Barnhart, 2009). Despite the fact that miscarriage is the most common complication of clinically evident pregnancies, ectopic pregnancy remains the leading cause of maternal deaths in the first trimester of pregnancy. This accounts for 0.5 deaths per 1000 pregnancies and 6% of all pregnancy related deaths (Barnhart, 2009). Early detection in conjunction with outpatient management has significant public health implications including: reducing maternal morbidity and mortality, preserving future fertility, and decreasing medical expenses that would otherwise be incurred with hospitalization and/or surgery (Barnhart, 2006).

PRESENTING SYMPTOMATOLOGY

As many as 18% of emergency visits for abdominal pain and/or vaginal bleeding are due to ectopic pregnancies (ACOG, 2008). Of these women, 40% to 50% are either misdiagnosed or not diagnosed following the initial presentation to the emergency setting (ACOG, 2008). Historically, the diagnosis of ectopic pregnancy was often made in the setting of rupture, which made this condition primarily a surgical issue. An increasing number of ectopic pregnancies are now being diagnosed well in advance of rupture, allowing for less invasive treatment options.

The vast majority of ectopic pregnancies will implant within the fallopian tube, with over 95% occurring in the ampullary region. Additional extrauterine implantation locations include the abdominal cavity, peritoneum, ovary, interstitium, uterine cornua, scar tissue, and cervix. The most common risk factor for developing an ectopic pregnancy is underlying tubal pathology. Hence, conditions that alter either tubal integrity or function, such as prior tubal surgery or sterilization, genital tract infections, and prior ectopic pregnancy, are all significant contrbuting factors. Additional risk factors include infertility, assisted reproductive technologies, and smoking. It is critical to note that half of all women who present with an ectopic pregnancy will have no known risk factors. This poses a diagnostic challenge when evaluating pregnant women who present with seemingly common symptoms such as lower abdominal cramping and/or vaginal spotting.

PHYSICAL EXAMINATION FINDINGS

Ectopic pregnancies can be fatal when misdiagnosed. Even the most conservative and vigilant approaches can fail to make a correct and timely diagnosis. Several factors that lead to misdiagnoses include poor patient reliability with respect to presenting symptoms, absent or nonspecific findings on physical exam, and the fact that almost 50% of women with an ectopic pregnancy have no apparent risk factors (Silva et al., 2006).

Vaginal bleeding is a common occurrence in early pregnancy. While approximately half of these pregnancies will go on to miscarry, the remainder will be either viable intrauterine pregnancies or ectopics. Thus, the risk of an ectopic pregnancy must be considered in any woman presenting with nonspecific symptoms such as lower abdominal cramping and vaginal bleeding. Unfortunately, the classic triad of pain, vaginal bleeding, and palpable adnexal mass is present in less than half of the cases. Regardless of pregnancy location or viability, all women presenting with vaginal bleeding in early pregnancy must have a blood type and screen obtained. In Rh negative women who have no evidence of sensitization, anti-D immune globulin should be administered.

Diagnosis relies on a combination of clinical, biochemical, and imaging findings. Ultimately, early diagnosis is facilitated by maintaining a high index of clinical suspicion in conjunction with a comprehensive approach to patient evaluation. It is recommended that all reproductive age women who have vaginal bleeding be evaluated for pregnancy, but determining the location of the pregnancy is of paramount importance. For women presenting with signs and symptoms of a ruptured ectopic pregnancy, this then becomes a surgical emergency. These symptoms include hemodynamic instability (hypotension, tachycardia) and rebound tenderness due to hemoperitoneum. Ideally, the treatment of these women is managed by an obstetrician and in more remote areas, a general surgeon. Fortunately, the vast majority of cases will present with symptoms prior to rupture. Hence, ectopic pregnancy is predominantly a nonsurgical entity with respect to both the diagnosis and subsequent management.

As previously noted, the vast majority of ectopic pregnancies occur in the ampullary region of the fallopian tube. However, there are several additional extrauterine locations worthy of specific mention. These unique extrauterine locations are particularly critical to note, given their tendency to be difficult to diagnose and their associated increased morbidity. Extrauterine locations include interstitial ectopic pregnancies as noted in Figures 3.1 A and B and a cervical pregnancy in Figure 3.2.

The terms interstitial and cornual pregnancies are commonly used interchangeably to describe an ectopic pregnancy that implants in the proximal segment of the tube that is embedded within the muscular wall of the uterus. However, the term "cornual" is best reserved for pregnancies occurring in one horn of a bicornuate uterus. True interstitial pregnancies comprise approximately 3% of ectopics (Dilbaz et al., 2005). These are at increased risk for rupture and subsequent hemorrhage given the tendency to present late in gestation (Dilbaz et al., 2005). A typical ultrasound finding of an interstitial ectopic pregnancy includes an eccentric position of the gestational sac, which lies within 5 mm of the uterine serosa. Heterotopic pregnancies occur when there is

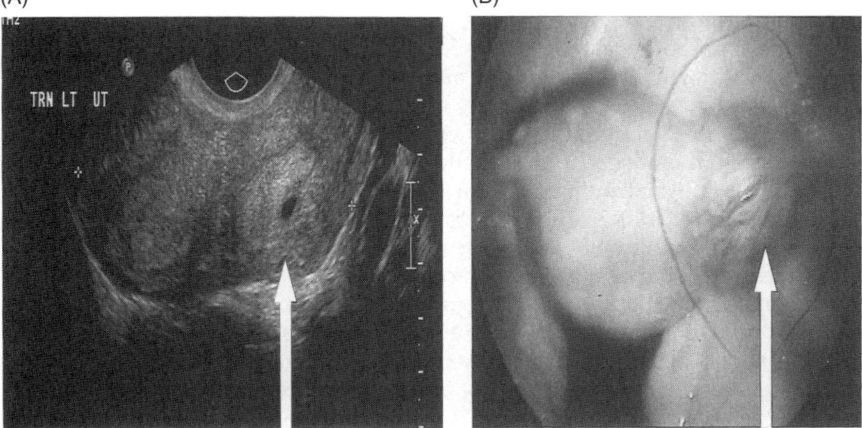

FIGURE 3.1 (A) Interstitial ectopic pregnancy on ultrasound imaging. (B) Interstitial ectopic pregnancy at the time of surgery.

Source: Courtesy of Department of Radiology, Women & Infants Hospital, Providence, RI.

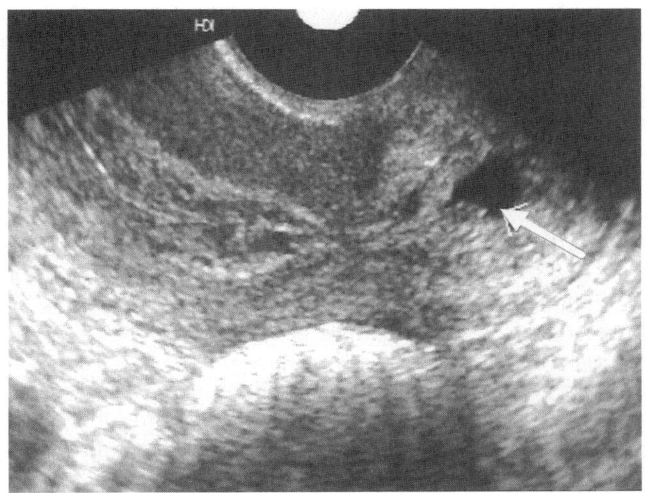

FIGURE 3.2 Cervical ectopic pregnancy. Sagittal view with fetal pole within gestational sac located in cervix.

Source: Courtesy of Department of Radiology, Women & Infants Hospital, Providence, RI.

simultaneously an intrauterine and an extrauterine pregnancy. These account for 1/4000 pregnancies in the general population and 1/100 cases for women undergoing assisted reproductive technology treatments (Barnhart, 2009).

Lastly, cervical pregnancies are an extremely rare form of ectopic pregnancy in which the ovum implants in the lining of the endocervical canal. This accounts for less than 1% of all ectopic pregnancies (Vela & Tulandi, 2007). These typically present with heavy vaginal bleeding that is often painless and, less commonly, with lower abdominal pain.

One final consideration is that of an abdominal pregnancy. Although exceptionally rare, the potential sequelae from this particular form of ectopic pregnancy can be devastating. Providers need to consider this in their diagnostic evaluation of all women with an unlocated pregnancy. Abdominal pregnancies can be a result of the direct implantation of the developing embryo on the abdominal viscera or peritoneal surface. Also, they may be due to the expulsion of an embryo from the fallopian tube. As a result of these variable locations, abdominal pregnancies are associated with a wide range of signs and symptoms. Unlike tubal pregnancies, they may go undetected until a very advanced gestational age. Thus it is imperative to maintain a high index of suspicion when making the diagnosis.

Symptoms of abdominal pregnancy range from nausea and vomiting from a pregnancy implanted on the bowel to an acute abdomen with subsequent shock due to massive intraabdominal hemorrhage. The differential diagnoses include any other form of extrauterine pregnancy, placental abruption, a true cornual pregnancy, and uterine rupture. Regardless of the gestational age at presentation, the primary treatment option is surgical.

LABORATORY AND IMAGING STUDIES

The first step in evaluating any female who presents with an early unlocated pregnancy is to determine whether it is a normal pregnancy, a failed pregnancy, or an extrauterine pregnancy. This can be accomplished with beta hCG values, as well as uterine curettage once a viable pregnancy has been ruled out. Without the use of uterine curettage, a presumed diagnosis of ectopic pregnancy will be inaccurate in almost half of cases (Barnhart et al., 2002).

Ultrasonographic Evaluation

Absolute criteria for a failed intrauterine pregnancy include a crown rump length greater than 5 mm with no fetal heartbeat or a menstrual age known to be greater than 6.5 weeks with no fetal heartbeat noted. If the diagnosis of a failed intrauterine pregnancy cannot be definitively made based on these absolute criteria, then an ectopic pregnancy must be a consideration. The sensitivity of transvaginal ultrasound for diagnosing an ectopic pregnancy ranges from 73% to 93% (Barnhart, 2009). This is dependent on several factors including gestational age, ultrasound equipment, and technical abilities of the ultrasonographer (Barnhart, 2009).

Ultrasound alone can be diagnostic of an ectopic pregnancy if an embryo with fetal cardiac activity is visualized in an extrauterine location. Unfortunately, this is often not the case. The most common finding for an ectopic pregnancy on transvaginal ultrasound is an adnexal mass, usually located between the uterus and ovary. However, not all adnexal masses are ectopic pregnancies. In fact, most represent hemorrhagic corpus luteum. A mass in the setting of an ectopic pregnancy may be a solid, complex, ring-like structure; but it can also be subtle and present as a mere asymmetry of ovarian size. Alternatively, a mass representing an ectopic may be mistaken for another benign structure such as adjacent bowel, a simple or paratubal cyst, endometrioma, or corpus luteum. Ultimately, the location of a corpus luteum is not helpful because contralateral implantation occurs in up to a third of the cases. An additional aspect to consider is the echotexture of the mass. For example, the relative echogenicity of a "tubal ring," as shown in Figure 3.3,

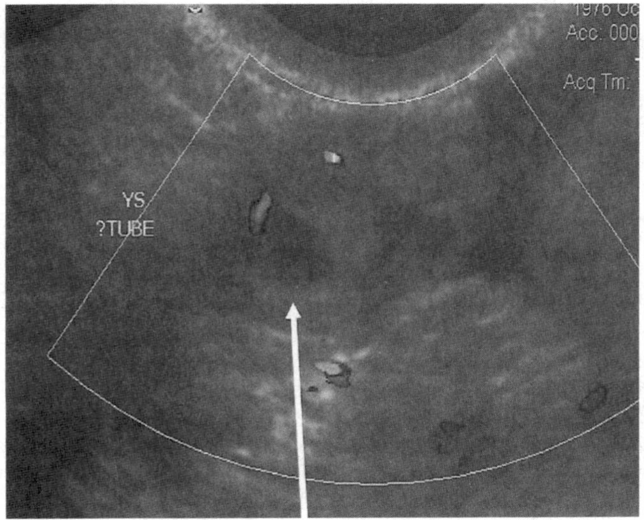

FIGURE 3.3 Tubal ring.

Source: Courtesy of Department of Radiology, Women & Infants Hospital, Providence, RI.

is a useful characteristic that can differentiate an ectopic pregnancy from a corpus luteum (Frates et al., 2001).

Furthermore, real-time ultrasound imaging with utilization of the probe and gentle pressure on the abdominal wall can facilitate movement of a mass to separate from the ovary. Lack of independent motion of an adjacent mass and ovary is strongly suggestive of no ectopic pregnancy (Blaivas & Lyon, 2005). Of note, if a transvaginal ultrasound is performed to rule out an ectopic pregnancy and is completely normal, an abdominal ultrasound must be performed to complete the evaluation.

While small amounts of free fluid can be seen on ultrasound in both ectopic and intrauterine pregnancies, moderate to large amounts of fluid increases the suspicion for an ectopic pregnancy. The presence of heterogeneous, echogenic fluid detected by transvaginal ultrasonography closely correlates with hemoperitoneum detected at the time of surgery in women with suspected ectopic pregnancies.

hCG Trends

Beta hCG levels play a critical adjunctive role in the early diagnosis of ectopic pregnancies. There is no single level of serum beta hCG that can reliably diagnose an intrauterine or ectopic pregnancy. However, there is a "discriminatory zone," which is the lowest level at which an intrauterine gestational sac can be reliably visualized on ultrasound. This discriminatory level for beta hCG has been reported to range between 1,500 and 2,000 mIU/mL for transvaginal ultrasound and 6,500 mIU/mL for transabdominal approaches (Seeber & Barnhart, 2006). However, this hCG level is institutionally dependent and varies based on multiple factors. These factors include the particular hCG assay utilized by the laboratory, the quality of the ultrasound equipment, the skill of the ultrasonographer, and the presence of physical factors (e.g., fibroids). It is critical that institutions adopt a collaborative process to maximize the sensitivity for diagnosing an ectopic pregnancy while minimizing the possibility of disrupting a normal intrauterine pregnancy. The absence of an intrauterine gestational sac at beta hCG levels above the discriminatory zone is suggestive of either an ectopic or nonviable pregnancy and warrants further evaluation (Creanga et al., 2011). However, regardless of an institution's particular discriminatory zone, clinical management is best guided by serial beta hCG levels, which are more accurate than any single measurement.

The minimal rise in beta hCG for a normal viable pregnancy is 24% at 1 day and 53% at 2 days (Barnhart et al., 2004). However, while 99% of viable intrauterine pregnancies will demonstrate this trend, 21% of ectopic pregnancies will demonstrate a similar rise (Silva et al., 2006). Conversely, 8% of ectopic pregnancies will demonstrate declining beta hCGs levels at the same rate as a spontaneous miscarriage (Silva et al., 2006). Furthermore, some normal pregnancies will not have a gestational sac on initial ultrasound despite either normally rising hormone levels or levels above the discriminatory zone. In such cases, it is appropriate to perform serial ultrasound, particularly in women with a desired pregnancy. Nonetheless, with beta hCG levels well above the discriminatory zone and no identifiable pregnancy on serial ultrasounds, it remains necessary to confirm the location of this likely nonviable gestation. Additionally, as many as 40% of ectopic diagnoses are incorrect without uterine curettage. Thus, once a pregnancy has been deemed to be nonviable, a reasonable diagnostic, as well as potentially therapeutic option is to perform a uterine curettage (Rivera, Nguyen, & Sit, 2009). In this

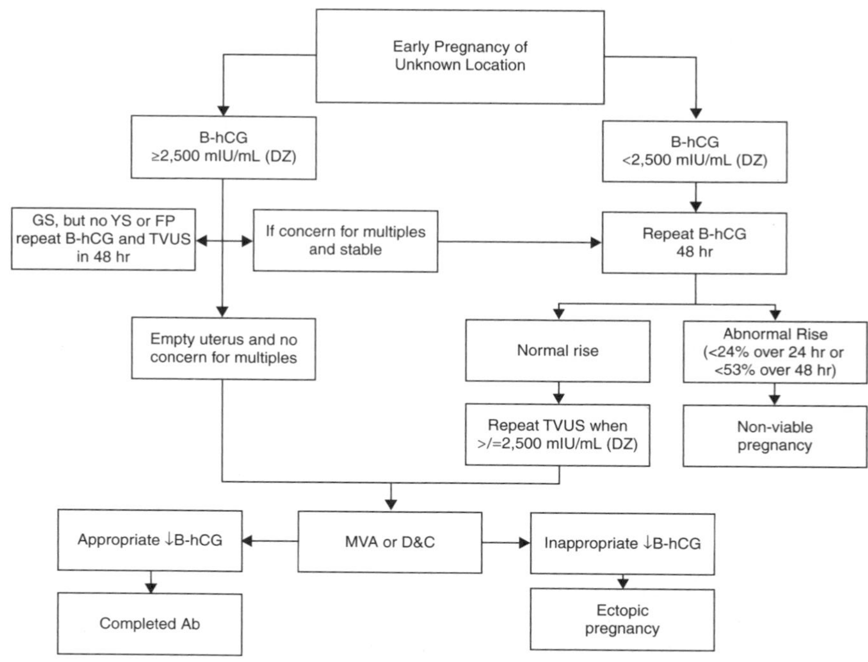

FIGURE 3.4 Management of the early unlocated pregnancy.

Source: Courtesy of Women & Infants Emergency Obstetrics and Gynecology Department, Providence, RI.

procedure, the uterus is evacua
of a pregnancy can be confirmed.
either the presence of chorionic villi
decline in follow-up beta hCG levels 12
ation. (Barnhart et al., 2002). Uterine evacua
cability based on provider skill and experien
equipment, and the potential for disruption of a
provides an algorithm for the management of the ea

CLINICAL MANAGEMENT AND FOLLOW-

Treatment options for ectopic pregnancies include expectant ma
medical therapy, and surgical intervention. Expectant management
serial beta hCG monitoring in conjunction with close outpatient follow-
ensure complete resolution of the ectopic pregnancy. Criteria for this ma
agement option include hemodynamic stability, absence of symptoms, beta hCG levels greater than 200 mIU/mL, a reliable patient, informed consent, and ability to comply with ongoing close observation. The ultimate decision regarding appropriate treatment is largely dependent on characteristics of both the patient, as well as clinical expertise of the provider.

MEDICAL MANAGEMENT

As the detection of ectopic pregnancies has increased over the past decade, minimally invasive therapy has become the standard of care. The key to successful conservative management lies in early diagnosis. Today, providers are far more likely to treat appropriate candidates in an outpatient setting with the use of methotrexate as described in Exhibit 3.1.

EXHIBIT 3.1

Methotrexate (MTX) Treatment Regimens

- **Pretreatment evaluation:** rule out failed intrauterine pregnancy
- **Baseline labs**: beta hCG, creatinine, liver function tests, complete blood count, blood type, and screen
- **Single dose protocol**: MTX 50 mg/m^2 IM on day 1 with hCG measurements on days 4 and 7. Expect 15% decline in hCG levels from day 4 to 7. Then follow weekly to nonpregnant levels. If inappropriate decline or levels plateau/increase, redose MTX
- **Sequential or two dose**: MTX 50 mg/m^2 IM on day 0 and day 4 with hCG measurements on days 4 and 7. Monitor decline as above. If inappropriate decline or levels plateau/increase, redose on days 7 and 11 and monitor for 15% decline
- **Fixed multidose**: MTX 1 mg/kg IM on days 1, 3, 5, and 7 with leucovorin rescue at 0.1 mg/kg IM on days 2, 4, 6, and 8. Measure hCG levels on MTX dose days and continue to monitor until 15% decline from initial level and then weekly until nonpregnant levels. Redose as per above protocol if inappropriate decline or levels plateau/increase

Source: Adapted from ACOG (2008).

binds to dihydrofolate
ily affects actively pro-
w, buccal and intestinal
c tissue. In addition to its
on rapidly dividing cells
of methotrexate as noted
oth a safe and appropriate
selected patient. There are
e overall success rates rang-
ingle-dose regimen is most
shown to be safe and cost-
women (Stovall et al., 1991).
ditional benefits of both con-
ecifically, this regimen can be
5,000 mIU/mL but allows for
"fixed multi-dose" regimen.
gnancies that can be treated
adnexal mass less than 3.5 to
y. Although the adnexal mass
ot demonstrate any signs of fur-
tored by both clinical symptoms
and ongo... hat individuals who have none of
the contraindications for ... in Exhibit 3.3, but otherwise have
a poor social situation (e.g., homeless) are not candidates for medical management unless appropriate follow-up can be assured.

Factors associated with failed medical management include initial beta hCG levels above 5,000 mIU/mL, ultrasonographic evidence of significant free fluid, presence of fetal cardiac activity, and a pretreatment beta hCG level that has increased more than 50% over a 48-hour period (Barnhart, 2009). In addition to the pretreatment laboratory evaluation, women opting for medical management require prolonged follow-up regardless of the particular methotrexate dosing regimen chosen. Women who have failed both expectant and medical management for an ectopic pregnancy ultimately require surgical intervention. Of note, interstitial, heterotopic, and cervical pregnancies can be treated medically with direct ultrasound-guided injection of either

EXHIBIT 3.2

Side Effects of Methotrexate

- Gastrointestinal symptoms (e.g., nausea, vomiting, and diarrhea)
- Stomatitis
- Macular rash
- Central nervous system symptoms (e.g., headache, dizziness, fatigue, and difficulty concentrating)
- Blood dyscrasias (e.g., anemia, macrocytosis)
- Alopecia
- Fever
- Hepatic, pulmonary, and renal toxicity

Source: Adapted from ACOG (2008).

EXHIBIT 3.3

Contraindications to Methotrexate Therapy

- **Absolute contraindications:** Known intrauterine pregnancy, blood dyscrasias (e.g., severe anemia, thrombocytopenia), immunodeficiency breastfeeding, prior sensitivity to methotrexate, active pulmonary disease, active peptic ulcer disease, liver disease (alcoholic or other chronic disease), and kidney disease
- **Relative contraindications:** Embryonic cardiac activity detected by transvaginal ultrasonography, patient declines blood transfusion, high initial hCG concentration (> 5,000 mIU/mL), ectopic pregnancy greater than 3.5 to 4.0 cm in size as imaged by transvaginal ultrasound, refusal to accept blood products, and inability to participate in follow-up

Source: Adapted from ASRM (2008) and ACOG (2008).

methotrexate or potassium chloride. This procedure is performed by a provider with appropriate clinical experience and training. Otherwise, these conditions are best treated surgically.

SURGICAL MANAGEMENT

Although the management approach for ectopic pregnancies has largely moved away from surgery, there are still women for whom surgery is indicated. Appropriate indications for surgical management include hemodynamic instability or ruptured ectopic pregnancy, coexisting intrauterine pregnancy, contraindications to methotrexate, desire for permanent sterilization, and those patients who have failed medical therapy.

The primary surgical approaches involve removing the entire tube via a salpingectomy versus removing the ectopic pregnancy from the affected tube while preserving the fallopian tube. Although no studies to date have directly compared the two procedures, there are similar outcomes with respect to operative morbidity and subsequent fertility rates. However, the obvious disadvantage of a salpingostomy is that it is less successful than either a salpingectomy or an open surgical approach because of the increased risk for a persistent or recurrent ectopic pregnancy in an already damaged fallopian tube. (Hajenius et al, 2007). If a salpingostomy is performed, it is critical to follow beta hCG levels to zero in order to prevent a persistent ectopic. In these cases, postoperative prophylactic single-dose methotrexate can be administered to reduce this risk (ASRM, 2008).

Either procedure can be performed laparoscopically, which is the standard and preferred surgical approach for ectopic pregnancy. However, conversion to an open laparotomy is appropriate under certain circumstances. The final decision to move toward an open surgical approach is based on the clinical status of the patient in conjunction with the clinical expertise and judgment of the surgeon and anesthesiologist. Regardless of the surgical approach chosen, there are similar recurrence and tubal patency rates following both medical and surgical intervention (Buster & Krotz, 2007).

REFERENCES

American College of Obstetricians and Gynecologists (ACOG). (2008). *Practice Bulletin: Medical Management of Ectopic Pregnancy, 94,* 1–7.

American Society for Reproductive Medicine, Birmingham, Alabama (ASRM). (2008). *The Practice Committee of the American Society for Reproductive Medicine, 90,* 206–212.

Barnhart, K. T, Hummel, A. C., Summel, M. D., Menon, S., Jain, J., & Chakhtoura, N. (2007).Use of "2 dose" regimen of methotrexate to treat ectopic pregnancy. *Fertility and Sterility, 87,* 250–256.

Barnhart, K. T., Katz, I., Hummel, A., & Garcia, C. R. (2002). Presumed diagnosis of ectopic pregnancy. *Obstetrics and Gynecology, 100,* 505–510.

Barnhart, K. T., Sammel, M. D., Rinaudo, P. F., Zhou, L., Hummel, A. C., & Wensheng, G. (2004). Symptomatic patients with an early viable intrauterine pregnancy: hCG curves redefined. *Obstetrics and Gynecology, 104,* 50–55.

Barnhart, K. T. (2006). Risk factors for ectopic pregnancies in women with symptomatic first trimester pregnancies. *Fertility and Sterility, 86,* 33–43.

Barnhart, K. T. (2009). Ectopic pregnancy. *The New England Journal of Medicine, 361,* 379–387.

Blaivas, M., & Lyon, M. (2005). Reliability of adnexal mass mobility in distinguishing possible ectopic pregnancy from corpus luteum cysts. *Journal of Ultrasound in Medicine, 24*(5), 599–603.

Buster, J. E. & Krotz, S. (2007). Reproductive performance after ectopic pregnancy. *Seminars in Reproductive Medicine, 25*(2), 131–133.

Creanga, A. A., Shapiro-Mendoza, S., Bish, C. L., Zane, S., Berg, C. J., & Callaghan, W. M. (2011). Trends in ectopic pregnancy mortality in the United States. *Journal of Obstetrics and Gynecology, 117,* 837–842.

Dilbaz, S., Katas, B., & Demir, B.(2005). Treating cornual pregnancy with a single methotrexate injection . A report of 3 cases. *Journal of Reproductive Medicine, 50,* 141.

Frates, M. C., Visweswaran, L., & Laing, F. C. (2001). Comparison of tubal ring and corpus luteum echogenicities: A useful differentiating characteristics. *Journal of Ultrasound in Medicine, 20*(1), 27–31.

Hajenius, P. J., Mol, F., Mol, B. W., Bossuyt, P. M., Ankum, W. M., & Van der Veen, F. (2007). Interventions for tubal ectopic pregnancy. *Cochrane Database of Systematic Reviews, 24*(1), CD000324.

Rivera, V., Nguyen, P. H., & Sit, A. (2009). Change in quantitative human chorionic gonadotropin after manual vacuum aspiration in women with pregnancy of unknown location. *American Journal of Obstetrics and Gynecology, 200*(5), 56–59.

Seeber, B. E, & Barnhart, K. T. (2006). Suspected ectopic pregnancy. *Obstetrics and Gynecology, 107,* 399–343.

Silva, C., Sammel, M. D., Zhou, L., Gracia, C., Hammel, A. C., & Barnhart, L. (2006). Human chorionic gonadotropin profile for women with ectopic pregnancy. *Journal of Obstetrics and Gynecology, 117,* 605–611.

Stovall, T. G., Ling, F. W., & Gray, L. (1991). Single dose methotrexate for treatment of ectopic pregnancy. *Journal of Obsterics and Gynecology, 77,* 754–757.

Vela, G., & Tulandi, T. (2007). Cervical pregnancy: The importance of early diagnosis and treatment. *Journal of Minimally Invasive Gynecology, 14,* 481.

4 Vaginal Bleeding in Early Pregnancy

Emily White

Vaginal bleeding in the first trimester of pregnancy is a common complaint seen in women who present to an emergency room. Approximately 25% of clinically relevant pregnancies have vaginal bleeding in the first trimester and half of these will eventually miscarry (Paspulati, Bhatt, & Nour, 2004). Vaginal bleeding may be caused by implantation of the embryo, subchorionic hematoma, miscarriage, gestational trophoblastic disease, or ectopic pregnancy. It is crucial for the clinician to assess for the more dangerous causes, especially ectopic pregnancy. Miscarriage is a common complication of early pregnancy, occurring in 15% to 20% of clinically relevant pregnancies (Wilcox et al., 1998). Ectopic pregnancy, the implantation of the embryo outside the uterine cavity, is a more rare but potentially life-threatening complication. The incidence of ectopic pregnancy is approximately 1.5% to 2% of pregnancies (Barnhart, 2009). The morbidity and mortality from ruptured ectopic pregnancies have decreased due to early detection and effective management strategies. However, 6% of maternal deaths are still caused from ruptured ectopic pregnancies, often because providers failed to recognize the early signs and symptoms of this condition (Barnhart, 2009).

PRESENTING SYMPTOMATOLOGY

The amount of vaginal bleeding in the first trimester can range from spotting to severe hemorrhage. The amount of bleeding alone is not indicative of the cause of bleeding. However, when a woman complains of vaginal bleeding, it is critical to quantify the amount of blood loss. If there has been heavy bleeding, anemia and even hemodynamic instability may ensue. Along with the bleeding, the woman may have noticed the passing of tissue, or even a fetus. If the tissue is available, it should be examined for chorionic villi or fetal parts. Temporal associations are also relevant. For example, if the bleeding only occurs when passing urine, it could be that the bleeding is from a urinary tract infection.

Vaginal bleeding may or may not be associated with abdominal pain. In a woman presenting with vaginal bleeding and abdominal pain, it is an ectopic pregnancy until proven otherwise. Additionally, symptoms of hemoperitoneum from a ruptured ectopic pregnancy include right shoulder pain, dizziness, and abdominal distension. The pace of a woman's evaluation will depend on the presenting history and symptomatology.

HISTORY AND DATA COLLECTION

Many women presenting with vaginal bleeding may not know if they are pregnant or whether there is even the possibility of pregnancy. Every sexually active, reproductive-aged woman who presents with irregular vaginal bleeding or abdominal pain needs a pregnancy test.

If known, the woman's last menstrual period (LMP) can be used to estimate the gestational age of the pregnancy. If the woman has irregular menses or an unsure LMP, basing gestational age on LMP may be inaccurate. If a woman has had a previous ultrasound in this pregnancy that documents an intrauterine pregnancy then this, in conjunction with the LMP, is the most accurate assessment of gestational age. A previous ultrasound documenting an intrauterine pregnancy also negates concern for ectopic pregnancy. The risk of heterotopic pregnancy, a concurrent pregnancy in the uterus and ectopic pregnancy, is extremely low in the general population, approximately 1/4000 (Deutchman et al., 2009).

If the location of the pregnancy is unknown, it is important to assess for any risk factors for an ectopic. These risk factors include previous ectopic pregnancy, tubal surgery, current intrauterine device, infertility treatments, history of pelvic inflammatory disease, age over 35 years, and smoking (Barnhart, 2009; Deutchman et al, 2009). Although conception after tubal ligation or with an intrauterine device in place is rare, if pregnancy does occur, there is an extremely high rate (25%–50%) of ectopic pregnancy (Barnhart, 2009).

Ectopic pregnancies most commonly implant in the fallopian tubes, accounting for over 95% of all ectopic pregnancies (Bouyer et al., 2002). However, those ectopic pregnancies that implant in the cervix, uterine cornua, cesarean section scar, ovaries, or abdominal cavity are more difficult to diagnose and manage, leading to higher morbidity.

PHYSICAL EXAMINATION

In addition to the history and symptomatology, the woman's vital signs and appearance are crucial to determine the pace and breadth of the workup. A woman may lose between 15% and 25% of blood volume before developing hypotension and tachycardia (Roberts, 2003). Acute blood loss leading to hemorrhagic shock can develop from a ruptured ectopic pregnancy or hemorrhage from a spontaneous abortion. Hemorrhagic shock is a rare, but serious condition in first trimester that needs to be treated urgently.

In stable women, the physical examination includes a careful abdominal examination. This examination is to palpate for uterine enlargement, tenderness, abdominal distension, and peritoneal signs.

A pelvic examination should be performed in all pregnant women complaining of vaginal bleeding. A visual inspection of external genitalia can identify nonobstetric causes of bleeding, such as hemorrhoids or trauma. A speculum examination is helpful in assessing amount of blood in the vault, as well as active bleeding. During the speculum examination, the cervix should be visualized. This may elicit other nonobstetric causes of bleeding, such as sexually transmitted infections or cervical polyps. Significant cervical dilation or visible products of conception are indicative of an inevitable abortion. Often removing these products of conception from the cervical os provides immediate relief of the woman's pain and limits the amount of bleeding. Uterine size and position should be evaluated by bimanual examination. This can provide an approximation of gestational age. The adnexa are palpated for masses and tenderness, which may indicate an ectopic pregnancy or other etiology, such as an ovarian cyst.

LABORATORY AND IMAGING STUDIES

The first measurable finding of a pregnancy is an elevated human chorionic gonadotropin (hCG) test. The hCG is detectable in the plasma of pregnant women 8 days after ovulation, at the time of implantation of the blastocyst. Home pregnancy tests can detect hCG as low as 25 mIU/mL International Reference Population (Deutchman et al., 2009). Currently, it is possible to detect a pregnancy even before a woman misses a menses.

A single hCG does not identify the location or viability of a pregnancy but can serve as an estimate for gestational age. The discriminatory zone is the hCG above which one expects to see a gestational sac (GS) on transvaginal ultrasound (TVUS). Failure to see a GS above this level suggests either an ectopic pregnancy or an abnormal intrauterine pregnancy. The discriminatory zone has been reported between 1500 and 3000 mIU (Barnhart, 2009). The discriminatory zone is not absolute. If a smaller number is used (e.g., 1500 mIU), the sensitivity for diagnosing an ectopic pregnancy increases, but the risk of mistaking a normal pregnancy as abnormal and interrupting the pregnancy also increases. A small collection of fluid in the uterus, or pseudosac, may appear as an anechoic structure similar to the GS. Due to this possible confusion, a GS is suggestive of an intrauterine pregnancy, but the presence of a yolk sac (YS) is necessary to definitely diagnose an intrauterine pregnancy.

TVUS is paramount in the evaluation of women with early gestational bleeding. Women presenting with vaginal bleeding benefit from an ultrasound to determine the viability and location of the pregnancy. If a pregnancy is not visualized, then the findings of the ultrasound need to be correlated to hCG measurement. The determination of viability and location of a pregnancy is not always possible in one emergency visit. TVUS is preferred to transabdominal in the first trimester because it can more clearly identify the parameters at an earlier gestational age (Table 4.1).

At 5 weeks' gestation, a GS is expected to be seen on TVUS and should measure at least 5 mm. Between 5 and 6 weeks, a YS develops and by the time the GS is 10 mm on TVUS, a YS should always be seen (Figure 4.1).

Around 6 weeks an embryo with fetal cardiac activity is visible on TVUS. By the time the GS reaches 18 mm, fetal cardiac activity should be present. These criteria should be used as guidelines. If the examination is difficult or equivocal, then a follow-up ultrasound should be obtained. There is

TABLE 4.1 First Trimester Scanning Milestones

PARAMETER	TRANSABDOMINAL ULTRASOUND	TRANSVAGINAL ULTRASOUND
Gestational sac (GS)	—	Present at 5 weeks (5 mm)
Yolk sac (YS)	Present GS > 20 mm	Present at 5.5 weeks Present GS > 10 mm
Cardiac activity	Present GS > 25mm	Present GS > 18 mm

Source: Adapted from Paspulati et al., 2004.

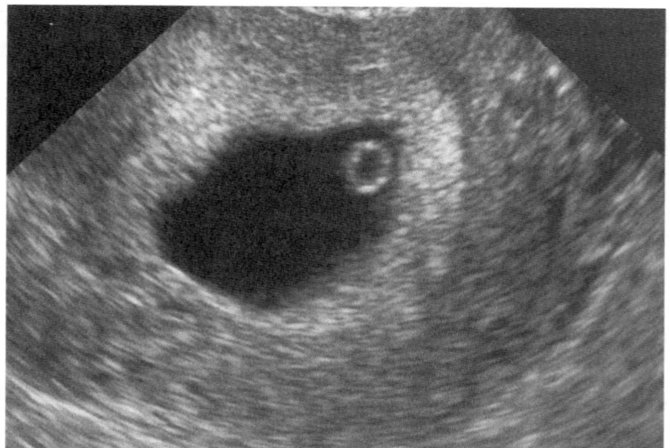

FIGURE 4.1 Yolk sac.

Source: Courtesy of Department of Radiology, Women & Infants Hospital, Providence, RI.

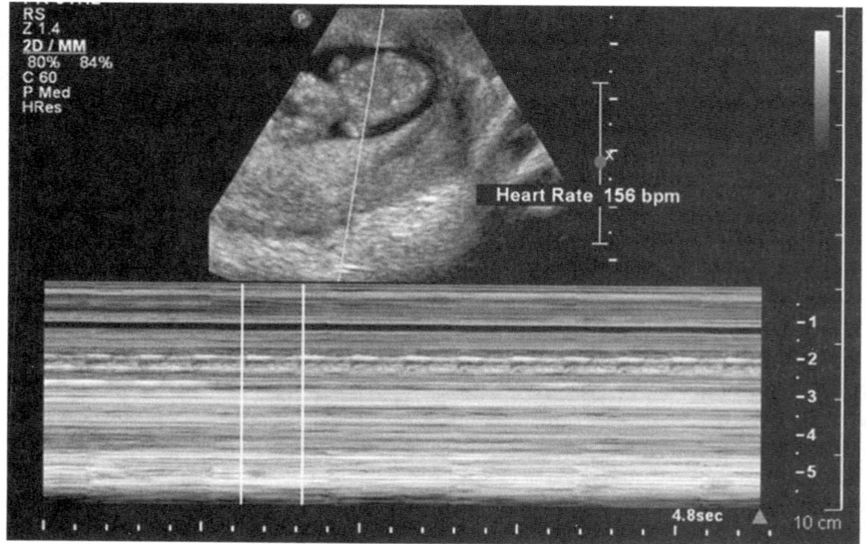

FIGURE 4.2 Fetal cardiac activity, M mode.

Source: Courtesy of Department of Radiology, Women & Infants Hospital, Providence, RI.

substantially higher energy output for Doppler than for imaging, which may have harmful effects on the developing fetus. The preferred method to assess cardiac activity in early pregnancy is M mode, which has lower energy output than Doppler (Figure 4.2).

DIFFERENTIAL DIAGNOSIS

The essential causes of first trimester bleeding are ectopic pregnancy, spontaneous abortion, and gestational trophoblastic disease. However, normal pregnancies may also have bleeding in the first trimester, often from a subchorionic hematoma, as pictured in Figure 4.3.

Subchorionic hematomas may occur in up to 20% of women with threatened abortions (Paspulati et al., 2004). When the hematoma is small, it may be physiologic; however, there may be a correlation between a large subchroinic hematoma and early pregnancy loss. An unfused amnion and chorion, as shown in Figure 4.4, should not be mistaken for a subchorionic hematoma.

There are various presentations and ultrasound findings of spontaneous abortions, depending on the gestational age of the pregnancy. One must be familiar with normal pregnancy development in order to recognize a failing pregnancy. An embryonic demise is characterized by a visible embryo without a heartbeat. Cardiac activity may not be visible in early normal embryo (crown rump length [CRL] < 5 mm) leading to the rule "alive after five." However, it has been suggested that there may be a high false positive rate using such a low cut-off, such as 5 mm. Some of these pregnancies may in fact be viable and develop normally and a more conservative estimate of CRL 7 mm should be used instead (Abdallah et al., 2011). A slow heart rate is a worrisome finding on ultrasound and these women would benefit from a repeat ultrasound in a week or so to assess for demise.

An anembryonic gestation is when the GS forms, but the embryo fails to develop. This is characterized on TVUS as a GS with a mean diameter greater than 18 mm without a YS or embryo (Paspulati et al., 2004). However, there is variation in the literature of what cut-off value of mean sac diameter defines miscarriage (Abdallah et al, 2011). The larger the sac size used, the greater the positive predictive value, and the least chance of interrupting a potentially viable pregnancy. With both anembryonic and failed embryonic pregnancies, correlation with expected gestational age and follow-up ultrasound may be useful in determining fetal viability. Waiting to repeat an ultrasound in 7 to 10 days is not likely to lead to any physical harm. Although not knowing the potential viability of the pregnancy may be difficult for the

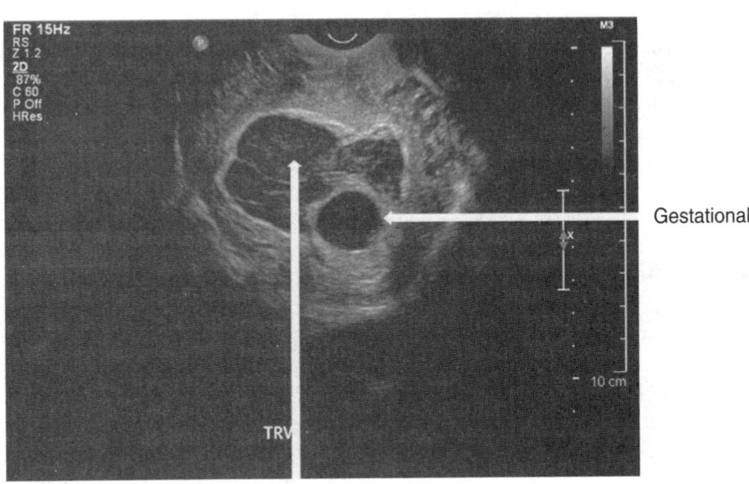

FIGURE 4.3 Subchorionic hematoma.

Source: Courtesy of Department of Radiology, Women & Infants Hospital, Providence, RI.

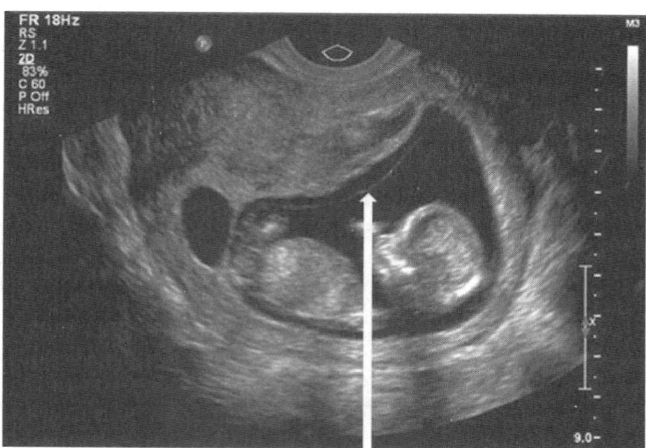

FIGURE 4.4 Unfused amnion and chorion.

Source: Courtesy of Department of Radiology, Women & Infants Hospital, Providence, RI.

woman, this should be balanced against potential inadvertent termination of a normal pregnancy. Gestational trophoblastic disease is characterized by markedly elevated hCG levels and ultrasound findings of a diffuse mixed echogenic pattern or "snowstorm" appearance, as seen in Figure 4.5. Cystic enlargement of the ovaries, theca lutein cysts may also be present. Early or partial moles may have subtle or no ultrasound findings.

Ectopic pregnancy is always on the differential until the pregnancy is located. An embryo with cardiac activity outside of the uterus confirms ectopic pregnancy shown in Figure 4.6. An adnexal mass without an embryo, as seen in Figure 4.7, or hemoperitoneum, shown in Figure 4.8, are highly concerning for an ectopic pregnancy.

The clinical scenario often arises when there is no definitive GS or ectopic pregnancy visible on ultrasound. This could potentially be a viable pregnancy, failed intrauterine pregnancy, or ectopic pregnancy. Close follow-up with hCG and TVUS is required until a definitive diagnosis can be made.

CLINICAL MANAGEMENT AND FOLLOW-UP

If the above evaluation has not confirmed pregnancy location, then serial measurements of hCG are often helpful. In a normal pregnancy, hCG rises in a predictable fashion during the first 8 weeks or so. Approximately 99% of viable intrauterine pregnancies will have a minimal rise of 53% in 2 days (Barnhart, 2009). A rise less than this or a decrease in hCG either reflect an ectopic pregnancy or a failed intrauterine pregnancy. Multiple gestations have a similar rise in hCG, but the absolute values are higher than singleton pregnancies. Therefore, multiple gestation pregnancies do not have the same discriminatory zone as singleton pregnancies, but a separate discriminatory zone has not yet been established.

In women with a miscarriage, hCG generally declines between 20% and 35% in 48 hours (Barnhart et al., 2004). However, lower initial hCG values

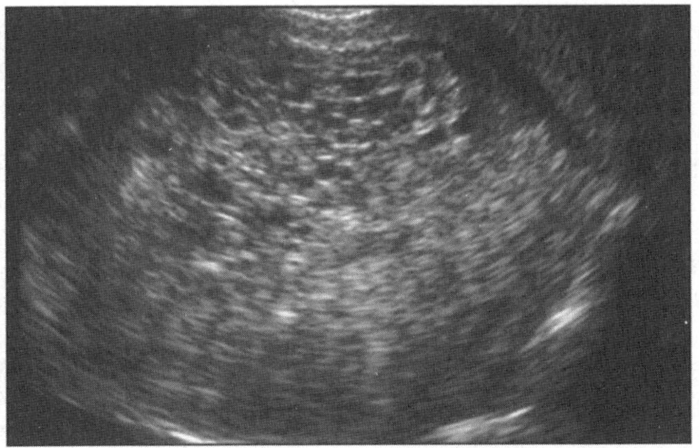

FIGURE 4.5 Gestational trophoblastic disease.

Source: Courtesy of Department of Radiology, Women & Infants Hospital, Providence, RI.

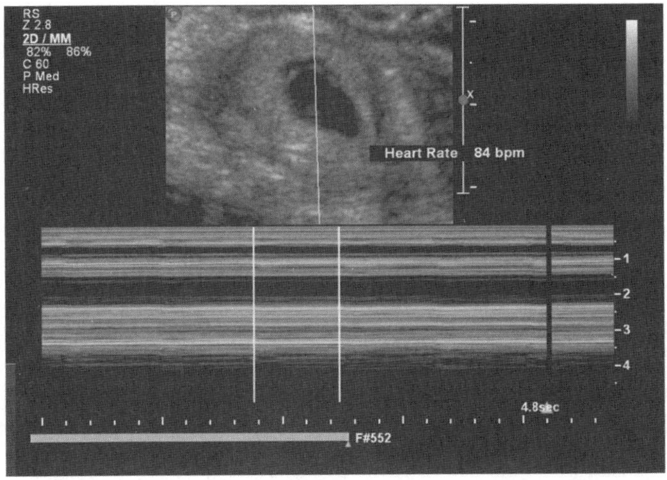

FIGURE 4.6 Adnexal mass with fetal cardiac activity.

Source: Courtesy of Department of Radiology, Women & Infants Hospital, Providence, RI.

decline at a slower rate. For example, a hCG of 50 mIU has a mean decline of 12% in 48 hours (Chung et al., 2006). When hCG values are declining at a rate that it is at least as high as expected, outpatient monitoring with serial hCG levels is appropriate until levels are undetectable.

Approximately half of ectopic pregnancies have rising hCG levels and the other half have declining levels. However, in 71% of ectopic pregnancies, the change in hCG is outside the normal range for normal pregnancies or spontaneous abortion (Silva et al., 2006). The other 30% of ectopic pregnancies have hCG curves that mimic normal gestations or miscarriages.

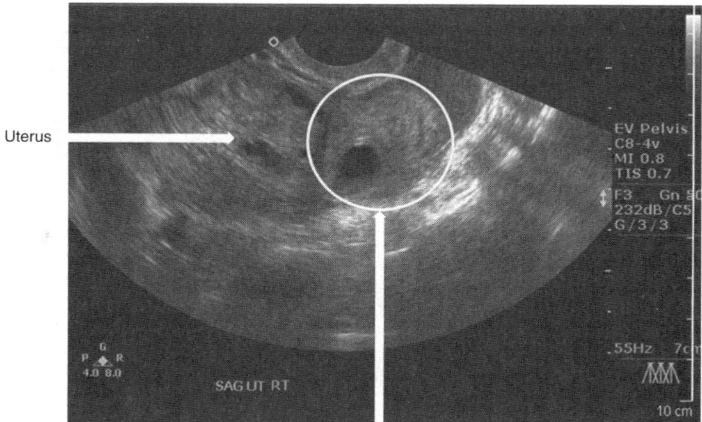

FIGURE 4.7 Right adnexal mass without an embryo.

Source: Courtesy of Department of Radiology, Women & Infants Hospital, Providence, RI.

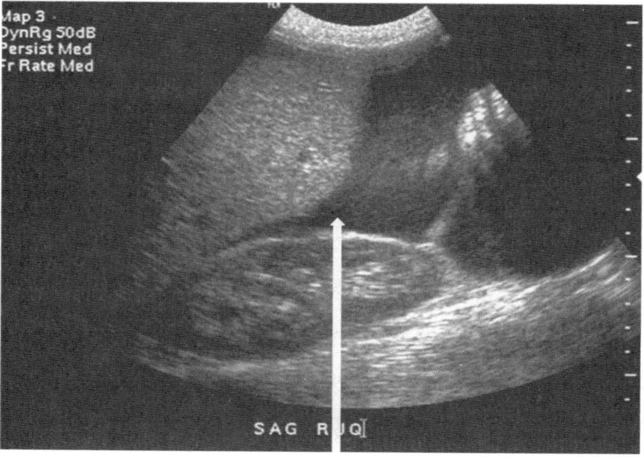

FIGURE 4.8 Hemoperitoneum.

Source: Courtesy of Department of Radiology, Women & Infants Hospital, Providence, RI.

There are times in early pregnancy when the pregnancy location is unknown. This can arise when the hCG is above the discriminatory zone without evidence of an intrauterine pregnancy. Another case may be that the hCGs are declining very slowly or rising less than the expected 53% in 48 hours. Tissue sampling with uterine evacuation is useful in these situations. If products of conception are identified on pathology, then the nonviable intrauterine pregnancy has been diagnosed and treated. Alternatively, a hCG obtained prior to the uterine evacuation can be compared to a repeat hCG obtained 12 to 24 hours after the procedure. If the hCG declines 20% or more in this time frame, then the trophoblastic cells were likely removed from the uterus, and there was a nonviable intrauterine pregnancy (Barnhart, 2009). The hCG level can then be monitored with serial measurements until it is undetectable. If the hCG fails to decline 20% after uterine evacuation, it strongly suggests that the trophoblasts are still present and an ectopic pregnancy exists. The woman then needs appropriate treatment of the ectopic pregnancy.

Women diagnosed with a miscarriage have a variety of options for clinical management. Often, these pregnancies are highly desired, and the provider needs to recognize the grief the woman and family may be experiencing. Most miscarriages occur spontaneously and completely and do not require any intervention. Historically, dilation and curettage was the treatment of choice for miscarriages.

If the woman has not completed the miscarriage, either expectant management or medical management with misoprostol may be safe and effective treatments. Incomplete abortions have a high treatment success rate, defined as complete expulsion of the pregnancy, with either expectant management (86%) or medical management (100%) (Bagratee et al., 2004). However, expectant management has drastically lower success rates with embryonic demise or anembryonic pregnancies. By day 7, expectant management only has a 29% success rate compared with 87% for medical management (Bagratee et al., 2004).

Although misoprostol is not approved by the United States Food and Drug Administration for use in treating miscarriage, a number of studies have shown its safety and efficacy (Zhang et al., 2005; Winikoff, 2005). Misoprostol has less gastrointestinal side effects when administered vaginally instead of orally. One protocol recommends that 800 mcg of misotoprostol be placed vaginally, and if the woman does not have complete expulsion by day 3, then this dose is repeated. Complete expulsion is defined as no GS and endometrial thickness greater than 3 cm on TVUS in a clinically stable woman. On day 8 if there is not complete expulsion, then uterine evacuation is performed (Zhang et al., 2005).

Counseling about the process and expectations is key to patient satisfaction with this process and preventing unnecessary revisits. Antibiotic prophylaxis is not necessary for expectant management or medical management (Achilles et al., 2011). Since there is a known intrauterine pregnancy following, hCG levels have no role in the management of these women.

Uterine evacuation of an incomplete, missed, or inevitable abortion can be completed with either a manual vacuum aspiration, or dilation and curettage. Manual vacuum aspiration has been shown to be as efficacious, safe, and as tolerable as dilation and curettage for evacuating the uterus in the first trimester (Wen et al., 2008). Antibiotic prophylaxis with doxycycline prior to surgical intervention is recommended (Achilles et al., 2011).

Women who present with vaginal bleeding in pregnancy must have a blood type and antibody screen. Women who do not carry the Rh D antigen are identified as Rh D negative and may become alloimmunized if exposed to Rh D positive blood from a fetomaternal hemorrhage. The administration of anti-D immune globulin drastically decreases the rate of alloimmunization. In the first trimester, the red cell mass of the fetus is small. The dose of anti-D immune globulin necessary to protect against sensitization by 2.5 mL of red blood cells is 50 mcg (ACOG, 1999).

REFERENCES

Abdallah, Y., Daemen, A., Kirk, E., Pexsters, A., et al. (2011). Limitations of current definitions of miscarriage using mean gestational sac diameter and crown-rump length measurements: A multicenter observational study. *Ultrasound in Obstetrics and Gynecology, 38*(5), 497–502.

Achilles, S. L., & Reeves, M. F., Society of Family Planning. (2011). Prevention of infection after induced abortion. *Contraception, 83*(4), 295–309.

Bouyer, J., Coste, J., Fernandez, H., et al. (2002). Sites of ectopic pregnancy: A 10 year population-based study of 1800 cases. *Human Reproduction, 17*(12), 3224–3330.

ACOG Practice Bulletin. (1999). Prevention of Rh D Alloimmunization. *International Journal of Gynecology and Obstetrics, 66*(1), 63–70.

Barnhart, K. (2009). Ectopic pregnancy. *The New England Journal of Medicine, 361*(4), 379–387.

Barnhart, K., Sammel, M. D., Chung, K., Zhou, L., et al. (2004). Decline in serum human chorionic gonadotropin and spontaneous complete abortion: Defining the normal curve. *Obstetrics and Gynecology, 104*(5), 975–981.

Bagratee, J. S., Khullar, V., Regan, L., Moodley, J., et al. (2004). A randomized controlled trial comparing medical and expectant management of first trimester miscarriage. *Human Reproduction, 19*(2), 266–271.

Chung, K., Sammel, M., Zhou, L., Hummel, A., et al. (2006). Defining the curve when initial levels of human chorionic gonadotropin in womans with spontaneous abortions are low. *Fertility and Sterility, 85*(2), 508–510.

Deutchman, M., Tubay, A. T., & Turok, D. K., (2009). First trimester bleeding. *American Family Physician, 79*(11), 985–992.

Paspulati, R. M., Bhatt, S., & Nour, S. (2004). Sonographic evaluation of first-trimester bleeding. *Radiology Clinics of North America, 42*, 297–314.

Roberts, S. (2003). Hypovolemic and cardiac shock. In G. Dildy (Ed.), *Critical Care Obstetrics* (4th Ed., pp. 554). Malden, MA: Blackwell Science.

Silva, C., Sammel, M. D., Zhou, L., Gracia, C., et al. (2006). Human chorionic gonadotropin profile for women with ectopic pregnancy. *Obstetrics and Gynecology, 107*(3), 605–610.

Wen, J., Cai, Q. Y., Deng, F., & Li, Y. P. (2008). Manual versus electronic vacuum aspiration for first-trimester abortion: A systemic review. *BJOG, 115*(1), 5–13.

Wilcox, A. J., Weinberg, C. R., O'Connor, J. F., et al. (1998). Incidence of early loss of pregnancy. *The New England Journal of Medicine, 319*(4), 189–194.

Winikoff, B. (2005). Pregnancy failure and misoprostol–time for a change. *The New England Journal of Medicine, 353*(8), 834–836.

Zhang, J., Giles, J. M., Barnhart, K., Creinin, M. D., et al. (2005). Management of early pregnancy failure trial: A comparison of medical management with misoprostol and surgical management for early pregnancy failure. *The New England Journal of Medicine, 353*(8), 761–769.

5 Recognition and Treatment of Postabortion Complications

Janet Singer

Over one million pregnancies are terminated each year in the United States. Serious complications are uncommon, and deaths are exceedingly rare (Paul & Stewart, 2009). Less than 1% of women terminating a pregnancy will experience a major complication, and most complications will be recognized in the immediate postabortion period and treated by the provider onsite (Cappiello, Beal, & Simmonds, 2011). Still, some abortion complications will emerge after discharge from an abortion facility or setting, and it is prudent for clinicians working in an emergency department or obstetric triage unit to recognize these complications.

Symptomatology, assessment, and clinical management are the most common complications of abortion, which include bleeding secondary to retained products of conception (POCs) and infection. Other rare complications, including uterine perforation and cervical lacerations, and a discussion of postabortion emotional issues will be included.

TYPES OF ABORTION TERMINATIONS

Early abortions can be accomplished with medication or aspiration. Early aspiration abortion, sometimes called surgical abortion, is accomplished with dilation and suction curettage. The incidence of complications from aspiration abortion is outlined in Exhibit 5.1. In medication abortion, mifepristone and misoprostol are the medications of choice, though sometimes misoprostol alone or methotrexate can be used. Exhibit 5.2 lists the incidence of complications from medication abortion. Later abortions involve performing dilation and evacuation of the pregnancy or labor induction.

PRESENTING SYMPTOMATOLOGY

Women with complications from abortion will most often present with bleeding and/or pain. It is crucial to distinguish between normal postabortion bleeding and pain, and other symptoms, such as fever, which suggest a postabortion complication.

EXHIBIT 5.1

Types and Incidences of Complications From Aspiration Abortion

- Incomplete abortion (0.3%–2.0%)
- Infection (0.1%–2.0%)
- Cervical laceration (0.6%–1.2%)
- Uterine perforation (<0.4%)
- Blood clots (<0.2%)
- Excessive bleeding (0.02%–0.3%)
- Death (0.0006%, 1 in 160,000 cases)

Source: National Abortion Federation (2006).

EXHIBIT 5.2

Types and Incidences of Complications From Medication Abortion

- Incomplete abortion (<3%)
- Continuing pregnancy (<1%)
- Excessive bleeding (<1%)
- Infections (0.09%–0.6%)
- Death from *Clostridium sordellii*-related toxic shock (<0.001%)

Source: Adapted from National Abortion Federation (2006, 2010), ACOG Practice Bulletin No. 67 (2005), and Paul & Stewart (2009).

Nearly all women experience bleeding postabortion, typically for several days followed by spotting for up to 4 weeks or longer (Davis, Westhoff, & DeNonno, 2000; Paul & Stewart, 2009). Bleeding with a medication abortion is often heavier than a normal period (Harper, Winikoff, Ellertson, & Coyaji, 1998). However, comparative studies of aspiration and medication abortion show total blood loss to be similar in the two methods, with bleeding resulting from a medication abortion having a longer duration (Jensen, Astley, Morgan, & Nichols, 1999; National Abortion Federation, 2010). Most women experience cramping pain after an abortion. With medication abortion, pain can range from mild to severe, usually resolving shortly after the abortion is complete (National Abortion Federation, 2010; Spitz, Bardin, Benton, & Robins, 1998). With aspiration abortion, most women experience only mild uterine cramping and this usually resolves within a few days.

HISTORY AND DATA COLLECTION

For any woman presenting postabortion, it is important to determine when the abortion occurred, what type was performed, and at what gestational age. The later in gestation that an abortion is performed, the more likely the woman is to experience a complication. It is critical to obtain a description of any bleeding the woman is experiencing, the rate at which the woman is saturating pads, and whether any clots or tissue have been passed. In assessing pain, it is important to distinguish between cramping, which can be associated with retained POCs and fundal tenderness, which can be associated with infection. Additional history would include whether the woman experienced any fevers, chills, lightheadedness, or any persistent pregnancy symptoms like breast tenderness, nausea, and vomiting. It is important to take a careful medication history. After an abortion, it is usual for women to receive antibiotics, commonly doxycycline, and uterotonics such as methergine. In gathering the history, it may be helpful to speak with the abortion provider to obtain details of the procedure and any immediate complications. Complete and compassionate care requires assessing each woman's emotional status, as the life situation that leads a woman to terminate a pregnancy can be complex and stressful. An assessment of the woman's social support and prior history of mental health issues will identify those most likely to need postabortion emotional support.

In addition, some women may present for care who have attempted a self-induced abortion. More than 2% of abortion patients, in one study, reported ingesting something in an attempt to end a pregnancy, most commonly misoprostol, but also herbs and vitamin C have been identified. This is twice as likely to occur with women who are foreign-born (Jones, 2011).

PHYSICAL EXAMINATION

Vital signs are obtained to assess for fever, tachycardia, and/or hypotension. An abdominal examination is performed to assess for tenderness and uterine tone/consistency and size, if the uterus is enlarged above the pubic symphysis. A speculum examination is an essential part of the physical assessment. During the speculum examination, an inspection for bleeding is performed. It is determined whether the bleeding is coming from the cervical os and whether there are any cervical or vaginal lacerations. The amount of bleeding is described in terms of scopettes used to wipe away the blood. The color of the blood, old brownish or frank red, is also described. Any POCs in the vagina or protruding from the cervical os are noted and any mucopurulent discharge identified. Gonorrhea and chlamydia cultures are obtained, if these have not already been collected just prior to the abortion. After the speculum examination, a bimanual examination is performed to assess the uterus for enlargement, tone, and tenderness.

LABORATORY AND IMAGING STUDIES

Blood type and antibody screen are obtained. Typically a woman who is Rh negative will have received Rh immune globulin from the abortion provider. However, any woman who is Rh negative and has self-induced an abortion will need Rh immune globulin. If bleeding is heavy, a complete blood count and coagulation studies are ordered. A urine beta human chorionic gonadotropin (beta hCG) level can be used in addition to physical examination findings to determine if the abortion is complete. A positive beta hCG alone does not mean that the woman is still pregnant or needs intervention. A beta hCG level declines steadily after first trimester aspiration abortion, halving at least every 48 hours. Because beta hCG levels are as high as 150,000 in early pregnancy, levels may still be high enough to cause urine pregnancy tests to remain positive for as long as 60 days postabortion (Fjerstad & Stewart, 2009). With medication abortion, beta hCG levels continue to increase after mifepristone is administered and then generally, but not always, decline rapidly after misoprostol is administered. Even women with a successful medication abortion may continue to have elevated beta hCG levels (Fjerstad & Stewart, 2009). Serial quantitative serum beta hCGs may be useful to follow for appropriate decline over time. A single value does not help in diagnosing an abortion complication.

Ultrasound is useful for determining if a gestational sac or fetal parts remain in the uterus. Determining endometrial thickness with ultrasound is *not* clinically useful postabortion, as there is no thickness that correlates consistently with the need to intervene (Cowett, 2004; Reeves, Lohr, Harwood, & Creinin, 2008). Ultrasound may be used to assess for intra-abdominal hematoma when uterine perforation is suspected in a woman exhibiting signs of hypovolemic shock.

POSTABORTION BLEEDING

DIFFERENTIAL DIAGNOSIS

When the presenting complaint is postabortion bleeding, uterine atony is the first diagnosis to be considered. Atony and the resulting abnormal postabortion bleeding are most often related to retained POCs/incomplete abortion. If atony is ruled out, lacerations are considered to be a likely cause of abnormal bleeding.

CLINICAL MANAGEMENT OF UTERINE ATONY AND RETAINED POCs

The first step in managing uterine atony is to massage the uterus and administer uterotonics (National Abortion Federation, 2011). Table 5.1 lists the appropriate uterotonics to administer. In addition, intravenous (IV) access and vital signs are monitored throughout. If uterotonics are unable to control the bleeding, intrauterine tamponade with Foley or Bakri balloon or packing may be attempted.

If on speculum examination, POCs are seen at the cervical os, they may be removed with a ring forceps. If POCs are identified in the uterus on ultrasound, and bleeding is heavy, aspiration may be indicated. If bleeding is *not* heavy and the woman shows *no signs of infection*, misoprostol is another option to bring about expulsion of the POCs (Paul & Stewart, 2009). If no POCs are seen on ultrasound, the decision to aspirate the uterus is based on the clinical findings, not on an ultrasound measurement of endometrial thickness (Reeves et al., 2008). After the uterus is emptied, specimens are rinsed in a strainer and identified. Specimens are sent to pathology for further identification and analysis as needed.

CLINICAL MANAGEMENT OF CERVICAL LACERATION

A cervical laceration is treated by tamponading the laceration with a ring forceps for several minutes, and/or applying silver nitrate or Monsel's solution. Suturing is necessary if the bleeding does not stop with these interventions or if the laceration is extensive (Lichtenberg & Grimes, 2009).

RARE COMPLICATIONS

If bleeding continues after the clinical management described above, other diagnoses must be considered. These include uterine perforation, coagulopathy, placenta accreta, and arteriovenous malformations.

TABLE 5.1 Standard Agents for Treating Postabortion Hemorrhage

MEDICATION	DOSAGE AND ROUTE	SIDE EFFECTS AND CONTRAINDICATIONS
Misoprostol	800–1,000 mcg per rectum or 800 mcg sublingual	Diarrhea and abdominal pain in >10%
Oxytocin	10 units IM or 10–40 units IV	Antidiuretic effect in high doses (rare)
Methergine (methylergonovine maleate)	0.2 mg po or IM. PO dose may be given 4 times/day for up to 1 week. IM dose may be repeated every 2–4 hr	Produces sustained contractions of smooth muscles. Contraindicated in patients with hypertension, and it is recommended not to give IV secondary to hypertensive crisis/stroke
Hemabate (carboprost tromethamine)	250 mcg IM. May be given every 15–90 min up to 8 doses	Diarrhea, nausea, and vomiting in 33%–66%. Contraindicated in patients with active cardiac, pulmonary, renal, or hepatic dysfunction. May cause transient pyrexia and elevated blood pressure

Source: Adapted from National Abortion Federation (2011).

POSTABORTION PAIN

DIFFERENTIAL DIAGNOSIS

Pain, by itself, is rarely a sign of an abortion complication. However, pain is concerning when it is accompanied by other signs or symptoms, such as fever or heavy bleeding. If pain persists, an evaluation to rule out retained POCs (see above for clinical management), endometritis, hematometra, or uterine perforation is necessary (National Abortion Federation, 2011).

CLINICAL MANAGEMENT OF ENDOMETRITIS

Postabortion endometritis with or without retained POCs must be considered in any woman who presents with lower abdominal pain postabortion. Other signs of endometritis include fever, enlarged tender uterus, abnormal bleeding, elevated white blood cell count, vaginal discharge, and malaise (Pau & Stewart, 2009). Typically, these signs occur in the first few days postabortion (Lichtenberg & Grimes, 2009).

IV access is maintained and vital signs monitored throughout. It is essential to treat endometritis with broad spectrum antibiotics, as infection is likely to be polymicrobial in nature (Lichtenberg & Grimes 2009). Exhibit 5.3 details the antibiotic treatment of endometritis. Women with mild infection may be treated with oral antibiotics on an outpatient basis and then re-examined in 3 days to assure substantial clinical improvement. IV antibiotic therapy is indicated in women with severe illness, suspected pelvic abscess, immunocompromise, inability to tolerate oral medication, or failed outpatient treatment (Centers for Disease Control and Prevention, 2010; Paul & Stewart, 2009).

CLINICAL MANAGEMENT OF HEMATOMETRA

Pain may also be due to clots remaining in the uterus. Women with hematometra will have an enlarged, tender uterus and minimal to no bleeding. Reaspiration and the administration of uterotonics are the indicated treatments, and symptoms usually resolve quickly (Paul & Stewart, 2009).

CLINICAL MANAGEMENT OF UTERINE PERFORATION/RUPTURE

Uterine perforation is a very rare complication of abortion. Clinically significant uterine perforations are likely to be suspected or recognized during the abortion procedure. The provider might note that an instrument has passed farther than the expected length of the uterus, more than the usual amount

EXHIBIT 5.3

Antibiotic Treatment of Postabortion Endometritis

Inpatient and Outpatient

Recommended Parenteral Regimen A
Cefotetan 2 g IV q 12 hr *OR* cefoxitin 2g IV q 6 hr *plus* doxycycline 100 mg PO or IV q 12

Recommended Parenteral Regimen B
Clindamycin 900 mg IV q 8 hr *plus* gentamicin loading dose IV *OR* IM (2 mg/kg of body weight) followed by a maintenance dose (1.5 mg/kg) q 8 hr. May substitute single daily dosing (3–5 mg/kg).

Alternative Parenteral Regimen
Ampicillin/sulbactam 3 g IV q 6 hr *plus* doxycycline 100 mg PO or IV q 12 hr

Outpatient Regimen

Ceftriaxone 250 mg IM × 1 *plus* doxycycline 100 mg PO bid × 14 days *with or without* metronidazole 500 mg PO bid × 14 days *OR*

Cefoxitin 2 g IM × 1 and probenecid 1g PO concurrently × 1 *plus* doxycycline 100 mg PO bid × 14 days *with or without* metronidazole 500 mg PO bid × 14 days *OR*

Other parenteral third-generation cephalosporins *plus* doxycycline 100 mg PO bid × 14 days *with or without* metronidazole 500 mg PO bid × 14 days

Source: Adapted from Centers for Disease Control and Prevention (2010).

of pain is experienced during and immediately after the procedure, and/or tissue other than pregnancy tissue is in the aspirate (National Abortion Federation, 2011). In managing a uterine perforation, IV access is maintained and vital signs are monitored throughout. Serial hematocrits are obtained. If a woman is transferred to the hospital with a suspected perforation but no abdominal pain or evidence of internal bleeding, observation without intervention may be appropriate. Uterine rupture requiring surgical intervention is more likely to occur during procedures performed later in gestation. It becomes a surgical emergency when trauma to organs other than the uterus is suspected. If there is suspicion of internal bleeding, surgery is needed to identify and repair the injury. Uterine rupture may also be suspected if the woman has a history of a cesarean section and misoprostol was used in a second trimester termination of pregnancy (Paul & Stewart, 2009). Uterine perforation that is not diagnosed in the perioperative period, may present as severe anemia or peritonitis, and those complications must be treated, in addition to evaluating the perforation itself.

RARE COMPLICATIONS

Medication abortion rarely results in infection. However, *Clostridium sordellii* has caused a few cases of fatal toxic shock syndrome in women undergoing medication abortion. Women with this atypical infection tend to be afebrile with little uterine tenderness and present with flu-like symptoms, tachycardia, hypotension, a marked increase in white blood cell count, and a high hemoglobin level.

Clinical Management of *C. sordellii* Infection

There is little information to guide treatment in cases of *C. sordellii* infection and death usually occurs rapidly. It is believed that initiating antibiotics that suppress toxin synthesis (i.e., clindamycin) could be helpful in addition to usual resuscitative measures. Emergency surgery to remove necrotic tissue is necessary (Aldapel, Bryant, & Stevens, 2006).

EMOTIONAL RESPONSE

In general, women terminate pregnancies because they do not desire to continue a particular pregnancy at a particular time. Such situations can cause distress and elicit feelings of sadness and loss (National Abortion Federation, 2006). Unwanted pregnancy and abortion correlate with conditions like poverty, exposure to violence, and drug use, which can all negatively affect mental health. It has been shown that abortion does not pose a threat to women's mental health. In fact, relief is the most commonly felt emotion after abortion. In a comprehensive review of the literature for the APA Task Force on Mental Health and Abortion, no significant difference was found between the psychological outcomes of women with unplanned pregnancies who terminated pregnancies and those who continued pregnancies (Major et al., 2008). Prior mental health status and the presence or absence of social supports are the strongest predictors of postabortion mental health status (Major et al., 2008).

REFERENCES

ACOG Practice Bulletin No. 67. (2005). Medical management of abortion. American College of Ob/Gyn. *Obstetrics and Gynecology*, 106 (4), 871–881.

Aldapel, M. J., Bryant, A. E., & Stevens, D. L. (2006). Clostridium sordellii infection: Epidemiology, clinical findings, and current perspectives on diagnosis and treatment. *Clinical Infectious Diseases, 43*(11), 1436–46.

Cappiello, J. D., Beal, M. W., & Simmonds, K. E. (2011). Clinical issues in post-abortion care. *The Nurse Practitioner, 36* (5), 35–40.

Centers for Disease Control and Prevention (CDC). (2010). Morbidity and mortality weekly report. sexually transmitted diseases treatment guidelines, 2010. Retrieved from http://cdc.gov/mmwr

Cowett, A. A., Cohen, L. S., Lichtenberg, E. S., & Stika, C. S. (2004). Ultrasound evaluation of the endometrium after medical termination of pregnancy. *Obstetrics and Gynecology, 103*(5), 871–875.

Davis, A., Westhoff, C., & DeNonno, L. (2000). Bleeding patterns after early abortion with mifepristone and misoprostol of manual vacuum aspiration. *Journal of American Medical Women's Association, 55*(*Suppl 3*), 141–144.

Fjerstad, M., & Stewart, F. (2009). Pregnancy testing and management of early pregnancy. In R. A. Hatcher, J. Trussell, A. L. Nelson, W. Cates, F. H. Steward, & D. Kowal (Eds.). *Contraceptive Technology* (19th ed., pp. 591–628). New York: Ardent Media, Inc.

Harper, C., Winikoff, B., Ellertson, C., & Coyaji, K. (1998). Blood loss with mifepristone/misoprostol abortion: measures from a trial in China, Cuba and India. *International Journal of Gynecology and Obstetrics, 63*(1), 39–49.

Jensen, J. T., Astley, S. J., Morgan, E., & Nichols, M. D. (1999). Outcomes of suction curettage and mifepristone abortion in the United States. *Contraception, 59*(3), 153–159.

Jones, R. K. (2011). How commonly do US abortion patients report attempts to self-induce? *American Journal of Obstetrics and Gynecology, 204*(1), 23.e1–23.e4.

Lichtenberg, E. S., & Grimes, D. A. (2009). Surgical complications: Prevention and management. In M. Paul, E. S. Lichtenberg, L. Borgatta, D. A. Grimes, P. G. Stubblefield, & M. D. Creinin (Eds.). *Management of unintended and abnormal pregnancy: Comprehensive abortion care* (pp. 224–251). Hoboken, NJ: Blackwell Publishing Ltd.

Major, B., Appelbaum, M., Beckman, L., Dutton, M., Russo, N. & West, C. (2008). *Report of the APA task force on mental health and abortion. APA task force on mental health and abortion*. Washington, DC. Retrieved from http://www.apa.org/pi/wpo/mental-health-abortion-report.pdf

National Abortion Federation. (2006). *Safety of abortion*. Retrieved from http://www.prochoice.org/about_abortion/facts/safety_of_abortion.html

National Abortion Federation. (2010). *Early options: A provider's guide to medical abortion*. Retrieved from http://www.prochoice.org/education/cme/online_cme/home.asp

National Abortion Federation. (2011). *Clinical policy guidelines*. Washington, DC: National Abortion Federation.

Paul, M., & Stewart, F. H. (2009). Abortion. In R. A. Hatcher, J. Trussell, A. L. Nelson, W. Cates, F. H. Steward, & D. Kowal (Eds.). *Contraceptive technology* (19th ed., pp 637–672). New York: Ardent Media, Inc.

Reeves, M. F., Lohr, P. A., Harwood, B. J., & Creinin, M. D. (2008). Ultrasonographic endometrial thickness after medical and surgical management of early pregnancy failure. *Obstetrics and Gynecology, 111*(*1*), 106–112.

Schmiege, S., & Russo, N. F. (2005). Depression and unwanted pregnancy: Longitudinal cohort study. *British Medical Journal, 331*(*7528*), 1303.

Spitz, I. M., Bardin, C. W., Benton, L., & Robins, A. (1998). Early pregnancy termination with mifepristone and misoprostol in the United States. *New England Journal of Medicine, 38*(*18*), 1241–1247.

6 Abdominal Pain and Masses in Pregnancy

Moune Jabre Raughley

Adnexal masses complicate between 1:81 and 1:8,000 pregnancies (Leiserowitz, 2006; Whitecar, Turner, & Higby, 1999). Of these, 1%–8% are malignant (Leiserowitz, 2006; Whitecar et al., 1999). Most adnexal masses in pregnancy are found incidentally on routine obstetric ultrasound (US) as they typically do not cause symptoms, and physical examination is limited by the gravid uterus (Leiserowitz, 2006). Pregnant women presenting with abdominal pain to an emergency department or obstetric triage setting frequently have a diagnostic US to assess the fetus, placenta, and adnexa.

The vast majority (50%–70%) of adnexal masses in pregnancy resolve spontaneously (Bernhard, Klebba, Gray, & Mutch, 1999; Bromley & Benacerraf, 1997; Hoover & Jenkins, 2011; Spitzer, Kaushal, & Benjamin, 1998; Zanetta et al., 2003). Those that persist into the second trimester pose greatest concern as they can be malignant, rupture, torse, or obstruct labor (Hoover & Jenkins, 2011). The actual risk of these complications, however, has been reported as less than 2% (Whitecar et al., 1999). In the symptomatic woman, one must determine if the adnexal mass necessitates emergent or urgent surgical intervention versus observation and pain management.

PRESENTING SYMPTOMATOLOGY

In the first trimester, symptomatic adnexal masses typically present with unilateral or bilateral pelvic cramping or pressure. Larger masses persisting into the second trimester tend to cause unilateral pelvic pain. Midline abdominal pain can occur if the mass is displaced to the midline by the gravid uterus. Severe pain may be associated with nausea and vomiting from peritoneal irritation. In rare cases, a ruptured mass can cause significant internal hemorrhage such that the woman reports dizziness in addition to pain. Uterine irritability or contractions may be seen in the late second and third trimester. In pregnant women, with pain secondary to an adnexal mass, vaginal bleeding, rupture of membranes, or impact on fetal status are exceedingly rare. However, symptoms may reflect other underlying obstetric conditions with the incidental finding of an adnexal mass.

HISTORY AND DATA COLLECTION

Obtaining a history in a pregnant woman with abdominal pain is similar to that of the nonpregnant patient. Important factors to ascertain are time of onset and duration of pain, inciting or mitigating factors, quality, severity, location, and radiation. Associated symptoms can include fever, nausea/vomiting, urinary symptoms, bowel changes, vaginal bleeding, leaking amniotic fluid, contractions, or flank pain. If nausea and/or vomiting are present, it is critical to assess if this is longstanding, in which case it could represent nausea and vomiting of pregnancy. If acute, then it could potentially be associated with the current clinical presentation. Accurate determination of gestational age is critical. Does the woman have a known intrauterine gestation or must ectopic pregnancy be excluded? Obtain the remaining history such as obstetrical, medical, surgical, and social history as per routine. Any recent USs need to be reviewed to help determine how long a mass has been present.

PHYSICAL EXAMINATION FINDINGS

Physiologic changes in pregnancy can affect vital signs. For example, mild tachycardia may be normal in the third trimester but would be atypical in early gestation. Likewise, blood pressure reaches its nadir in the second trimester. Tachycardia and hypotension can also result from significant internal hemorrhage.

In addition to routine cardiopulmonary examination, abdominal examination and assessment for costovertebral angle tenderness, a sterile speculum and vaginal examination are performed to evaluate for adnexal or uterine tenderness, cervical dilation, and potential rupture of membranes. Further examination is performed as directed by history. At 6 weeks gestation, the uterus is similar in size to the nonpregnant state and the adnexa may be palpable in a nonobese patient. By 12 weeks, the uterine fundus is at the level of the pubis symphysis then up to the umbilicus at 20 weeks. Clinical examination of the adnexa is extremely limited after 12 weeks' gestation.

LABORATORY AND IMAGING STUDIES

If a mass is suspected, US is the preferred imaging modality as it allows for optimal characterization of the mass and determination of its malignant potential (Hoover & Jenkins, 2011; Whitecar et al., 1999). Several studies have shown that antenatal US correctly diagnosed all the malignant tumors in these series (Schmeler et al., 2005; Hoover & Jenkins, 2011; Whitecar et al., 1999). US can be used to examine the kidneys and to assess for free fluid in the pelvic cul-de-sac, abdominal ascites in Morison's pouch, and hemoperitoneum. US has the additional benefit of being cheaper and faster to obtain in most circumstances than other modalities.

Magnetic resonance imaging (MRI) can be employed if additional imaging is needed and is especially useful to delineate the extent and nature of masses that are too large to visualize completely on US (Hoover & Jenkins, 2011). MRI should also be considered if appendicitis is suspected. As with US, MRI avoids maternal and fetal exposure to radiation.

Nonobstetric causes of abdominal pain are best evaluated by computed tomography (CT), as it provides better resolution imaging of the gastrointestinal tract. CT is generally considered relatively safe in pregnancy, but it is recommended that CT only be performed when absolutely necessary, as it does expose the mother and fetus to 2–4 rads per abdominopelvic study (Hoover & Jenkins, 2011). With regards to the use of iodinated contrast media for CT and gadolinium for MRI, both the American College of Radiology and American College of Obstetricians and Gynecologists (ACOG) note the limited data on safety in pregnancy and advise limiting use to when benefits greatly outweigh risks (Jaffe, Miller, & Merkle, 2007).

Laboratory testing includes a complete blood count to asses for leukocytosis and/or anemia as these may be present in the setting of torsion or ruptured ovarian cyst. Urinalysis may help exclude urinary tract causes of pain.

Serum tumor markers are of limited utility in the initial assessment of pregnant women as CA-125 levels are normally elevated in pregnancy with a peak in the first trimester (range, 7–251 units/mL) followed by steady decrease. CA-125 may be elevated in several benign conditions and other serum tumor markers such as alpha-fetoprotein (AFP), beta human chorionic gonadotropin (beta hCG), and lactate dehydrogenase (LDH) are significantly affected by pregnancy (Hoover & Jenkins, 2011). Tumor markers are largely used to follow disease progression and control in women in whom a malignancy has already been diagnosed (ACOG, 2007; Hoover & Jenkins, 2011).

DIFFERENTIAL DIAGNOSIS

In addition to the adnexal mass as the source of abdominal pain, the differential diagnosis of abdominal pain in pregnant women must include other obstetric and nonobstetric causes of pain. Common sources of pain, unrelated to adnexal masses, include physiologic abdominal pain of early pregnancy, spontaneous abortion, round ligament pain, appendicitis, gastroenteritis, nephrolithiasis, urinary tract infections, and pyelonephritis. Ectopic pregnancy must be included in the differential diagnosis in women with unlocated pregnancies.

Functional cysts such as corpus luteum are among the most common adnexal mass in pregnancy (Hoover & Jenkins, 2011). Other benign masses include mature cystic teratoma, serous or mucinous cystadenoma, endometrioma, paraovarian cysts, and leiomyoma. Malignant tumors are rare (3.6%–6.8% incidence). The most common types are germ cell, stromal, or epithelial tumors of low malignant potential (ACOG, 2007). See Exhibit 6.1 for incidence of common adnexal masses.

CLINICAL MANAGEMENT AND FOLLOW-UP

The fundamental question in the acute management of pregnant women with adnexal masses is whether to observe or intervene surgically (and when to do so emergently). Factors to consider include the following: degree of suspicion for malignancy, hemodynamic stability, concern for torsion, and pain severity. Most hemodynamically stable women presenting to an emergency department without evidence of torsion may be observed acutely then managed on an outpatient basis. This allows time to obtain additional imaging or subspecialist consultation, as needed. Abdominopelvic pain may be treated with acetaminophen or oral narcotics in the interim.

Given the inherent risks of surgery, there is a growing body of evidence to support observation and delay of surgery until the postpartum period. The

EXHIBIT 6.1

Incidence of Common Adnexal Masses in Pregnancy

TYPE OF MASS	PERCENTAGE (%)
Mature cystic teratoma	25
Corpus luteum and functional cysts	17
Serous cystadenoma	14
Mucinous cystadenoma	11
Endometrioma	8
Carcinoma	2.8
Low malignant potential tumor	3
Leiomyoma	2
Paraovarian cysts	<5
Pelvic kidney	<0.1

Source: Hoover & Jenkins (2011) and Cinman, Okeke, & Smith (2007).

vast majority of adnexal masses noted in pregnancy spontaneously resolve, thus obviating the need for surgical intervention (Schmeler et al., 2005; Hoover & Jenkins, 2011; Whitecar et al., 1999).

Surgery may increase the risk of spontaneous abortion, preterm labor, and rupture of membranes. Observation can increase risk of torsion, rupture of the mass, peritonitis, hemorrhage, delay in diagnosis of cancer, and obstruction of delivery. Compared with pregnant women not undergoing surgery, the overall risk of premature delivery increased by 22% in those who had surgery, regardless of the surgical approach (Hoover & Jenkins, 2011). There is conflicting evidence as to whether emergent versus scheduled surgery carries an increased risk of fetal adverse effects.

Whitecar et al. (1999) reviewed 130 cases of pregnant women with adnexal masses that required laparotomy. Of these, 16 were emergent. They found that laparotomy at less than 23 weeks' gestational age was associated with significantly fewer adverse pregnancy outcomes greater than 23 weeks, but there were no significant differences in maternal morbidity or fetal outcomes between emergent and scheduled laparotomy. Adverse fetal outcomes in emergent surgery are more likely to be related to the underlying condition that necessitated surgery rather than the surgery itself (Hoover & Jenkins, 2011).

A study by Schmeler et al. (2005) reviewed 127,177 deliveries and identified 59 women (0.05%) with an adnexal mass ≥5 cm. Median gestational age at diagnosis was 12 weeks and 80% were diagnosed on US, the rest, at time of cesarean section. Seventeen women (29%) underwent surgery. Of these, the majority were planned laparotomies for suspected malignancy. The few emergent surgeries were performed for torsion. One woman in the surgical group had preterm premature rupture of membranes at 23 weeks with subsequent delivery at 28 weeks. No other adverse fetal outcomes were reported. Forty-two women in the observation group were observed expectantly in the antenatal period and then had surgery either intrapartum or postpartum. The median gestational age at delivery for all women was 39 weeks. The authors observed no statistically significant difference in obstetrical outcomes between the surgical and observation groups. All the malignant masses had concerning sonographic findings that prompted antenatal surgery. The authors concluded that the risk of malignancy is less than 1% in pregnant women with incidentally identified masses with low-risk features on US. This is similar to rates in nonpregnant women. As such, expectant management may be a reasonable option in appropriately selected women.

In 2010, the Society for Radiologists in Ultrasound (SRU) released a consensus statement on the recommended management and follow-up for adnexal masses that are incidentally seen on US in asymptomatic, nonpregnant women (Levine et al., 2010). Although the guidelines are intended for masses in the nonpregnant population, other studies have utilized similar management in pregnant women (Hoover & Jenkins, 2011; Platek, 1995; Schmeler et al., 2005; Zanetta et al., 2001).

The SRU guidelines allow stratification of adnexal masses into those that require further follow-up and those that do not based on the presence of features suggestive of malignancy or benignity. The guidelines for premenopausal women include the following: normal ovaries are typically less than 3 cm in size, round or oval with thin smooth walls, anechoic spaces, and no flow seen on color Doppler US. Ovaries may contain multiple physiologic follicles or simple cysts that are considered normal if measure less than 3 cm. The corpus luteum appears as a thick-walled cyst with or without crenulated inner margins, measures less than 3 cm and often has internal echoes with a peripheral ring of vascularity on color Doppler US. Physiologic cysts (Figure 6.1) and corpus luteum cysts (Figure 6.2) do not require further follow-up.

Simple cysts as noted in Figure 6.3 that are anechoic with smooth thin walls measuring 5 to 7 cm without any features of complexity may be followed with annual repeat imaging in premenopausal women. Those measuring greater than 7 cm can be further evaluated with additional imaging or surgical evaluation if clinically indicated.

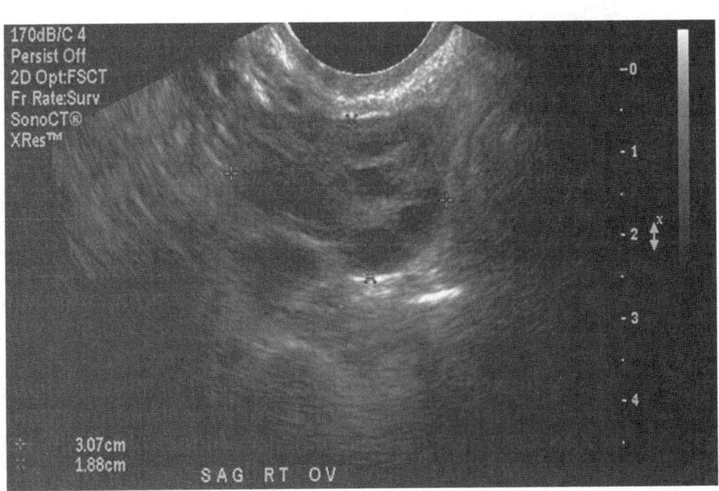

FIGURE 6.1 Normal ovary with physiologic follicles.

Source: Courtesy of the Department of Radiology, Women & Infants Hospital, Providence, RI.

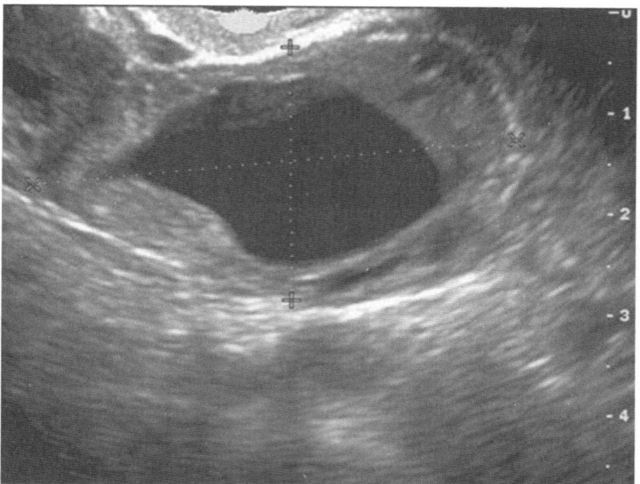

FIGURE 6.2 Corpus luteum cyst.

Source: Courtesy of the Department of Radiology, Women & Infants Hospital, Providence, RI.

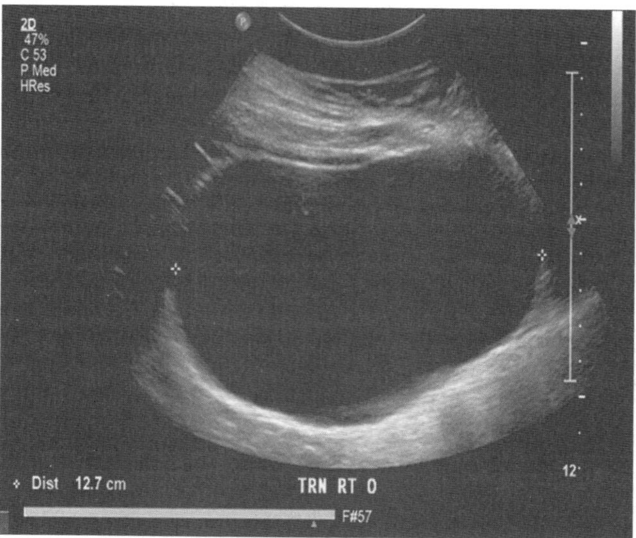

FIGURE 6.3 Simple cyst.

Source: Courtesy of the Department of Radiology, Women & Infants Hospital, Providence, RI.

Hemorrhagic cysts (Figure 6.4) have a reticular pattern of internal echoes or multiple irregular hyperechoic structures within the cyst. They may have solid-appearing areas with concave margins without internal flow on color Doppler US. No follow-up is necessary for hemorrhagic cysts measuring less than 5 cm but those greater than 5 cm should be reimaged at 6 to 12 weeks to document resolution.

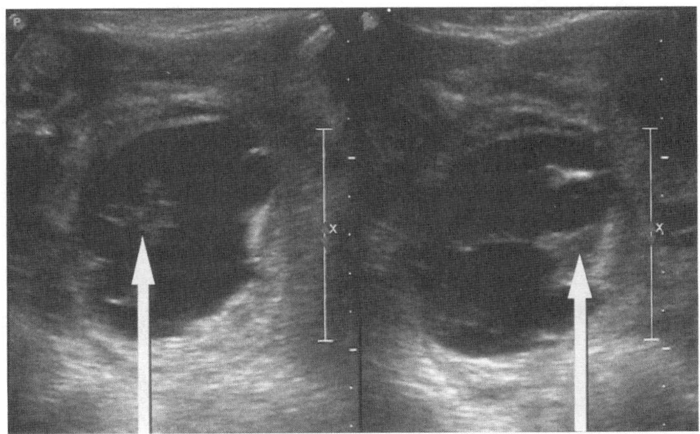

FIGURE 6.4 Hemorrhagic cyst.

Source: Courtesy of the Department of Radiology, Women & Infants Hospital, Providence, RI.

Endometriomas (Figure 6.5) have homogenous low-level internal echoes that give the classic "ground glass" appearance. Although they do not have a solid component, endometriomas can have small echogenic foci in the walls. Mature cystic teratomas (Figure 6.6) have a focal or diffuse hyperechoic component and may have hyperechoic lines or dots as well as areas of acoustic shadowing. Both endometriomas and mature cystic teratomas should be followed annually to document stability if not surgically removed. Peritoneal inclusion cysts and hydrosalpinx can be reimaged as clinically indicated.

Sonographic features concerning for neoplasm include nodularity, calcifications, and septations. Thin septations and solitary nodules without flow are likely to be benign neoplasms, whereas thick septations or nodules with blood flow are worrisome for malignancy. Such findings warrant additional imaging with MRI and possibly surgical evaluation (Levine et al., 2010).

When emergent surgical intervention is warranted, the surgical approach must be determined. If suspicion for malignancy is high, pre, or intraoperative, gynecologic oncology consult and frozen pathology must be considered. Frozen-section accuracy varies between 72% and 89% (ACOG, 2007).

It is unclear whether a laparoscopic or laparotomic approach is preferable in the gravid woman. A recent review article by Hoover noted concerns with laparoscopy including the paucity of data on effects of pneumoperitoneum, potential for fetal acidosis from maternal conversion of insufflated carbon dioxide gas to circulating carbonic acid, injection of carbon dioxide into the uterus and potential for uterine injury (Veress needle, trochar; Hoover & Jenkins, 2011). Laparoscopy has several significant advantages, however, such as shorter recovery period with faster postoperative ambulation, less postoperative pain requiring less narcotic use, less need for uterine retraction, and thus less uterine irritability (Hoover & Jenkins, 2011).

In 2008, the Society of American Gastrointestinal and Endoscopic Surgeons issued guidelines for use of laparoscopy in pregnant women (Yumi, 2008), which are as follows: laparoscopy is safe at any gestational age, though 16–20 weeks is optimal. A woman is placed in the left lateral decubitus position to minimize vena caval compression. The open (Hasson) technique can be safely performed for initial abdominal access though use of the Veress

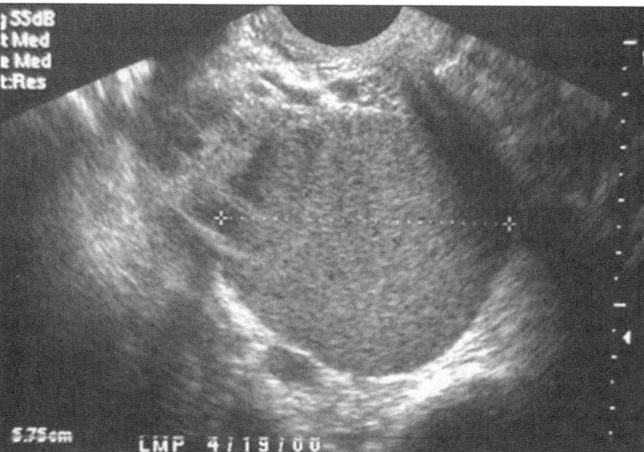

FIGURE 6.5 Endometrioma.

Source: Courtesy of the Department of Radiology, Women & Infants Hospital, Providence, RI.

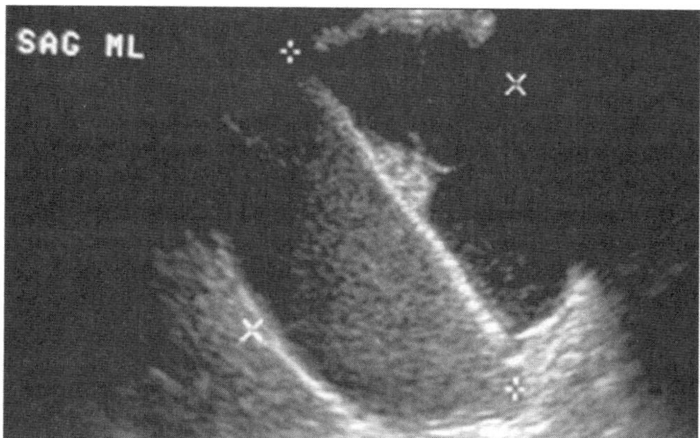

FIGURE 6.6 Mature cystic teratoma (dermoid).

Source: Courtesy of the Department of Radiology, Women & Infants Hospital, Providence, RI.

needle may be considered if performed under US guidance, and the location is adjusted to the fundal height (at least 6 cm above or in left upper quadrant). Intra-abdominal pressure of 10 to 15 mmHg with Trendelenburg position may be safely used. Capnography should be used for intraoperative CO_2 monitoring. Routine blood gas monitoring is not indicated. Pneumatic compression devices can be used during and after surgery along with early ambulation for prophylaxis against deep venous thrombosis. Though prophylactic tocolysis is not indicated, it may be considered perioperatively for signs of preterm labor. The fetal heart is monitored pre- and postoperatively in emergent abdominal surgery.

Based on the existing evidence, ACOG recommends evaluating the pregnant woman with an adnexal mass similarly to the premenopausal woman. US should be the first imaging modality followed by MRI if further imaging is necessary. CA-125 levels are usually mildly elevated in pregnancy (<250 units/mL) and not typically associated with malignancy. Persistent, large adnexal masses are frequently surgically removed in the second trimester to prevent emergent intervention at a later time for torsion or rupture, though there is a lack of supporting data for this. Given the low risk for both malignancy and acute complications, expectant management can be considered in pregnant women with adnexal masses.

REFERENCES

American College of Obstetricians and Gynecologists (ACOG). (2007). Practice bulletin: Management of adnexal masses. *Obstetrics & Gynecology, 110*(1), 201–214.

Bernhard, L. M., Klebba, P. K., Gray, D. L., & Mutch, D. G. (1999). Predictors of persistence of adnexal masses in pregnancy. *Obstetrics & Gynecology, 93*(4), 585–589.

Bromley, B., & Benacerraf, B. (1997). Adnexal masses during pregnancy: Accuracy of sonographic diagnosis and outcome. *Journal of Ultrasound in Medicine, 16*(7), 447–452.

Cinman, N. M., Okeke, Z., & Smith, A. D. (2007). Pelvic kidney: Associated diseases and treatment. *Journal of Endourology, 21*(8), 836–842.

Hoover, K., & Jenkins, T. R. (2011). Evaluation and management of adnexal masses in pregnancy. *American Journal of Obstetrics & Gynecology, 205*(2), 97–102.

Jaffe, T. A., Miller, C. M., & Merkle, E. M. (2007). Practice patterns in imaging of the pregnant patient with abdominal pain: A survey of academic centers. *American Journal of Roentgenology, 189*(5), 1128–1134.

Leiserowitz, G. (2006). Managing ovarian masses during pregnancy. *Obstetrical & Gynecological Survey, 61*(7), 463–470.

Levine, D., Brown, D. L., Andreotti, R. F., Benacerraf, B., Benson, C. B., Brewster, W. R. . . . Smith-Bindman, R. (2010). Management of asymptomatic ovarian and other adnexal cysts imaged at US Society of Radiologists in Ultrasound Consensus Conference Statement. *Radiology, 256*(3), 943–954.

Schmeler, K., Mayo-Smith, W., Peipert, J., Weitzen, S., Manuel, M., & Gordinier, M. (2005). Adnexal masses in pregnancy: Surgery compared with observation. *Obstetrics & Gynecology, 105*(5 Pt 1), 1098–1103.

Spitzer, M., Kaushal, N., & Benjamin, F. (1998). Maternal CA-125 levels in pregnancy and the puerperium. *Journal of Reproductive Medicine, 43*(4), 387–392.

Whitecar, P., Turner, S., & Higby, K. (1999). Adnexal masses in pregnancy: A review of 130 cases undergoing surgical management. *American Journal of Obstetrics & Gynecology, 181*(1), 19–24.

Yumi, H. (2008). Guidelines for diagnosis, treatment, and use of laparoscopy for surgical problems during pregnancy. *Surgical Endoscopy, 22*(4), 849–861.

Zanetta, G., Mariani, E., Lissoni, A., Ceruti, P., Trio, D., Strobelt, N., & Mariani, S. (2003). A prospective study of the role of ultrasound in the management of adnexal masses in pregnancy. *British Journal of Obstetrics and Gynecology, 110*(6), 578–583.

Zanetta, G., Rota, S., Chiari, S., Bonazzi, C., Bratina, G., & Mangioni, C. (2001). Behavior of borderline tumors with particular interest to persistence, recurrence, and progression to invasive carcinoma: a prospective study. *Journal of Clinical Oncology, 19*(10), 2658–2664.

Pregnancy Loss Prior to Viability

7

Luu Cortes Doan and Robyn A. Gray

Pregnancy loss prior to viability refers to spontaneous abortions occurring at less than 23 completed weeks of gestation (Seri & Evans, 2008). This phenomenon will affect approximately 15% of clinically recognized pregnancies (Saraiya et al., 1999). Most of these pregnancy losses will occur early in the first trimester, prior to 13 weeks' gestation. However, at least 13% of spontaneous abortions will occur in the second trimester between 13 and 20 weeks' gestation (Saraiya et al., 1999). Causes for pregnancy loss in the second trimester include previable premature rupture of membranes (previable PROM), previable preterm labor, cervical insufficiency, and intrauterine fetal demise (IUFD) as noted in Table 7.1.

The diagnosis of pregnancy loss in the second trimester and the clinical presentation in the obstetric triage or emergency setting will be reviewed. Definitive treatment plans will frequently involve consultation with a neonatologist or maternal/fetal medicine specialist depending on gestational age. Initial treatment options will be reviewed.

THRESHOLD OF FETAL VIABILITY

Occasionally, a pregnant woman with a viable fetus will present with premature rupture of membranes or preterm labor at the threshold of viability or 24 weeks' gestation. When there is an imminent delivery of a fetus with cardiac activity prior to 23 completed weeks of gestation and an estimated fetal weight of less than 500 g, the extremely low chance of neonatal survival precludes intervention on behalf of the fetus (Seri & Evans, 2008). Conversely, neonates born at or beyond 25^0 weeks, with a birth weight of greater than 600 g, have a greater than 50% chance of survival without severe permanent disability and warrant full resuscitative efforts (Seri & Evans, 2009). The gestational age of 23^0 to 24^6 is described as the threshold of viability in which survival and morbidity are uncertain. Gestational age must be confirmed by last menstrual period and ultrasound dating. If delivery is not imminent, an ultrasound can be used to estimate fetal weight and determine the sex of the fetus—two factors that can influence neonatal survival. A multidisciplinary team approach is used in discussing prognosis for fetuses on the threshold of viability.

TABLE 7.1 Second Trimester Pregnancy Loss

	PREVIABLE PROM	PREVIABLE PRETERM LABOR	CERVICAL INSUFFICIENCY	INTRAUTERINE FETAL DEMISE
Clinical presentation	Leakage of vaginal fluid or increased vaginal discharge	Abdominal/ back/or pelvic pain or discomfort Vaginal bleeding or spotting	Pelvic pressure Vaginal discharge Cramping/ backache Spotting Mild contractions	Absent fetal movement Vaginal bleeding Contractions
Risk factors	Prior PPROM History of cervical conization Second trimester vaginal bleeding Connective tissue disorder Low BMI Cigarette smoking	Prior preterm labor Infection Abruption PPROM Multiple gestations Uterine anomalies	History recurrent/ prior preterm delivery, mid trimester loss Cervical injury Exposure, DES congenital LEEP/CKC	Advanced maternal age Obesity Multiple gestation Tobacco Abruptio placenta HTN DM Infection
Physical examination findings	Amniotic fluid pool pH > 7 Ferning on dry slide	Cervical dilation or effacement Cervical change over 30 to 60min	Cervical dilation > 4 cm Membranes through cervical os	Nonspecific
Ultrasound findings	+/- Low AFI		Cervical length < 25 mm in women with previous preterm birth and singleton gestation; otherwise, < 15 mm	Absent cardiac activity

Source: Adapted from ACOG (2003), (2007), (2009); Althuisius et al., (2001); Beghella et al., (2011); Gabbe et al., (2007); Goldenberg et al., (2008); Seri & Evans (2008); Owen (2009).

PREVIABLE PREMATURE RUPTURE OF MEMBRANES (PREVIABLE PROM)

PRESENTING SYMPTOMATOLOGY

A pregnant woman with previable PROM may present with a variety of symptoms. She may experience a distinct gush of fluid from the vagina or give a history of several days of increased vaginal discharge and spotting. Intraamniotic infection often precedes previable PROM (Gabbe et al., 2007). Women with infections may also present with fever, nausea or vomiting, exquisite abdominal or pelvic pain, and/or foul-smelling vaginal discharge.

HISTORY AND DATA COLLECTION

A thorough history specifically addressing the maternal risk factors for previable PROM are obtained, including the following: prior history of preterm premature rupture of membranes (PPROM), history of second trimester vaginal bleeding, history of cervical conization or shortened cervix, amniocentesis, low body mass index, low socioeconomic status, cigarette smoking, connective tissue disorder, and multiple gestations (ACOG, 2007). The color, amount, and odor of fluid are noted. Timing of the last sexual intercourse should also be elicited.

PHYSICAL EXAMINATION

Vital signs are imperative. Fever, hypotension, tachycardia, and tachypnea, all may be signs of an infectious process. The abdominal examination may reveal significant tenderness to palpation. Exquisite fundal tenderness, rebound tenderness, and guarding are all concerns for an infectious process.

On speculum exam, rupture of membranes can be determined by the presence of an amniotic fluid pool in the posterior fornix. Amniotic fluid will have approximately a pH of 7 and when left to dry on a slide, a ferning pattern will be seen through the microscope. During the speculum examination, the cervix is visualized to ascertain whether the cervix is dilated. Occasionally, a prolapsed cord or fetal part may be found protruding through the cervical os. Finally, the presence of purulent vaginal discharge or fever will raise the provider's suspicion for septic abortion. If a speculum exam is negative or equivocal for ruptured membranes, a wet mount can be performed to evaluate for bacterial vaginosis, candidiasis, or trichomoniasis. If the status of amniotic membranes is unclear, the speculum examination can also be repeated in 1 hour to reevaluate the fluid for evidence of ferning.

LABORATORY AND IMAGING STUDIES

Laboratory studies include a complete blood count (CBC) to evaluate for any leukocytosis suggesting infection and to establish a baseline hemoglobin level. Rh status is also collected and a urinalysis is obtained.

A transabdominal ultrasound reveals whether the amniotic fluid volume is grossly normal or if oligohydramnios is present. Fetal cardiac activity is noted. If a woman is near the threshold of viability, estimated fetal weight should be obtained.

DIFFERENTIAL DIAGNOSIS

In the second trimester, the differential diagnosis of vaginal discharge or leaking includes PPROM, cervicitis or vaginitis, or recent intercourse. Urinary tract infections or incontinence may also lead to the sensation of leaking fluid.

CLINICAL MANAGEMENT AND FOLLOW-UP

Previable PROM is a devastating diagnosis for pregnant women to receive. Perinatal morbidity and mortality are commonly seen. Neonatal outcomes in the setting of previable PROM may include pulmonary hypoplasia and fetal deformation, particularly when rupture occurs early in the second trimester or lasts more than 2 weeks. A study by Manuck et al., (2009) followed 152 expectant managed women with PPROM less than 24 weeks' gestation. Approximately 41% ended with IUFD, previable delivery, or neonatal death. Of the 59% who survived to hospital discharge, half of these experienced serious neonatal morbidity. Expectant management can be pursued as an outpatient prior to 24 weeks as long as the woman is counseled regarding signs of infection (ACOG, 2007). Administration of antenatal steroids is controversial, and a maternal fetal medicine specialist should be consulted.

In women who are proven to have ruptured membranes, yet are hemodynamically stable and without evidence of infection, there is no urgency to move toward an immediate management decision. Time ought to be allowed for the mother and partner to have all questions addressed, speak in private, and process the importance of what has occurred. Management options include expectant management, induction of labor, or dilatation and evacuation (D&E). Expectant management is offered only to those women with PROM prior to viability who demonstrate no evidence of infection or significant hemorrhage from abruption. Expectant management, however, does carry the risk of delivery outside a clinical facility, infection, and rarely, coagulopathy and hemorrhage. Therefore, women may be managed as outpatients only if they are able to return for emergency care quickly. Active management requires consultation by experienced obstetric providers at appropriately equipped facilities. These women are typically managed by dilatation and evacuation or by labor induction with misoprostol (Paul et al., 2009).

In the setting of septic abortion, fluid resuscitation, broad spectrum antibiotic therapy, and surgical uterine evacuation must be administered expeditiously. Intravenous antibiotic regimens include clindamycin 900 mg IV q 8 hours with gentamicin 5 mg/kg IV q 24 hours with or without ampicillin 2 gm IV q 6 hours (Stubblefield & Grimes, 1994). Antibiotic therapy is continued for 48 hours after the last temperature elevation.

PREVIABLE PRETERM LABOR

PRESENTING SYMPTOMATOLOGY

Preterm labor is defined by uterine contractions leading to cervical dilation and effacement prior to 37 weeks' gestation (ACOG, 2003). When this occurs prior to 23 completed weeks' gestation, it can be described as previable preterm labor. These women will present with pain, ranging from intermittent menses-like cramping or pelvic pressure to painful uterine contractions. Vaginal spotting and an increase in vaginal discharge may be associated symptoms.

HISTORY AND DATA COLLECTION

Infection is a common trigger for preterm labor; therefore, a thorough review of systems and documentation of the presence or absence of fever, chills, abdominal pain, purulent vaginal discharge, dysuria, flank pain, nausea, vomiting, and diarrhea is needed. Other risk factors for preterm labor include abdominal trauma, placental abruption, history of preterm birth, multiple gestation, premature rupture of membranes, uterine fibroids, tobacco use, low body mass index, low socioeconomic status, and Black race (Goldenberg et al., 2008).

PHYSICAL EXAMINATION

Evaluation of vital signs and a physical examination are performed to rule out infection or other causes of preterm labor. The diagnosis of preterm labor is made when there are regular contractions with active cervical change.

LABORATORY AND IMAGING STUDIES

Recommended labs include a CBC, type and screen, and urinalysis. Gonorrhea and chlamydia testing are appropriate for women at high risk for infection. An example of a shortened cervix with funneling on transvaginal ultrasound is seen in Figure 7.1. If the fetus is approaching viability, biometry is performed to obtain an estimated fetal weight.

DIFFERENTIAL DIAGNOSIS

The differential diagnosis includes obstetric/gynecologic causes such as preterm contractions (without cervical change or dilatation), round ligament pain, degenerating fibroids, ovarian cyst rupture, or torsion. Gastrointestinal, musculoskeletal, and genitourinary causes must also be considered.

CLINICAL MANAGEMENT AND FOLLOW-UP

If there is no evidence of an intrauterine infection, a pregnant woman can be offered expectant management and be allowed to progress through labor without intervention. Women who desire active management can be admitted

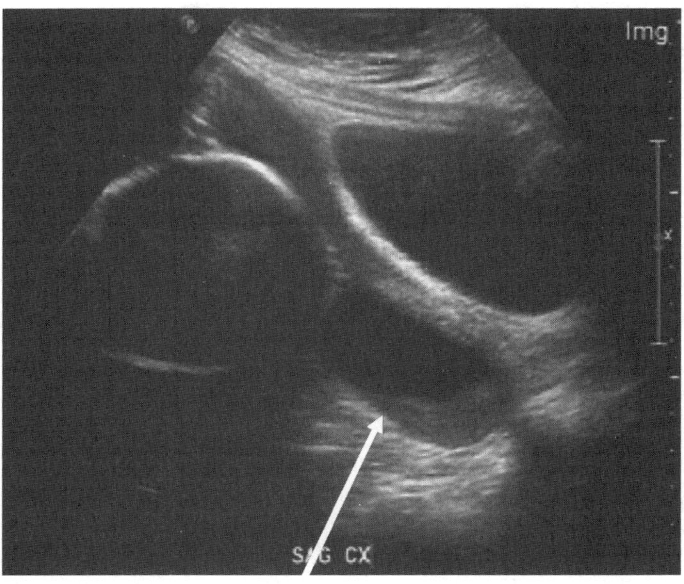

FIGURE 7.1 Cervical shortening with funneling.

Source: Courtesy Department of Radiology, Women & Infants Hospital, Providence, RI.

to the labor floor and augmented with prostaglandins, such as misoprostol. In both scenarios, women should be offered adequate pain control.

CERVICAL INSUFFICIENCY

PRESENTING SYMPTOMATOLOGY

The classic study defining cervical insufficiency uses the following criteria: advanced cervical dilation (≥ 4 cm and effacement ≥ 80% before 28 weeks' gestation) in the absence of painful contractions, vaginal bleeding, rupture of membranes, and infection (Olah & Gee, 1992). There may be a history of repeated mid-trimester losses or progressively earlier deliveries in prior pregnancies.

Classically, cervical insufficiency presents with complaints of vague, mild symptoms, which are often thought to be "normal" changes of pregnancy. These include pelvic pressure, premenstrual-like cramping or backache, and increased vaginal discharge with a change in color (pink, tan, or spotting) and consistency (thin or watery). When women present late for evaluation, they are usually found to have advanced cervical dilatation on examination, spotting, rupture of membranes, or contractions, which can be frequently mild.

HISTORY AND DATA COLLECTION

Gestational age of the pregnancy is determined early in gestation. A history of prior or recurrent preterm delivery, especially second trimester loss, between 15 and 28 weeks' gestation may raise the risk for cervical insufficiency.

Screening for anatomic causes includes those that are both congenital and acquired, although most are idiopathic. Congenital causes include collagen disorders, such as Ehlers–Danlos syndrome (Leduc & Wasserstrum, 1992) and type I collagen expression disorders (Iwahashi et al., 2003). Exposure to diethylstilbestrol (DES) in utero has been linked to pregnancy loss from cervical insufficiency (Kaufman et al., 2000). Acquired causes of cervical insufficiency include prior obstetric trauma (cervical laceration), mechanical (curettage, termination of pregnancy), and management of cervical dysplasia (LEEP: electrosurgical excision procedure, cold knife conization (Kyrgiou et al., 2006).

PHYSICAL EXAMINATION

Vital signs are documented with attention to presence of fever with or without abdominal tenderness. Sterile speculum examination is performed testing for chlamydia, gonorrhea, and for any rupture of membranes. Visualization of the cervix may reveal membranes prolapsing through the cervical os. If premature rupture of membranes is excluded, sterile digital examination of the cervix is performed for dilatation and effacement.

Assessment for contractions can help to differentiate between preterm labor, abruptio placenta, and cervical insufficiency. Documentation of the presence of a fetal heart rate needs to be performed; however, continuous fetal monitoring is not indicated in previable pregnancies.

LABORATORY AND IMAGING STUDIES

In the obstetric triage setting, CBC, hold tube, and urinalysis are obtained. When there is evidence for infection or a high suspicion for infection, then amniocentesis is indicated.

If membranes are not visualized on physical examination, then transvaginal ultrasound is performed to evaluate for cervical length, dilatation, and funneling. During transvaginal ultrasound, fundal pressure may be applied for better visualization of the internal os. When funneling occurs from this increased intraabdominal pressure, or occurs spontaneously, it has been shown that it does not define cervical insufficiency or the predictive value of cervical length on preterm delivery (Berghella et al., 2007). Ultrasound can also be used to assess the state of fetal membranes, extrachorionic hemorrhage, cervical polyps, uterine/cervical anomalies, or intraamniotic debris.

DIFFERENTIAL DIAGNOSIS

The differential diagnosis for women presenting with these complaints and findings include previable preterm labor, previable premature rupture of membranes, abruptio placenta, and chorioamnionitis. Gynecologic conditions such as cervicitis and sexually transmitted diseases need to be considered.

CLINICAL MANAGEMENT AND FOLLOW-UP

Women with a prior preterm birth and a current singleton pregnancy with a cervical length of less than 25 mm may be offered cerclage (Berghella et al., 2011). Those with no prior history of any preterm birth or other risk factors can be offered a cerclage if the cervical length is less than 15 mm (Althuisius et al., 2011; Owen, 2009).

If cervical length is less than 25 mm before 23 weeks' gestation with a prior preterm birth, discussion must take place regarding options for cerclage, especially in the setting of progesterone prophylaxis. It was shown in the cervical incompetence prevention randomized cerclage trial (CIPRACT), that with cervical length less than 25 mm before 28 weeks' gestation, that therapeutic cerclage and bed rest improved preterm delivery before 34 weeks, and decreased neonatal morbidity and mortality (Althuisius et al., 2001). It is appropriate to begin management with progesterone in women with suspected cervical insufficiency, with one study indicating significant benefit in reducing the risk of delivery in women with a history of a prior preterm birth (Meis et al., 2003; ACOG, 2008). Reduction in the risk of preterm birth in women with short cervix (DeFranco et al., 2007) and those without a history of preterm birth (Fonseca et al., 2007, Hassan et al., 2011) have also been reported with progesterone use.

The above approach is supported by the vaginal ultrasound cerclage trial (VUCT), (Owen et al., 2009) and by a meta-analysis by Berghella et al (2011). In VUCT, women were randomized to cerclage or no cerclage, all had histories of prior preterm birth between 16 and 34 weeks and a cervical length on ultrasound below 25 mm. This study did not show a significant reduction in preterm birth less than 35 weeks, except in women with cervical lengths less than 15 mm. Berghella et al (2007) showed that cerclage for cervical shortening in women with prior preterm birth had significant reductions in neonatal morbidity and mortality, at lengths below 25 mm and 15.9 mm. In a meta-analysis, it was shown that women with singleton gestations with prior preterm birth can be safely monitored with ultrasound surveillance, and placement of cerclage only when indicated for true cervical shortening (Berghella & Mackeen, 2011).

When cervical shortening is found incidentally and there is no history of prior preterm delivery (especially mid-trimester loss), evidence supports use of vaginal progesterone with improved neonatal outcomes and prolonged pregnancy (Hassan et al., 2011). The data are similar for all women whether there was a prior history of preterm delivery or not. For these women with incidental cervical shortening, the data do not show reduction in preterm delivery less than 35 weeks with cerclage (Berghella et al., 2005) or reduction in maternal or perinatal morbidity/mortality (To et al., 2004).

However, Romero et al. (2012) have reported that vaginal progesterone support in asymptomatic women with cervical shortening found on ultrasound resulted in significant reductions in preterm delivery at all gestational ages less than 35 weeks, with improved neontatal outcomes, showing a composite reduction in morbidity and mortality of 43% (Romero et al., 2012). These findings were found with vaginal progesterone dosing of 90–200 mcg/day, with no changes in efficacy.

Women can be offered a rescue or emergent cerclage when cervical dilatation and fetal membranes are visible, and gestational age is less than 24 weeks in an attempt to prolong pregnancy and improve outcomes. In this setting, there can be no evidence of infection, rupture of membranes, vaginal bleeding, or signs of labor. If there is a concern for subclinical infection, then amniocentesis is highly recommended.

INTRAUTERINE FETAL DEMISE/STILLBIRTH

PRESENTING SYMPTOMATOLOGY

When fetal demise is diagnosed prior to viability, it is often found incidentally on ultrasound. Occasionally, women will present to the obstetric triage setting with complaints of decreased or absent fetal movement, vaginal bleeding, or uterine contractions.

HISTORY AND DATA COLLECTION

The prenatal record and all ultrasounds are reviewed, as well as any significant medical and surgical history in the setting of an IUFD. Questions regarding chromosomal abnormalities, history of infections during the pregnancy, abnormal fetal testing, known intrauterine growth restriction, or illicit drug use must be addressed. The possible risk factors for fetal demise are extensive, as shown in Exhibit 7.1.

PHYSICAL EXAMINATION

Routine vital signs and an overall evaluation are performed once the woman has been diagnosed with a fetal demise. If vital signs are stable without evidence of preeclampsia, abruptio placenta, or disseminated intravascular coagulopathy (DIC), then it is appropriate to limit the initial physical examination and perform the pelvic exam once the woman has had time to process the diagnosis. On speculum examination, any vaginal bleeding is evaluated and a bimanual

EXHIBIT 7.1

Risk Factors and Causes of Stillbirth

- Non-Hispanic Black race
- Nulliparity
- Advanced maternal age (AMA)
- Obesity
- Smoking
- Drug and alcohol use
- Comorbidities:
  - Hypertension, preeclampsia
  - Diabetes mellitus
  - Thrombophilia
  - History of thromboembolism
  - Systemic lupus erythematous
  - Renal disease
  - Thyroid disease
  - Cholestasis of pregnancy
- Multiple gestation
- Congenital anomalies
- Growth restriction
- Infection (parvovirus B19, syphilis, listeria)

Source: Adapted from ACOG (2009).

exam is performed to determine cervical dilation and effacement. With no complaint of bleeding, a bimanual exam is performed to determine cervical dilatation and effacement.

LABORATORY AND IMAGING STUDIES

When fetal demise is suspected, it is recommended that a bedside ultrasound confirmation of absent cardiac activity, with two providers present, be performed. If a woman requests a further ultrasound, this can be performed for confirmation of findings, as necessary.

The American College of Obstetricians & Gynecologists (2009) recommends the following evaluation at the time of demise: CBC, lupus anticoagulant, anticardiolipin antibodies, human parvovirus B19 IgG/IgM antibodies, thyroid stimulating hormone. In cases with severe growth restriction, maternal thrombosis, or abnormal placental pathology, testing should include Factor V Leiden mutation, prothrombin mutation, anti-thrombin III levels, and protein C and S activity. Routine testing for thrombophilias is controversial and may lead to unnecessary additional interventions. In selected cases, additional studies could include indirect Coombs, glucose screening, evaluation for preeclampsia, which would include creatinine, liver functions, uric acid, and a urine protein:creatine ratio.

DIFFERENTIAL DIAGNOSIS

When a woman presents with the complaint of decreased/absent fetal movement, findings may indicate oligohydramnios or anterior placenta. In addition, medical etiologies such as chronic hypertension, preeclampsia, diabetes mellitus, gestational diabetes, and thrombophilia must be considered.

CLINICAL MANAGEMENT AND FOLLOW-UP

The timing of delivery is dependent on the gestational age at which the fetal demise occurred, maternal preference, and history of prior uterine scar. Often, pregnant women will desire an expeditious delivery due to the emotional burden. However, timing is not critical, and coagulopathies associated with fetal demise are still very rare. Maternal medical indications for immediate intervention include abruptio placenta, intrauterine infection, preeclampsia, and disseminated intravascular coagulation (DIC).

For women with a second trimester fetal loss, dilatation and evacuation can be offered. Fetal autopsy would no longer be an option with this form of management. Labor induction before 28 weeks' gestation is often performed with vaginal misoprostol and appears to be the most efficient regardless of the Bishop score (Tang et al., 2004). The most common dose for misoprostol is 200 to 400 mcg vaginally every 4 to 12 hours. Dickinson (2005) showed that misoprostol was still an acceptable choice for women with previous uterine scar between 24 and 28 weeks, with dosing of 400 mcg every 6 hours. In a Cochrane review, Neilson et al (2006) reviewed several randomized trials showing the efficacy of vaginal misoprostol for nonviable pregnancies/stillbirths less than 24 weeks' gestation.

Fetal autopsy is offered to women with the understanding that it will provide information in 30% of cases (ACOG, 2009). Other options include external evaluation by a trained perinatal pathologist, imaging, tissue sample, and fetal karotype after delivery with only a 30% yield (ACOG, 2009). The placenta should always be sent after stillbirth for evaluation of infection, both viral and bacterial, and for evidence of abruption.

BEREAVEMENT ISSUES

Pregnancy loss in the second trimester is devastating and quite often unexpected. If there are no signs of infection or hemodynamic instability, women must be given adequate time to process loss and review options. Social services or chaplain services may be helpful in supporting women through their decision-making process. The woman must be educated regarding local bereavement services and support groups to assist in the grieving process over the long term.

REFERENCES

Althuisius, S. M., Dekker, G. A., Hummel, P., Bekedam, D. J. & van Geijn, H. P. (2001). Final results of the Cervical Incompetence Prevention Randomized Cerclage Trial (CIPRACT): Therapeutic cerclage with bed rest versus bed rest alone. *American Journal of Obstetrics and Gynecology,185*(5),1106–1112.

American College of Obstetricians and Gynecologists (ACOG). (2003). ACOG practice bulletin number 43: Management of preterm labor. *Obstetrics & Gynecology, 82*(1), 127–135.

American College of Obstetricians and Gynecologists (ACOG). (2007). ACOG practice bulletin number 80: Premature rupture of membranes. *Obstetrics & Gynecology, 109*(4), 1007–1019.

American College of Obstetricians and Gynecologists (ACOG). (2008). ACOG committee opinion 419: Use of progesterone to reduce preterm birth. *Obstetrics & Gynecology, 112*, 963.

American College of Obstetricians and Gynecologists (ACOG). (2009). ACOG practice bulletin number 102: Management of stillbirth. *Obstetrics & Gynecology, 113*(3), 748–761.

Berghella, V., & Mackeen, A. D. (2011). Cervical length screening with ultrasound-indicated cerclage compared with history-indicated cerclage for prevention of preterm birth: A meta-analysis. *Obstetrics & Gynecology, 118*(1), 148–155.

Berghella, V., Odibo, A. O., To, M. S., Rust, O. A., & Althuisius, S. M. (2005). Cerclage for short cervix on ultrasonography: Meta-analysis of trials using individual patient-level data. *Obstetrics & Gynecology, 106*, 181–189.

Berghella, V., Owen, J., MacPherson, C., Yost, N., Swain, M., Dildy, G. A., . . . Maternal-Fetal Medicine Units Network. (2007). Natural history of cervical funneling in women at high risk for spontaneous preterm birth. *Obstetrics & Gynecology, 109*, 863–869.

Berghella, V., Rafael, T. J., Szychowski, J. M., Rust, O. A., & Owen, J. (2011). Cerclage for short cervix on ultrasonography in women with singleton gestations and previous preterm birth: A meta-analysis. *Obstetrics & Gynecology, 117*(3), 663–671.

DeFranco, E. A., O'Brien, J. M., Adair, C. D., Lewis, D. F., Hall, D. R., Fusey, S., . . . Creasy, G. W. (2007). Vaginal progesterone is associated with a decrease in risk of early preterm birth and improved neonatal outcome in women with a short cervix: A secondary analysis from a randomized, double-blind, placebo-controlled trial. *Ultrasound in Obstetrics & Gynecology, 30*, 697–705.

Dickinson, J. E. (2005). Misoprostol for second trimester pregnancy termination in women with a prior cesarean section. *Obstetrics & Gynecology, 105*, 352–356.

Fonseca, E. B., Celik, E., Parra, M., Singh, M., & Nicolaides, K. H. (2007). Progesterone and risk of preterm birth among women with short cervix *New England Journal of Medicine, 357*, 462–469.

Gabbe, S. G., Niebyl, J. R., & Simpson, J. L. (2007). *Obstetrics: Normal and problem pregnancies* (5th ed.). Philadelphia, PA: Churchill Livingstone Elsevier.

Goldenberg, R. L., Culhane, J. F., Iams, J. D., & Romero, R. (2008). The epidemiology and causes of preterm birth. *The Lancet, 371*(9606), 75–84.

Hassan, S. S., Romero, R., Vidyadhari, D., Fusey, S., Baxter, J. K., Khandelwal, M., . . . Creasy, G. W. (2011). Vaginal progesterone reduces the rate of preterm birth in women with sonographic short cervix: A multicenter, randomized, double blind, placebo-controlled trial. *Ultrasound in Obstetrics & Gynecology, 38*, 18–31.

Iwahashi, M., Muragaki, Y., Ooshima, A., & Umesaki, N. (2003). Decreased type I collagen expression in human uterine cervix during pregnancy. *The Journal of Clinical Endocrinology and Metabolism, 88*, 2231–2235.

Kaufman, R. H., Adam, E., Hatch, E. E., Noller, K., Herbst, A. L., Palmer, J. R., & Hover, R. N. (2000). Continued follow-up of pregnancy outcomes in diethylstilbestrol-exposed offspring. *Obstetrics & Gynecology, 96*(4), 483–489.

Kyrgiou, M., Koliopoulos, G., Martin-Hirsch, P., Arbyn, M., Prendiville, W., & Paraskevaidis, E. (2006). Obstetric outcomes after conservative treatment for intraepithelial or early invasive cervical lesions: Systematic review and meta-analysis. *Lancet, 367*, 489–498.

Leduc, L., & Wasserstrum, N. (1992). Successful treatment with the Smith-Hodge pessary of cervical incompetence due to defective connective tissue in Ehlers-Danlos syndrome. *American Journal of Perinatology, 9*, 25–27.

Manuck, T. A., Eller, A. G., Esplin, M. S., Stoddard, G. J., Varner, M. W., & Silver, R. M. (2009). Outcomes of expectantly managed preterm premature rupture of membranes occurring before 24 weeks gestation. *Obstetrics and Gynecology, 114*(1), 29–37.

Meis, P. J., Klebanoff, M., Thom, E., Dombrowski, M. P., Sibai, B., Moawad, A. H., . . . National Institute of Child Health and Human Development Maternal-Fetal Medicine Units Network. (2003). Prevention of recurrent preterm delivery by 17 alpha-hydroxyprogesterone caproate. *The New England Journal of Medicine, 348*, 2379–2385.

Neilson, J. P., Hickey, M., & Vazquez, J. (2006). Medical treatment for early fetal death (less than 24 weeks) *Cochrane Database of Systematic Review, 3*, CD002253.

Olah, K. S. & Gee, H. (1992). Prevention of preterm delivery–can we afford to continue to ignore the cervix? *British Journal of Obstetrics and Gynaecology, 99,* 278–280.

Owen, J., Hankins, G., Iams, J. D., Berghella, V., Sheffield, J. S., Perez-Delboy A,... Hauth, J. C. (2009). Multicenter randomized trial of cerclage for preterm birth prevention in high-risk women with shortened mid-trimester cervical length. *American Journal of Obstetrics and Gynecology, 201,* 375.e1–8.

Paul, M., Lichtenberg, E. S., Borgatta, L., Grimes, D. A., Stubblefield, P. G., & Creinin, M. D. (2009). *Management of unintended and abnormal pregnancy: Comprehensive abortion care.* West Sussex, UK: Wiley Blackwell.

Romero, R., Nicolaides, K., Conde-Agudelo, A., et al. (2012). Vaginal progesterone in women with an aysmptomatic sonographic short cervix in the midtrimester decreases preterm delivery and neonatal morbidity: A systematic review and metaanalysis of individual patient data. *American Journal of Obstetrics and Gynecology,* 206,124.e1–19.

Seri, I., Evans, J. (2008). Limits of viability: Definitions of the gray zone. *Journal of Perinatology, 28,* S4–S8.

Stubblefield, P. G., & Grimes, D. A. (1994). Septic abortion. *The New England Journal of Medicine, 331*(5), 310–314.

Saraiya, M., Berg, C. H., Shulman, H., Green, C. A., & Atrash, H. K. (1999). Estimates of the annual number of clinically recognized pregnancies in the United Sates, 1981–1991. *American Journal of Epidemiology, 149,* 1025–1029.

Tang, O. S., Lau, W. N., Chan, C. C., & Ho, P. C. (2004). A prospective randomized comparison of sublingual and vaginal misoprostol in second trimester termination of pregnancy. *BJOG, 111,* 1001–1005.

To, M. S., Alfirevic, Z., Heath, V. C., Cicero, S., Cacho, A. M., Williamson, P. R.,... Fetal Medicine Foundation Second Trimester Screening Group. (2004). Cervical cerclage for prevention of preterm delivery in women with short cervix: Randomized controlled trial. *Lancet,* 363, 1849–1853.

Early Complications of Multiple Gestations

8

Karen Archabald

The incidence of multiple gestations has increased over time, with data from the 2008 Centers for Disease Control National Vital Statistics revealing a twin birth rate of 32.6 per 1,000 and a triplet or higher order birth rate of 1.47 per 1,000 live births. These percentages correlate to 138,660 twin, 5,877 triplet, 345 quadruplet, and 46 quintuplet or higher births in the United States annually (Martin et al., 2010). The increase in multiple gestations is attributed to increased use of assisted reproductive technology, as well as an increasing number of women becoming pregnant at an advanced maternal age. Given the continued increasing prevalence of multiple gestations, associated complications are very likely to present to a general obstetric triage unit.

The focus will be on complications specific to multiple gestations. Complications from partial pregnancy loss due to spontaneous or planned fetal reduction, shortened cervix, preterm premature rupture of membranes (PPROM), and preterm labor will be addressed.

SPONTANEOUS OR ELECTIVE FETAL REDUCTION

Both spontaneous and elective fetal reductions are common in women with multiple gestations. Spontaneous reduction is more likely to occur in the first trimester, while planned elective fetal reduction is commonly performed between 10 and 14 weeks' gestation (Stone et al., 2008).

PRESENTING SYMPTOMATOLOGY

The majority of women will be asymptomatic when spontaneous fetal reduction is noted. A retrospective cohort study found 5.3% of 38 women who experienced spontaneous fetal reduction had vaginal bleeding, compared to 8.3% of controls (Steinkampf, Whitten, & Hammond, 2005). Women who have undergone a planned fetal reduction have an approximate 5% chance of miscarriage prior to 24 weeks (Stone et al., 2008), which is not significantly higher than the baseline risk of miscarriage in twins (Yaron et al., 1999).

HISTORY AND DATA COLLECTION

Gestational age is established by either last menstrual period, transfer date, or early ultrasound. The number of fetuses, as well as the chorionicity and amnionicity are documented if possible. If the pregnant woman has recently undergone a planned multifetal reduction, the procedure note will note any complications. If vaginal bleeding occurs, the duration and amount, as well as associated uterine cramping need to be documented.

PHYSICAL EXAMINATION

If the woman presents with vaginal bleeding, a complete pelvic exam is warranted. A speculum examination will allow quantification of the amount of vaginal bleeding, as well as the presence of any active bleeding. Visual inspection of the cervix will allow assessment of cervical dilation, as well as any bleeding from the cervical stroma. A bimanual examination will allow assessment of cervical dilation and uterine tenderness.

LABORATORY AND IMAGING STUDIES

Documentation of blood type and screen, as well as RH antigen status is critical. If the amount of vaginal bleeding is significant, a complete blood count (CBC) is warranted. A transvaginal ultrasound is necessary to assess fetal viability and to establish chorionicity and amnionicity if not previously established. In the first trimester, two separate placentas confirm the diagnosis of dichorionicity. If only one placenta is visualized, the presence of the "twin peak" or "lambda" sign is highly predictive of dichorionicity. Sonographically, the groove between the dividing membranes as they insert into the placenta appears thickened because this potential space is filled with amniotic and chorionic mesoderm unlike in monochorionic pregnancies

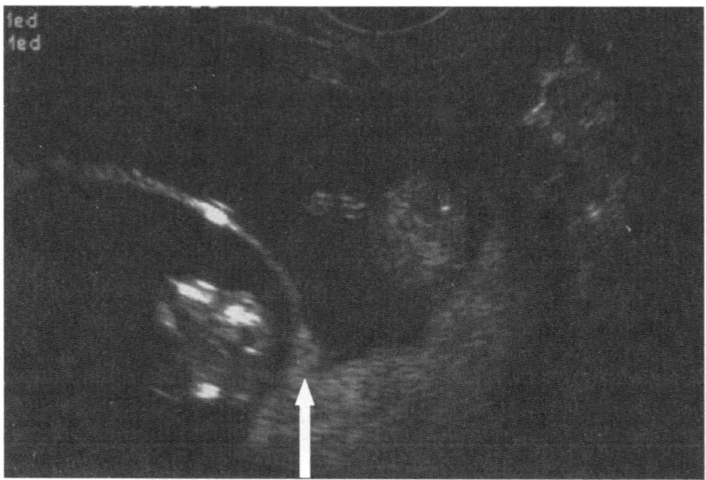

FIGURE 8.1 Twin peak or lambda sign in dichorionic gestation.

Source: Courtesy of the Department of Radiology, Women & Infants Hospital, Providence, RI.

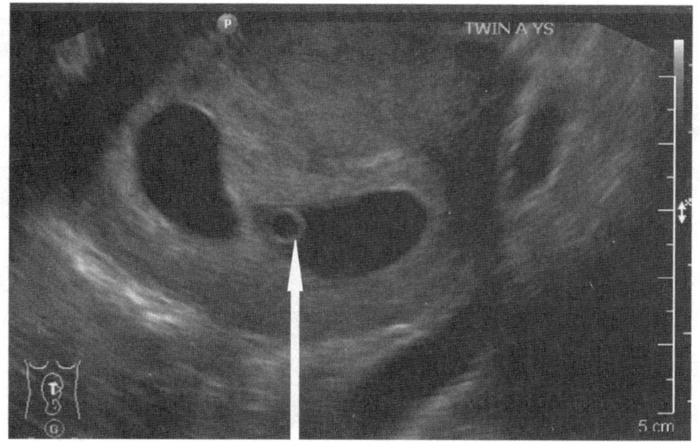

FIGURE 8.2 Vanishing twin with only one yolk sac visible.

Source: Courtesy of the Department of Radiology, Women & Infants Hospital, Providence, RI.

where the space remains empty. Please see Figure 8.1 for a sonographic image of the lambda sign.

If the woman has undergone a fetal reduction, it is imperative to carefully note which fetuses have cardiac activity. Imaging may reveal two gestational sacs with only one sac with a yolk sac or fetus as noted in Figure 8.2.

CLINICAL MANAGEMENT AND FOLLOW-UP

Spontaneous reduction of twin or higher order multiple gestation is common. The majority of data on spontaneous reduction comes from a large retrospective study in a fertility clinic that followed pregnancies from 5.5 to 6 weeks every 2 weeks with transvaginal ultrasound. At 12 weeks, 62% of twin pregnancies conceived naturally and 31% of twin pregnancies conceived with assisted reproductive technology had spontaneously reduced to singleton pregnancies (Dickey, 2005). In the same cohort, spontaneous reduction of one or more gestational sacs and/or embryos occurred before the 12th week of gestation in 53% of triplet (95% CI, 44%–61%), and 65% of quadruplet (95% CI, 46%–85%) pregnancies (Dickey et al., 2002). Prognosis of the pregnancy is overall good; however, observational studies show a decrease in length of pregnancy and lower birth weight in infants born to women whose pregnancies spontaneously reduced compared with unreduced pregnancies (Dickey, 2005; Pinborg, Lidegaard, Freiesleben, & Andersen, 2007). The practitioner should be prepared to provide emotional support to the woman and family as loss of a fetus, even with a remaining viable pregnancy, can be devastating.

In women who have undergone multifetal reduction, the miscarriage rate is not elevated from baseline (Evans & Britt, 2008). Regardless, women are encouraged to follow up with their provider or to seek care in an obstetric triage unit for worsening vaginal bleeding or uterine cramping. Women may experience increased anxiety after multifetal reduction, making emotional support and reassurance important throughout the pregnancy (Garel et al., 1997).

Women with multiple gestations routinely undergo serial ultrasonographic examinations. Whether the cervical length is a planned part of the evaluation, or a shortened cervix is noted incidentally, women may arrive in obstetric triage for evaluation and management of a shortened cervix. Shortened cervix is defined as a cervix measuring less than 25 mm, which is smaller than the 10% expected reduction (Iams et al., 1996).

PRESENTING SYMPTOMATOLOGY

Shortened cervix noted incidentally on ultrasound is often asymptomatic. However, it may also be associated with symptoms of preterm labor.

HISTORY AND DATA COLLECTION

The gestational age must be established by either last menstrual period, transfer date, or early ultrasound. A careful obstetric history is obtained focusing on history of any deliveries prior to 37 weeks or second trimester losses. History of a cold knife cone biopsy or loop electrosurgical excision procedures is obtained as these have been associated with shortened cervix in the midtrimester (Fischer, Sveinbjornsson, & Hansen, 2010) and preterm delivery (Ørtoft, Henriksen, Hansen, & Petersen, 2010).

PHYSICAL EXAMINATION

Determining the presence of uterine contractions on tocometry is helpful for distinguishing preterm labor from asymptomatic shortened cervix. If the fetuses are viable, a non stress test (NST) will provide information regarding fetal well-being. An abdominal examination with particular attention to the fundus is completed to evaluate for chorioamnionitis. A sterile speculum examination with visual assessment of the cervix will provide information on rupture of membranes, and if no rupture, then dilation and effacement. A confirmatory digital examination will provide further information if there is no evidence of ruptured membranes.

LABORATORY AND IMAGING STUDIES

If there is concern for chorioamnionitis, a CBC is indicated. Ultrasonographic evaluation of the cervix has already been completed in this clinical scenario; however, the exam can be confirmed in the triage unit if a practitioner is available who is comfortable with evaluation of ultrasonographic cervical measurement. Cervical length is measured with an empty maternal bladder via the transvaginal approach. The probe is placed in the anterior fornix of the vagina until the cervix is visualized and a sagittal long axis view of the endocervical canal is obtained. The probe is then withdrawn until the image is blurred, then advanced with enough pressure to restore the image. The cervical length is measured from the internal to the external os along the endocervical canal.

A shortened cervix between 20 and 24 weeks was shown in a recent meta-analysis to have a pooled positive likelihood ratio of 9.6 to predict preterm delivery prior to 28 weeks in twins (Conde-Agudelo, Romero, Hassan, & Yeo, 2010). Although data on triplets are limited, a study of 51 triplet gestations found a cervical length of less than 2.5 cm between 21 and 24 weeks' gestation had an 86% sensitivity for prediction of spontaneous delivery at less than 28 weeks' gestation (Guzman et al., 2000).

Despite the predictive value of a shortened cervix for preterm delivery, options for intervention are minimal. Cerclage in the asymptomatic patient with twins and a shortened cervix in the mid-trimester have been shown to have no impact on preterm delivery or birth weight in one analysis (Newman, Krombach, Myers, & McGee, 2002). A meta-analysis of four randomized trials found cerclage to actually increase preterm delivery at less than 35 weeks in twin gestations (RR: 2.15; 95% CI: 1.15–4.01) (Berghella, Odibo, To, Rust, & Althuisius, 2005). In triplets, a randomized controlled trial of 24 women with triplet gestation and shortened cervix, defined as less than 25 mm showed no impact on birth weight or gestational age at delivery (Moragianni, Aronis, & Craparo, 2011). Cerclage for the asymptomatic shortened cervix in multifetal gestation is not recommended.

In a series of 413 women with asymptomatic shortened cervix measuring less than 15 mm at 20 to 25 weeks ultrasound, 200 mg micronized vaginal progesterone daily from 24 to 34 weeks significantly decreased preterm delivery (RR: 0.56; 95% CI: 0.36–0.86). This same study included 24 women with twin pregnancy; however, the trend toward decreased preterm birth was not significant (Fonseca, Celik, Parra, Singh, & Nicolaides, 2007). When used prophylactically, neither vaginal progesterone (Norman et al., 2009) nor intramuscular injection of 17 hydroxyprogesterone caproate (Rouse et al., 2007) have been found to decrease preterm birth rates in twins. The 17 hydroxyprogesterone caproate has not been found to decrease preterm birth rates in triplets (Combs, Garite, Maurel, Das, & Porto, 2010). There is no indication for vaginal or intramuscular progesterone when asymptomatic shortened cervix is identified in multiple gestations.

Therefore, when pregnant women with multiple gestation and asymptomatic shortened cervix present to the obstetric triage unit, once preterm labor and PPROM have been ruled out, no acute intervention is necessary. Consultation with a maternal fetal medicine specialist can be arranged to discuss outpatient management. Depending on gestational age, discussion with neonatology regarding neonatal outcomes may be helpful.

PRETERM PREMATURE RUPTURE OF MEMBRANES

PPROM is more common in twin pregnancies than in singleton pregnancies, complicating up to 8% of twin pregnancies compared to approximately 4% of singleton pregnancies (Mercer, Crocker, Pierce, & Sibai, 1993). Previable PPROM that presents a management challenge in twin gestation, accounts for a disproportionately higher percentage (14%–21%) of twin PPROM (Dinsmoor, Bachman, Haney, Goldstein, & MacKendrick, 2004; Falk et al., 2004). The impact of management decisions in multifetal gestation is complicated by the outcome of not only the fetus with ruptured membranes, but also the remaining fetuses as well.

PRESENTING SYMPTOMATOLOGY

Women with multiple gestations present with similar complaints when compared to women with PPROM in singleton gestations. Women may report a gush of fluid, but may also report intermittent or continuous leakage of clear or yellow fluid.

HISTORY AND DATA COLLECTION

A careful history regarding the timing of possible rupture of membranes, the color of the amniotic fluid, and any signs of chorioamnionitis including fever, general malaise, or abdominal tenderness will help guide management.

PHYSICAL EXAMINATION

Documentation of maternal temperature and pulse, as well as fetal heart rate is important when evaluating for chorioamnionitis. In viable fetuses, heart rate monitoring will provide information on fetal well-being and tocometry will provide information regarding signs of preterm labor. Assessment of uterine tenderness can be completed by abdominal examination. A sterile speculum examination will confirm ruptured membranes by the findings of pooling of the amniotic fluid in the posterior fornix or direct egress from the cervical os, pH of vaginal fluid of 7.0 to 7.3 by nitrazine paper, and ferning.

LABORATORY AND IMAGING STUDIES

If ruptured membranes are confirmed, recommendations for laboratory assessment include CBC, type and screen. Ultrasonographic evaluation can be helpful in determining which fetus has ruptured its membranes, as the presenting twin is not always the twin that is ruptured. A study of 291 women with PPROM evaluating the impact of oligohydramnios on pregnancy outcomes found that 67% of singletons had oligohydramnios by amniotic fluid index (AFI) less than 5.0 and 46.9% by maximum vertical pocket (MVP) of less than 2.0 at the time of diagnosis (Mercer et al., 2006). Although no studies exist in twins, it can be assumed that ultrasongraphic evidence of rupture can help differentiate the twin with the ruptured sac. In addition to evaluating the amniotic fluid, the ultrasonographic evaluation can document fetal growth, as well as presentation of all fetuses in order to help counsel on mode of delivery.

CLINICAL MANAGEMENT AND FOLLOW-UP

In PPROM between 24 and 34 weeks, options for management in twin pregnancy are similar to those for singletons. The latency period from the time of PPROM to the time of delivery appears to be shorter with a median latency of less than 24 hours and only 16% to 50% of pregnancies remaining undelivered in 48 hours (Sela & Simpson, 2011). In the obstetric triage unit, a) antenatal steroids, b) latency antibiotics, and c) magnesium sulfate (Rouse et al., 2008) for neuroprophylaxis can all be initiated if gestational age is less than 32 weeks and delivery appears imminent. Use of tocolytic medications to allow time for administration of antenatal steroids is controversial, but can be considered at early gestation if there is no evidence of infection. Inpatient management until delivery is recommended. Given the short latency period, observation on the labor floor for 24 hours to monitor for signs of labor with subsequent transfer to the antepartum unit if the woman is stable is reasonable.

Management of previable PPROM is complicated in multifetal gestation. Neonatal survival of twins and triplets with PPROM at less than 24 weeks gestation (24%) is similar to singletons (25%) (Falk et al., 2004). In cases of previable rupture, management is complicated by the impact of management decisions on the fetus or fetuses with intact membranes. Depending on gestational age, admission with the administration of broad-spectrum antibiotics and observation for signs of developing chorioamnionitis or labor are recommended. The woman can then be managed as either an inpatient or outpatient until viability at which point administration of corticosteroids can be discussed (Waters & Mercer, 2009). Delivery of the ruptured twin with delayed interval delivery of the remaining fetus or fetuses has been shown to improve one year survival from 24% to 56% (Zhang, Hamilton, Martin, & Trumble, 2004); however, improved survival rates are accompanied by increased maternal morbidity (Roman et al., 2011). Decisions for such nontraditional management should be made in consultation with a maternal fetal medicine specialist.

PRETERM LABOR

Preterm contractions and subsequent preterm delivery are common in twin and higher order multiple pregnancies. Data from the National Vital Statistics System for 2008 reveal that 59% of the 138,660 twin pregnancies were delivered before 37 weeks, 11.6% were born before 32 weeks, and 4% before 28 weeks. Of triplet pregnancies, 93% of the 6,268 triplet or higher gestations were born before 37 weeks, 39.7% before 32 weeks and 12% prior to 28 weeks (Martin et al., 2010). Appropriate evaluation of the woman with multiple gestations complaining of preterm contractions in obstetric triage is essential to ensure appropriate disposition.

PRESENTING SYMPTOMATOLOGY

Symptoms of preterm labor can be varied. The range of symptoms includes uterine contractions, menstrual type cramping, low back pain, pelvic or vaginal pressure, increased discharge, or blood tinged discharge with associated passing of a "mucous plug."

HISTORY AND DATA COLLECTION

Women with multiple gestations are at increased risk for preterm labor due to increased uterine distension. However, other known risk factors for preterm birth may also contribute to the preterm birth rate. Documentation of gestational age is essential. A thorough obstetric history must be obtained focusing specifically on risk factors for preterm labor and any history of cervical surgery or preterm birth as these increase the patient's risk for preterm delivery. Any history suggestive of abdominal trauma or abruption, signs or symptoms of infection either uterine or urinary must be elicited. Duration and frequency of contractions, if present, must be documented, as well as signs and symptoms of PPROM.

PHYSICAL EXAMINATION

External fetal monitoring will provide valuable information on uterine contractions and fetal well-being. An abdominal examination will help to assess for uterine tone and tenderness, or the presence of another intraabdominal process. A sterile speculum examination is performed to assess for PPROM, as well as to obtain swabs for labs (see below). If rupture is ruled out, a digital examination to assess cervical dilation and effacement can be performed. Continued external fetal monitoring and repeat cervical exam will help differentiate preterm labor from preterm contractions.

LABORATORY AND IMAGING STUDIES

Infection as a possible cause for preterm labor can be evaluated with a urinalysis, urine culture, and cervical swabs for gonorrhea and chlamydia. A swab should also be obtained for Group B streptococcus. If the woman has not had intercourse, vaginal bleeding, or a vaginal exam in the previous 24 hours, a fetal fibronectin (FFN) collected from the posterior fornix will also help guide management. Ultrasound is utilized to evaluate presentation of each of the fetuses and for estimated fetal weight if delivery appears imminent.

CLINICAL MANAGEMENT AND FOLLOW-UP

Women with documented cervical change by digital examination require admission to the labor floor, as well as a) antenatal steroids, b) tocolytics, and c) magnesium sulfate for neuroprophylaxis if gestational age is less than 32 weeks and delivery appears imminent.

In women with twins without evidence of cervical change with preterm contractions, FFN has been shown to be an effective method to predict preterm birth. A meta-analysis of three studies with 168 women with symptoms of preterm labor with twin pregnancies found that women with a negative FFN had only 1.6% probability of delivering within the next 7 days, compared to 24.5% with a positive FFN (Conde-Agudelo & Romero, 2010). Among women with preterm contractions and twins, the measurement of CL had a minimal predictive accuracy for preterm birth less than 34 and 37 weeks' gestation (pooled positive and negative likelihood ratios between 1.2–1.9 and between 0.65–0.69, respectively) (Conde-Agudelo et al., 2010). We therefore recommend FFN for triage of women with multiple gestations and symptoms of preterm contractions, but no cervical change. If the woman has no documented cervical change and a negative FFN, she can be safely discharged home with close follow-up. The disposition of a woman with a positive FFN is less clear, as the positive predictive value is only 24.5%. However, given the increased risk of preterm delivery, depending on gestational age, inpatient observation can be considered.

REFERENCES

Berghella, V., Odibo, A., To, M., Rust, O., & Althuisius, S. (2005). Cerclage for short cervix on ultrasonography: Meta-analysis of trials using individual patient-level data. *Obstetrics and Gynecology, 106*(1), 181–189.

Combs, C. A., Garite, T., Maurel, K., Das, A., & Porto, M. (2010). Failure of 17-hydroxyprogesterone to reduce neonatal morbidity or prolong triplet pregnancy: A double-blind, randomized clinical trial. *American Journal of Obstetrics and Gynecology, 203*(3), 248.e1–248.e9.

Conde-Agudelo, A., & Romero, R. (2010). Cervicovaginal fetal fibronectin for the prediction of spontaneous preterm birth in multiple pregnancies: A systematic review and meta-analysis. *The Journal of Maternal-Fetal & Neonatal Medicine, 23*(12), 1365–1376.

Conde-Agudelo, A., Romero, R., Hassan, S. S., & Yeo, L. (2010). Transvaginal sonographic cervical length for the prediction of spontaneous preterm birth in twin pregnancies: A systematic review and metaanalysis. *American Journal of Obstetrics and Gynecology, 203*(2), 128.e1–128.e12.

Dickey, R. P. (2005). Embryonic loss in iatrogenic multiples. *Obstetrics and Gynecology Clinics of North America, 32*(1), 17–27.

Dickey, R. P., Taylor, S. N., Lu, P. Y., Sartor, B. M., Storment, J. M., Rye, P. H.,... Matulich, E. M. (2002). Spontaneous reduction of multiple pregnancy: Incidence and effect on outcome. *American Journal of Obstetrics and Gynecology, 186*(1), 77–83.

Dinsmoor, M. J., Bachman, R., Haney, E. I., Goldstein, M., & MacKendrick, W. (2004). Outcomes after expectant management of extremely preterm premature rupture of the membranes. *American Journal of Obstetrics and Gynecology, 190*(1), 183–187.

Evans, M., & Britt, D. (2008). Fetal reduction 2008. *Current Opinion in Obstetrics Gynecology, 20*(4), 386–393.

Falk, S., Campbell, L., Lee Parritz, A., Cohen, A., Ecker, J., Wilkins Haug, L., & Lieberman, E. (2004). Expectant management in spontaneous preterm premature rupture of membranes between 14 and 24 weeks' gestation. *Journal of Perinatology, 24*(10), 611–616.

Fischer, R. L., Sveinbjornsson, G., & Hansen, C. (2010). Cervical sonography in pregnant women with a prior cone biopsy or loop electrosurgical excision procedure. *Ultrasound in Obstetrics and Gynecology, 36*(5), 613–617.

Fonseca, E. B., Celik, E., Parra, M., Singh, M., & Nicolaides, K. H. (2007). Progesterone and the risk of preterm birth among women with a short cervix. *New England Journal of Medicine, 357*(5), 462–469.

Garel, M., Stark, C., Blondel, B., Lefebvre, G., Vauthier-Brouzes, D., & Zorn, J. R. (1997). Psychological reactions after multifetal pregnancy reduction: A 2-year follow-up study. *Human Reproduction, 12*(3), 617–622.

Guzman, E. R., Walters, C., O'Reilly-Green, C., Meirowitz, N. B., Gipson, K., Nigam, J., & Vintzileos, A. M. (2000). Use of cervical ultrasonography in prediction of spontaneous preterm birth in triplet gestations. *American Journal of Obstetrics and Gynecology, 183*(5), 1108–1113.

Iams, J. D., Goldenberg, R. L., Meis, P. J., Mercer, B. M., Moawad, A., Das, A.,... Roberts, J. M. (1996). The length of the cervix and the risk of spontaneous premature delivery. *New England Journal of Medicine, 334*(9), 567–573.

Martin, J. A., Hamilton, B. E., Sutton, P.D., Ventura, S. J., Mathews, T. J., Kirmeyer, S., & Osterman, M. J. (2010). Births: Final data for 2007. *National Vital Statistics Report, 58*(24), 1–85.

Mercer, B. M., Crocker, L. G., Pierce, W. F., & Sibai, B. M. (1993). Clinical characteristics and outcome of twin gestation complicated by preterm premature rupture of the membranes. *American Journal of Obstetrics and Gynecology, 168*(5), 1467–1473.

Mercer, B. M., Rabello, Y. A., Thurnau, G. R., Miodovnik, M., Goldenberg, R. L., Das, A. F.,... McNellis, D. (2006). The NICHD-MFMU antibiotic treatment of preterm PROM study: Impact of initial amniotic fluid volume on pregnancy outcome. *American Journal of Obstetrics and Gynecology, 194*(2), 438–445.

Moragianni, V. A., Aronis, K. N., & Craparo, F. J. (2011). Biweekly ultrasound assessment of cervical shortening in triplet pregnancies and the effect of cerclage placement. *Ultrasound in Obstetrics & Gynecology, 37*(5), 617–618.

Newman, R. B., Krombach, R. S., Myers, M. C., & McGee, D. L. (2002). Effect of cerclage on obstetrical outcome in twin gestations with a shortened cervical length. *American Journal of Obstetrics and Gynecology, 186*(4), 634–640.

Norman, J., Mackenzie, F., Owen, P., Mactier, H., Hanretty, K., Cooper, S., . . . Norrie, J. (2009). Progesterone for the prevention of preterm birth in twin pregnancy (STOPPIT): A randomised, double-blind, placebo-controlled study and meta-analysis. *Lancet, 373*(9680), 2034–2040.

Ørtoft, G., Henriksen, T., Hansen, E., & Petersen, L. (2010). After conisation of the cervix, the perinatal mortality as a result of preterm delivery increases in subsequent pregnancy. *BJOG: An International Journal of Obstetrics & Gynaecology, 117*(3), 258–267.

Pinborg, A., Lidegaard, O., Freiesleben, N. l. C., & Andersen, A. (2007). Vanishing twins: A predictor of small-for-gestational age in IVF singletons. *Human Reproduction, 22*(10), 2707–2714.

Roman, A., Fishman, S., Fox, N., Klauser, C., Saltzman, D., & Rebarber, A. (2011). Maternal and neonatal outcomes after delayed-interval delivery of multifetal pregnancies. *American Journal of Perinatology, 28*(2), 91–96.

Rouse, D. J., Caritis, S. N., Peaceman, A. M., Sciscione, A., Thom, E. A., Spong, C. Y., . . . Anderson, G. (2007). A trial of 17 alpha-hydroxyprogesterone caproate to prevent prematurity in twins. *New England Journal of Medicine, 357*(5), 454–461.

Rouse, D. J., Hirtz, D. G., Thom, E., Varner, M. W., Spong, C. Y., Mercer, B. M., . . . Roberts, J. M. (2008). A randomized, controlled trial of magnesium sulfate for the prevention of cerebral palsy. *The New England Journal of Medicine, 359*(9), 895–905.

Sela, H., & Simpson, L. (2011). Preterm premature rupture of membranes complicating twin pregnancy: Management considerations. *Clinical Obstetrics and Gynecology, 54*(2), 321–329.

Steinkampf, M., Whitten, S., & Hammond, K. (2005). Effect of spontaneous pregnancy reduction on obstetric outcome. *Journal of Reproductive Medicine, 50*(8), 603–606.

Stone, J., Ferrara, L., Kamrath, J., Getrajdman, J., Berkowitz, R., Moshier, E., & Eddleman, K. (2008). Contemporary outcomes with the latest 1000 cases of multifetal pregnancy reduction (MPR). *American Journal of Obstetrics and Gynecology, 199*(4), 406.e1–406.e4.

Waters, T. P., & Mercer, B. M. (2009). The management of preterm premature rupture of the membranes near the limit of fetal viability. *American Journal of Obstetrics and Gynecology, 201*(3), 230–240.

Yaron, Y., Bryant-Greenwood, P. K., Dave, N., Moldenhauer, J. S., Kramer, R. L., Johnson, M. P., & Evans, M. I. (1999). Multifetal pregnancy reductions of triplets to twins: Comparison with nonreduced triplets and twins. *American Journal of Obstetrics and Gynecology, 180*(5), 1268–1271.

Zhang, J., Hamilton, B., Martin, J., & Trumble, A. (2004). Delayed interval delivery and infant survival: A population-based study. *American Journal of Obstetrics and Gynecology, 191*(2), 470–476.

9 Nausea, Vomiting, and Hyperemesis of Pregnancy

Amy L. Snyder

Nausea and vomiting of pregnancy (NVP) is quite common, affecting between 70% and 85% of pregnant women (Jewell & Young, 2003). Rarely do pregnant women experience severe nausea and frequent vomiting known as hyperemesis gravidarum (HG), a condition that affects 2% to 5% of pregnant women (Eliakim, Abulafia, & Sherer, 2000). Although there is no single, commonly agreed definition for HG, most diagnostic criteria include the following: severe nausea and persistent vomiting, resulting in dehydration (as indicated by ketonuria and elevated urine specific gravity), electrolyte abnormalities (e.g., hypokalemia), and 5% or greater weight loss. NVP may lead to loss of work, interruption of family life, and stress but it typically represents a benign condition. HG can cause severe morbidity for both fetus and mother. Pregnancies complicated by HG are at higher risk for adverse outcomes, including premature birth and/or birth weight below the 10% for gestational age (Roseboom, Ravelli, van der Post, & Painter, 2011).

Attard and colleagues (2002) found that, in their sample of 223 women, those who suffered HG were slightly younger, more often primiparous, of lower socioeconomic status, and prone to substance abuse. They had more often conceived through assisted reproduction techniques, and more often had preexisting hypertension, metabolic conditions (e.g., diabetes mellitus) or psychological conditions than women who did not suffer from HG.

PRESENTING SYMPTOMATOLOGY

Pregnant women may present with nausea, vomiting, retching, fatigue, mild abdominal pain, heartburn, dyspepsia, hyperptyalism, and lightheadedness, if dehydration has occurred. These symptoms can persist throughout the day. Syncopal episodes or weight loss represents other common complaints that prompt patients to seek medical care. Abdominal pain not associated with retching, or a fever must prompt the provider to search for a diagnosis, other than NVP.

The proximal symptoms of HG include weight loss, dehydration, and electrolyte abnormalities, all of which require immediate medical attention and all of which may adversely affect the health of both the mother and infant. Extreme cases of HG have lead to other medical complications including peripheral neuropathies secondary to vitamin B_6 and B_{12} deficiencies,

Wernicke's encephalopathy (WE), splenic avulsion, esophageal rupture, pneumothorax, and acute tubular necrosis (ACOG, 2004).

HISTORY AND DATA COLLECTION

A thorough history is taken relative to onset of symptoms. Symptoms often begin from 4 weeks after the last menstrual period (LMP) and peak at 9 weeks from LMP. Sixty percent of symptoms resolve by the end of the first trimester and 91% resolve by 20 weeks' gestation (Niebyl, 2010). Knowing the duration of symptoms is crucial, as Wernicke's encephalopathy has been reported after 4 weeks of chronic, intense vomiting. Wernicke's is a neurologic condition that results from a depletion of vitamin B_6. Women should be questioned about other symptoms such as abdominal pain, fever, hematemesis, dysuria, hematuria, flank pain, diarrhea, and headache. Nausea and vomiting may cause mild upper abdominal pain from retching. Pain other than this should alert the clinician to seek an alternative diagnosis. A history of weight loss will help determine the severity. Recent travel and exposure to food borne illness must be documented, as well as remedies attempted and the results of such interventions.

PHYSICAL EXAMINATION

The physical examination in the obstetric triage or emergency room setting for women with NVP is typically benign. Mild epigastric pain may be present due to retching; however, the abdominal examination is otherwise normal without guarding, rebound, or organomegaly. Costovertebral angle tenderness may indicate renal pathology as the primary cause of the symptoms. The patient is typically afebrile, with a normal neurologic examination and no goiter palpable. Mucous membranes and skin turgor are useful in determining the severity of dehydration. Orthostatic vital signs are recorded, as well as weight. An increase in pulse of 20 beats per minute or a drop in blood pressure from sitting to standing indicates a hypovolemic state. This will help identify those women who will benefit from intravenous (IV) fluid administration.

LABORATORY TESTING AND IMAGING STUDIES

Laboratory testing includes urinanalysis and electrolyte evaluation. A complete blood count, liver function tests, amylase, lipase, and thyroid function tests are helpful in ruling out other causes of nausea and vomiting. Findings typically include suppressed thyroid stimulating hormone (TSH) levels and elevated free thyroxine, which resolves by 20 weeks' gestation. This is believed to be due to stimulation of the thyroid gland by human chorionic gonadotropin. Elevated free thyroxine and free triiodothyronine can be measured to test for true hyperthyroidism. Thyroid function tests are not indicated in a patient with no goiter palpable on physical examination. Other common changes seen are elevated transaminases (usually < 300 U/L) likely due to a combination of dehydration, malnutrition, and lactic acidosis. Levels in the 1000s are atypical and may indicate viral hepatitis as the primary diagnosis. Elevated bilirubin (< 4 mg/dl) and mildly elevated amylase and lipase, up to five times greater than normal are common findings. Amylase levels may be increased due to increased secretion of saliva, not from pancreatic production. If levels are 5 to 10 times greater than average, pancreatitis must be considered as a diagnosis and further imaging and gastroenterology consult obtained. Hematocrit and hemoglobin levels may be elevated due to hypovolemia or decreased from vitamin deficiency anemia (vitamin B_6 and B_{12}). A leukocytosis may indicate that infection is the underlying cause. Cholecystitis, pancreatitis, or pyelonephritis all need to be carefully considered. Electrolyte imbalances are common including hypokalemia, hyponatremia, and hypochloremic alkalosis. Ultrasound is not required, but it may disclose a potential cause of symptoms, such as multiple pregnancy or molar pregnancy.

DIFFERENTIAL DIAGNOSIS

NVP is a diagnosis of exclusion. Other causes of vomiting must be carefully considered. These include various infectious, neurologic, and gastrointestinal causes for nausea and vomiting. Table 9.1 notes these differential diagnoses.

CLINICAL MANAGEMENT AND FOLLOW-UP

The goal of therapy is to reduce symptoms, correct the consequences of vomiting such as dehydration and electrolyte imbalances, and prevent serious complications to the woman and fetus. Dehydration and electrolyte imbalances are corrected by IV fluids and electrolyte replacement. Antiemetics are used to reduce symptoms, and vitamins are replaced to prevent more serious deficiencies.

MEDICATION MANAGEMENT

If a patient appears to be dehydrated either by elevated specific gravity, findings on physical examination or orthostatic vital signs, IV fluids should be

TABLE 9.1 Differential Diagnoses for Nausea and Vomiting of Pregnancy

CONDITIONS/CAUSES	DIFFERENTIAL DIAGNOSES TO CONSIDER
Conditions related to pregnancy	Acute fatty liver of pregnancy, preeclampsia, premature contractions, hyperemesis gravidarum
Metabolic conditions	Addison's disease, diabetic ketoacidosis, hyperthyroidism, porphyria, thyrotoxicosis
Gastrointestinal causes	Achalasia, appendicitis, biliary tract disease, diaphragmatic hernia, gastroenteritis, gastroparesis, cholecystitis, cholelithiasis, hepatitis, intestinal obstruction, pancreatitis, stomach cancer, stomach or duodenal ulcer
Urogenital tract conditions	Degenerative uterine fibroids, nephrolithiasis, pyelonephritis, uremia, ovarian torsion
Neurological disorders	Acute alcohol withdrawal, migraine headache, vestibular disorders, central nervous system tumours, pseudotumor cerebri, Wernicke's encephalopathy
Miscellaneous conditions	Drug toxicities, food poisoning, iron imbalance, psychogenic causes

Source: Adapted from Jueckstock, Kaestner, & Mylonas (2010) and ACOG (2004).

initiated. Sodium chloride .9% is the preferred solution; 1.8% sodium chloride is not advised even in the setting of hyponatremia as rapid correction may lead to central pontine myelinolysis. Thiamine should be administered along with glucose if vomiting has persisted for longer than 3 weeks as thiamine depletion can result in WE. Wernicke's is diagnosed as the triad of ataxia, confusion, and ophthalmoplegia. This complication carries a 10% to 20% mortality rate and can cause persistent neurologic findings. About 100 mg of thiamine IV followed by daily oral supplementation is recommended. The shortest duration of vomiting, which has been shown to result in Wernicke's encephalopathy is 4 weeks (Togay-Isikay, Yigit, & Mutluer, 2001).

Bendectin was removed from the U.S. market in 1983 due to the cost of defending legal accusations of congenital malformations. To date, none of these allegations has been confirmed. The combination of doxylamine and vitamin $B_{6,}$ the two ingredients in Bendectin, (Diclectin is the Canadian sustained release form) reduce nausea up to 70 % (Niebyl, 2010). Doxylamine is an antihistamine that blocks binding of histamine at the H1 receptor site. This combination can still be obtained by using over-the-counter (OTC) Unisom, ½ of the 25 mg tablet along with Vitamin B_6 (10–25 mg) taken together 3 to 4 times per day. This is considered a first line treatment option by the American College of Obstetrics and Gynecology (ACOG). The most common side effects are drowsiness, dry mouth, blurred vision, constipation, and urinary retention. Diclectin is to be taken twice at bed, once in the morning, and once in the afternoon. Women are encouraged to continue usage as results may be delayed for several days. Trials have also shown efficacy of using vitamin B_6 alone to treat nausea with good results (Sahakian, Rouse, Sipes, Rose, & Niebyl, 1991; Niebyl & Goodwin, 2002).

Several dopamine antagonists may be used to treat NVP. Promethazine (phenergan) and prochlorperazine (compazine) are two commonly used agents. Both agents have demonstrated efficacy, as well as little or no risk for major malformations of offspring (Magee, Mazzotta, & Koren, 2002). In a trial comparing promethazine with metoclopramide, both were found to have similar results in treating nausea and vomiting and increasing overall well-being; however, promethazine had more side effects including drowsiness, dry mouth, headaches (30.2%), and dystonia (14%) for promethazine versus metoclopramide (4%) (Tan, Kline, Vallikkannu, & Omar, 2010). Compazine is available as a buccal tablet, which is associated with less drowsiness. Other side effects include extra pyramidal symptoms and parkinsonian-like symptoms usually seen with higher doses or extended usage. These symptoms can be treated with diphenhydramine or lorazepam.

Metoclopramide, a Food and Drug Administration (FDA) category B, is a dopamine antagonist with prokinetic properties. It is highly effective as described in the above study and accepted by most pregnant women. Usage for more than 12 weeks has been linked to tardive dyskinesia. No increase in malformations or poor obstetric outcomes has been seen in studies done to date, including an Israeli study of 3,458 women exposed to metoclopramide in the first trimester (Matok et al., 2009). Metoclopramide stimulates smooth muscle in the intestine and should be avoided in those women with bowel obstruction, perforation, or gastrointestinal bleeding.

Ondansetron is a HT3 antagonist commonly used to treat nausea and vomiting. Einarson and colleagues (2004) demonstrated the safety of ondansetron in a study comparing ondansetron to other antiemetics in a prospective comparative observational study. IV ondansetron has not been found to have greater efficacy than IV promethazine (Ebrahimi et al., 2010).

Gastroesophageal reflux symptoms such as heartburn, acid reflux, regurgitation, belching, flatulence, bloating, and indigestion are common during pregnancy and can compound symptoms of nausea and vomiting. Women with these symptoms perceived their nausea to be more severe. Acid reducing agents such as antacids, H-2 histamine blockers, and proton pump inhibitors are considered safe and effective in pregnancy. Antacids containing aluminium, calcium, and magnesium have all been found to be safe in pregnancy, though high dose, prolonged usage of magnesium trisilicate (Gaviscon, Genaton) is associated with nephrolithiasis, hypotonia, and respiratory distress in the fetus. (Ebrahimi et al., 2010). The link between *Helicobater pylori* and HG (Goldberg, Szilagyi, & Graves, 2007) has been documented. In a recent study, *H. pylori* was diagnosed by serum *H. pylori* IgG antibody in 71 of 80 patients with HG versus 24 controls (Mansour & Nashaat, 2011). Endoscopy was performed on women with severe symptoms and *H. pylori* was confirmed by histopathology. Cases of confirmed infection were treated with ranitidine 150 mg twice daily, metronidazole 500 mg twice daily, and ampicillin 1,000 mg twice daily for 2 weeks. Improvement was seen in 6 of 8 women. Screening for *H. pylori* must be considered in severe cases of hyperemesis and in women not responding to routine treatment regimens.

Methylprednisolone is used in refractory cases of hyperemesis. A randomized trial comparing methylprednisolone 16 mg three times daily for 3 days followed by a 2 week taper compared to oral promethazine showed equal rates of improvement among hospitalized patients but higher rates of readmission with the promethazine group. A later study did not replicate these findings. Several studies have shown a link between steroid usage and oral clefts (Carmichael & Shaw, 1999) (ACOG, 2004). ACOG recommends usage after 10 weeks' gestational age and in pregnant women who are being considered for enteral or parenteral feeding. The usual dosage is 48 mg daily for 3 days either IV or PO with a 2 week taper period. If symptoms recur, the woman may restart on the effective dose for up to 6 weeks.

A summary of treatment options is contained in Table 9.2.

Ginger

A review by Borrelli and Cappasso (2005), of six controlled trials, supported the efficacy of ginger use for the treatment of emesis, without any significant side effects. Ginger showed beneficial effects on women after admission for hyperemesis when compared to placebo. About 250 mg four times daily by tablet and syrup both showed beneficial effects. In syrup form, nausea decreased by 77% in the ginger group versus 20% in the placebo group. Sixty percent of the ginger group and 20% of the placebo group stopped vomiting after 6 days of usage. No negative outcomes for pregnancy or fetus were reported. When compared to vitamin B_6, ginger had equal reductions in nausea and number of vomiting episodes. Side effects of ginger were minor, i.e., reflux and heartburn.

Acupressure and Acupuncture

Acupressure is related to acupuncture and aims to heal by applying pressure to designated points throughout the body. Pressure to P6 or Neiguan is located 3 fingers or 4.5 cm above the wrist and is thought to treat nausea. Use of wrist bands and electrical stimulation of P6 for treatment show conflicting results (Matthew, Dowswell, Haas, Doyle, & O'mathuna, 2010). There are no consistent data to support acupuncture. A trial comparing acupuncture, sham acupuncture, and

TABLE 9.2 Treatment Options for Nausea and Vomiting in Pregnancy

MEDICATION DOSAGE	SIDE EFFECTS
Antihistamines	
Doxylamine 12.5 mg PO 3 or 4 x per day	Drowsiness, thickened bronchial secretions.
Diphenhydramine 25 to 50 mg PO q 4 to 6 hr 10 to 50 mg IV q 4 to 6 hr	Anticholinergic effects (tachycardia, constipation, confusion, urinary retention, decreased sweating, xerostomia)
Meclizine 25 mg PO q 4 to 6 hr	
Dimenhydrinate 25 to 50 mg PO q 4 to 6 hr 50 mg IV over 20 min 50 to 100 mg PR q 4 to 6 hr	
Dopamine antagonists	
Prochlorperazine 5 to 10 mg PO, IV, IM q 6 hr 25 mg PR bid	Dystonic reactions, akathisia, pseudoparkinsonism, tardive dyskinesia, neuroleptic malignant syndrome, drowsiness
Metoclopramide 10 mg PO, IV, IM q 6 to 8 hr	Dystonic reactions, akathisia, diarrhea
Promethazine 12.5 to 25 mg PO, IM, pr q 4 hr	Sedation, dystonic reactions, decreased seizure threshold
Serotonin antagonists	
Ondansetron 4 to 8 mg PO, IM q 8 hr	Headache, fatigue, constipation, drowsiness, QT prolongation
IV fluids 2 L lactated Ringers or normal saline over 3 to 5 hr	
Vitamins and minerals	
Thiamine 100 mg IV with initial fluids then 100 mg PO qd Multivitamin (MVI) 10 mL plus .6 mg folic acid in one liter and B_6 25 mg in every liter	

PO = orally, IV = intravenous, m = miligram, x = times, hr = hours, q = every, PR = rectally, IM = intramuscular.
Doxylamine is more efficacious when taken with pyridoxine vitamin B_6 25 mg 3 to 4 x per day.
Promethazine contraindicated for IV usage.

Source: Adapted from Clinical Pharmacology (2011).

no acupuncture showed a decrease in nausea for both sham and acupuncture groups; however, no change in vomiting (Smith, Crowther, & Bellby, 2002).

MANAGEMENT OF TREATMENT FAILURE FOR HG

For those women who continue to have symptoms and weight loss, despite adequate treatment with antiemetics, consideration may be given to parenteral or enteral feeding support. Many life-threatening risks are associated with parental feeding such as infections, thrombosis or endocarditis. In a study that looked at 85 pregnant women with central catheters, 25% developed serious complications (Jueckstock et al., 2010). Enteral tube feeding is the preferable route if tolerated by the pregnant woman.

Bariatric Surgery

As the obesity epidemic continues in the United States, bariatric surgery has become an increasingly more common procedure. The two most prevalent procedures are the gastric bypass and gastric banding. Women comprise 80% of the patients and half of those are of reproductive age (ACOG, 2009). Post-operative complications specific to this group include anastomotic leaks, bowel obstruction, internal hernias, ventral hernias, band erosion, and band migration. Dumping syndrome can occur after bypass procedures. Loads of refined sugars or high glycemic carbohydrate rapidly empty from the small stomach pouch to the small intestine resulting in fluid shifts from the intravascular space to the lumen of the bowel. The woman experiences bloating, cramps, nausea, vomiting, and diarrhea. Hyperinsulinemia and hypoglycemia can also be seen. Women presenting to an emergency room who provide this history need to be evaluated for these complications.

REFERENCES

ACOG Committee on Practice Bulletins. (2004). Nausea and vomiting of pregnancy. Clinical management guidelines for obstetrician-gynecologists, practice bulletin No. 52. *Obstetrics & Gynecology, 103*, 803–815.

ACOG Practice Bulletins. (2009). Bariatric surgery and pregnancy. Clinical management guidelines for obstetrician-gynecologists, practice bulletin No. 105, June 2009.

Attard, C. L., Kohli, M. A., Coleman, S., Bradley, C., Hux, M., Atanackovic, G., & Torrance, G. W. (2002). The burden of illness of severe nausea and vomiting of pregnancy in the United States. *American Journal of Obstetrics & Gynecology, 186,* S220–S227.

Borrelli, F., & Capasso, R. (2005). Effectiveness and safety of ginger in the treatment of pregnancy-induced nausea and vomiting. *Obstetrics & Gynecology, 105,* 849–856.

Carmichael, S. L., & Shaw, G. M. (1999) Maternal corticosteroid use and risk of selected congenital anomalies. *American Journal of Medical Genetics, 86,* 242–244.

Clinical Pharmacology. (2011). Retrieved from http://www.clinicalpharmacology-ip.com.revproxy.brown.edu/default.aspx

Ebrahimi, N., Maltepe, C., & Einarson, A. (2010). Optimal management of nausea and vomiting of pregnancy. *International Journal of Womens Health, 2,* 241–248.

Eliakim, R., Abulafia, O., & Sherer, D. M. (2000). Hyperemesis gravidarum: A current review. *American Journal of Perinatology, 17,* 207–218.

Einarson, A., Maltepe, C., Navloz, Y., Kennedy, D., Tan, M. P., & Koren, G. (2004). The safety of ondeansetron for nausea and vomiting of pregnancy: A prospective comparative study. *BJOG, 111,* 940–943.

Goldberg, D., Szilagyi, A., & Graves, L. (2007). Hyperemesis gravidarum and Helicobacter pylori infection: A systematic review. *Obstetrics and Gynecology. 110*(3), 695–703.

Jewell, D., & Young, G. (2003). Interventions for nausea and vomiting in early pregnancy (Cochrane Review). In: The Cochrane Library (Issue 4). Chichester, UK.: John Wiley & Sons, Ltd.

Jueckstock, J. K., Kaestner, R., & Mylonas, I. (2010). Managing hyperemesis gravidarum: A multimodal challenge. *BMC Medicine, 8,* 46. Retrieved from http://www.biomedcentral.com/1741–7015/8/46

Magee, L. A, Mazzotta, P., & Koren, G. (2002). Evidence-based view of safety and effectiveness of pharmacologic therapy for nausea and vomiting of pregnancy. *American Journal of Obstetrics and Gynecology, 186,* S256–S261.

Mansour, G. M., & Nashaat, E. H. (2011). Role of Helicobacter pylori in the pathogenesis of hyperemesis gravidarum. *Archives of Gynecology and Obstetrics, 284*(4), 843–847.

Matthew, A., Dowswell, T., Haas, D. M., Doyle, M., O'mathuna, D. P., (2010). Interventions for nausea and vomiting in early pregnancy. *Cochrane database of systemic reviews,* 9.

Matok, I., Gorodischer, R., Koren, G., Sheiner, E., Wiznitzer, A., & Levy, A. (2009). The safety of metoclopramide use in the first trimester of pregnancy. *The New England Journal of Medicine, 360,* 2528–2535.

Niebyl, J. R. (2010). Nausea and vomiting in pregnancy. *The New England Journal of Medicine, 363,* 16.

Niebyl, J. R., Goodwin, T. M. (2002). Overview of nausea and vomiting of pregnancy with an emphasis on vitamins and ginger. *American Journal of Obstetrics and Gynecology, 186,* S253–S255.

Roseboom, T. J., Ravelli, A. C. J., van der Post, J. A., & Painter, R. C. (2011). Maternal characteristics largely explain poor pregnancy outcome after hyperemesis gravidarum. *European Journal of Obstetrics & Gynecology and Reproductive Biology, 156,* 56–59.

Sahakian, V., Rouse, D., Sipes, S., Rose, N., & Niebyl, J. (1991). Vitamin B6 is effective therapy for nausea and vomiting of pregnancy: A randomized, double blind placebo-controlled study. *Obstetrics & Gynecology, 78,* 33–36.

Smith, C., Crowther, C., & Bellby, J. (2002). Acupuncture to treat nausea and vomiting in early pregnancy: A randomized controlled trial. *Birth, 29,* 1–9.

Tan, P. C., Khine, P. P. Vallikkannu, N., & Omar, S. Z. (2010). Promethazine compared with metoclopramide for hyperemesis gravidarum: A randomized controlled trial. *Obstetrics & Gynecology, 115,* 975–981.

Togay-Isikay, C., Yigit, A., & Mutluer, N. (2001). Wernicke's encephalopathy due to hyperemesis gravidarum: An under-recognised condition. *Australian* and *New Zealand Journal of Obstetrics and Gynaecology, 41,* 453–456.

Medical Conditions in Early Pregnancy

10

Asha J. Heard and Agatha S. Critchfield

Medical conditions can occur in early pregnancy and, although rare, can cause significant maternal and fetal morbidity. Often, women with these diseases can initially present to an obstetric triage or emergency room setting and may even necessitate referral to a tertiary care center. Prompt recognition and treatment of medical conditions during pregnancy can help to optimize maternal and fetal outcomes. The focus will be on a few medical conditions that can present in early pregnancy, which are as follows: pyelonephritis, nephrolithiasis, and pancreatitis. Pregnancy is a risk factor for pyelonephritis, which can occur due to lack of treatment or incomplete treatment of bacteriuria. Nephrolithiasis and pancreatitis often present with nonspecific symptoms such as abdominal pain, nausea, and vomiting that can mimic other conditions seen in early pregnancy and should be part of the differential when evaluating pregnant women in an obstetric triage or emergency room setting.

PYELONEPHRITIS

PRESENTING SYMPTOMATOLOGY

Pyelonephritis complicates approximately 1% to 2% of all pregnancies and can lead to significant maternal and fetal morbidity (Hill, Sheffied, McIntire, & Wendel, 2005). This can include sepsis, acute respiratory distress syndrome, preterm birth, anemia, and renal insufficiency. Pregnant women are thought to be more susceptible to pyelonephritis due to compression of the ureters by the gravid uterus, progesterone-mediated smooth muscle relaxation, increased glomerular filtration rate, and increased risk of bacteriuria during pregnancy. Approximately 21% of pyelonephritis during pregnancy occurs in the first trimester (Hill et al., 2005).

Pregnant women with pyelonephritis often have a history of a urinary tract infection or asymptomatic bacteriuria. Women with asymptomatic bacteriuria have an approximately 20- to 30-fold increased risk of developing pyelonephritis compared to women without bacteriuria (Jolley & Wing, 2010). Other risk factors for pyelonephritis include a previous history of pyelonephritis, sickle cell disease/trait, and diabetes. Approximately 13% of women with pyelonephritis in pregnancy may have at least one maternal risk factor (Hill et al., 2005).

Pregnant women with pyelonephritis may present with any of the following symptoms: fever, flank pain, dysuria, urinary frequency, costovertebral angle tenderness (CVAT), chills, nausea, or vomiting. In severe cases, they may present with signs and symptoms of septic shock including hypotension, tachycardia, shortness of breath, or multisystem organ failure. In contrast, women with a simple urinary tract infection may be asymptomatic or complain of localized symptoms only such as frequency, urgency, or dysuria.

PHYSICAL EXAMINATION

The diagnosis of acute pyelonephritis can be made on the clinical findings of fever (>38°C), flank pain, and CVAT with the laboratory finding of bacteriuria (Jolley & Wing, 2010). However, women with a simple urinary tract infection usually do not have any significant physical examination findings.

LABORATORY AND IMAGING STUDIES

A urinalysis can confirm that bacteriuria is present (>8–12 white blood cells/high power field) in a clean catch specimen (<2–4 epithelial cells). A urine culture obtained from a midstream clean catch specimen can isolate the microorganism and confirm the diagnosis by looking for greater than 100,000 colony forming units (Jolley & Wing, 2010). The most common pathogens associated with pyelonephritis are listed in Exhibit 10.1.

Other laboratory evaluation includes a complete blood count and serum chemistry evaluation. Elevation of the white blood cell count may be seen. In addition, there may be electrolyte abnormalities and transient renal insufficiency (Hill et al., 2005). The utility of obtaining blood cultures in the setting of pyelonephritis has been debated in the literature. Wing, Park, DeBuque, and Millar (2000) demonstrated that a change in management due to bacteremia alone occurred in only 1% of cases. There does not seem to be evidence that the presence of bacteremia is associated with a worse prognosis in the setting of pyelonephritis. However, blood cultures may be considered if the woman shows signs or symptoms of sepsis or has medical comorbidities.

EXHIBIT 10.1

Occurrence of Pathogens Associated With Pyelonephritis in Pregnancy

- *Escherichia coli* (83%)
- Group B streptococcus and other Gram-positive organisms (11.6%)
- *Klebsiella* or *Enterobacter* (3.5%)
- *Proteus* (2.2%)

Source: Adapted from Hill et al. (2005).

■ DIFFERENTIAL DIAGNOSIS

The differential diagnosis for pyelonephritis in pregnancy includes other disorders of genitourinary, gastrointestinal, and pulmonary systems. Other conditions that can present in a similar fashion include acute cystitis, nephrolithiasis, viral syndrome, renal failure, pneumonia, pancreatitis, appendicitis, and gastroenteritis.

■ CLINICAL MANAGEMENT AND FOLLOW-UP

Unlike a simple urinary tract infection or asymptomatic bacteriuria, which can be managed as an outpatient with oral antibiotics, the standard management of pyelonephritis in pregnancy is admission to the hospital for inpatient management. Archabald, Friedman, Raker, & Anderson (2009) found that maternal morbidity and obstetric outcomes did not differ between first-trimester pyelonephritis compared with second-/third-trimester pyelonephritis. Given this data, it is recommended that all pregnant women with pyelonephritis, regardless of trimester, be admitted for parenteral antibiotics, antipyretics, and intravenous hydration.

Cephalosporins are recommended as first-line therapy for pyelonephritis during pregnancy (Jolley & Wing, 2010) due to the increasing resistance of *Escherichia coli* to ampicillin. An appropriate initial regimen is ceftriaxone 2 g intravenously every 24 hours. Aminoglycosides (i.e., gentamicin) can be considered in cases of cephalosporin allergy, but it has been associated with ototoxicity following prolonged fetal exposure (Le, Briggs, McKeown, & Bustillo, 2004). Fluoroquinolones are avoided in pregnancy.

Parenteral antibiotics can be continued until the pregnant woman has shown clinical improvement and has been afebrile for 24 to 48 hours. Due to the risk of capillary endothelial damage due to bacteria-mediated endotoxins and subsequent risk of respiratory insufficiency and acute respiratory distress syndrome (ARDS), aggressive hydration during this time should be used with caution and urine output should be monitored closely. Treatment with oral antibiotics tailored to the sensitivity of the microorganism should be continued for 14 days following intravenous treatment. A post treatment urine culture as a test of cure should be sent.

If there is no clinical improvement seen in 48 to 72 hours, further evaluation for bacterial resistance, urolithiasis, renal abscess, and urinary tract abnormalities can be considered. At this point, consider broadening antibiotic coverage and imaging the urinary tract system with ultrasound or magnetic resonance imaging (MRI).

Recurrent pyelonephritis can occur in 6% to 8% of women with pyelonephritis in pregnancy (Lenke, VanDorsten, & Schifrin, 1983). Suppressive therapy is recommended for the duration of the pregnancy and up to 6 weeks postpartum with either nitrofurantoin 100 mg orally or cephalexin 250 to 500 mg orally at bedtime. Suppressive therapy may be considered in subsequent pregnancies.

NEPHROLITHIASIS

■ PRESENTING SYMPTOMATOLOGY

Symptomatic nephrolithiasis affects approximately 1 in 244 to 1 in 2,000 pregnancies (Srirangam, Hickerton, & Van Cleynenbreugel, 2008; Rosenberg et al., 2011). As noted previously, changes in the urinary tract during pregnancy include an increased glomerular filtration rate, compression of the ureters due to the gravid uterus, and progesterone-mediated smooth muscle relaxation. Despite these changes, the prevalence of nephrolithiasis is thought to be similar to the nonpregnant population (Rosenberg et al., 2011). This may be due to increased production of citrate and magnesium during pregnancy, which are thought to be urinary stone inhibitors (Meria, Hadjadj, Jungers, Daudon, & Members of the French Urological Association Urolithiasis Committee, 2010). Symptomatic nephrolithiasis presents in the second or third trimesters in approximately 80% to 90% of cases (Butler, Cox, Eberts, & Cunningham, 2000).

Pregnant women with symptomatic nephrolithiasis may present with back or flank pain, lower abdominal pain, dysuria, or hematuria. Nausea and/or vomiting may also be present. Flank or abdominal pain is the most common symptom, occurring in approximately 85% to 100% of patients (Srirangam et al., 2008). Pain is often described as intermittent and colicky in nature. Frank hematuria is reported to occur in 15% to 30% of cases (Srirangam et al, 2008). Microscopic hematuria may not be present in up to 25% of women with diagnosed calculi (Travassos et al., 2009). Women may report a history of nephrolithiasis in the past.

On physical examination, pregnant women may appear uncomfortable and in visible pain. Tachycardia may be present as part of the pain response. CVAT may be present.

A urinalysis and urine culture can assess for hematuria and pyuria, which may suggest an underlying infection. A complete blood count may indicate evidence of systemic infection. A baseline creatinine may be helpful to confirm normal renal function. Straining the urine of pregnant women with suspected nephrolithiasis may demonstrate the spontaneous passage of stones.

Imaging of the renal system may be helpful in confirming the diagnosis of renal calculi. Renal ultrasonography is often used as the first-line imaging modality. However, the sensitivity of ultrasound in confirming urolithiasis ranges from 34% to 86% (Srirangam et al., 2008). In addition, ultrasound may be unable to distinguish from an obstruction due to calculi or physiologic hydronephrosis. In the setting of symptoms that are not improving or worsening, other imaging modalities that can be considered include an abdominal flat plate x-ray, MRI, or single-shot intravenous pyelography.

The differential diagnosis of nephrolithiasis includes other genitourinary and gastrointestinal disorders as well as conditions related to pregnancy itself. The differential diagnoses for nephrolithiasis are listed in Exhibit 10.2.

If there is a clinical suspicion for nephrolithiasis in pregnancy, the first steps are aggressive hydration and pain control. Pregnant women may need to be admitted to the hospital for pain management. Opiates, either intravenously or orally, can be used for analgesia in pregnancy. Nonsteroidal antiinflammatory drugs (NSAIDs) are to be avoided, especially in the third trimester, due to risks of oligohydramnios and premature closure of the ductus arteriosus. If a superimposed infection is suspected, antibiotic therapy can be initiated while awaiting final urine culture results. Antiemetics can also be given if the woman's symptoms include nausea or vomiting. Approximately 64% to 84% of renal calculi pass spontaneously (Srirangam et al., 2008). Again, urine should be strained to assess for passage of calculi.

In approximately 15% to 30% of cases, further intervention may be needed (Srirangam et al., 2008). A urology consultation and/or further

EXHIBIT 10.2

Differential Diagnosis of Nephrolithiasis in Pregnancy

- Pyelonephritis
- Urinary tract infection
- Labor
- Diverticulitis
- Appendicitis
- Pancreatitis
- Round ligament pain
- Gastroenteritis
- Abruption
- Ectopic pregnancy

Source: Adapted from Srirangam et al. (2008).

imaging with ultrasound or MRI may be considered for symptoms that are not improving with conservative management, evidence of compromised renal function, or concern for superimposed pyelonephritis. Surgical interventions for persistent nephrolithiasis with obstruction during pregnancy include percutaneous nephrostomy, ureteral stent insertion, or ureteroscopy with stone retrieval (Srirangam et al., 2008). A recent series of ureteroscopy in pregnant women showed a 100% success rate without any complications (Travassos et al., 2009).

In pregnant women with nephrolithiasis, pregnancy outcomes including spontaneous abortion and preeclampsia were not significantly different compared to women without nephrolithiasis (Butler et al., 2000). Similarly, the risk of congenital anomalies is not increased in women with nephrolithiasis in pregnancy (Bánhidy, Acs, Puhó, & Czeizel., 2007). Swartz, Lydon-Rochelle, Simon, Wright, and Porter (2007), however, did find an increased risk of preterm birth in women admitted to the hospital for nephrolithiasis.

PANCREATITIS

PRESENTING SYMPTOMATOLOGY

Acute pancreatitis is estimated to occur in approximately 1 in 1,000 to 1 in 12,000 pregnancies (Eddy, Gideonsen, Song, Grobman, O'Halloran, 2008) and can initially present with nausea and vomiting, similar to hyperemesis of pregnancy. Therefore, it is important to consider when evaluating for nausea and vomiting of pregnancy. Approximately 57% of pancreatitis during pregnancy is estimated to occur in the first or second trimesters (Eddy et al., 2008).

Pancreatitis in pregnancy commonly presents with abdominal pain, that is classically located in the epigastric region with radiation to the back. Other significant symptoms include nausea and vomiting, which can also occur secondary to pregnancy itself. In severe cases, pregnant women may present with signs of sepsis, including fever, tachycardia, hypotension, and hyperventilation.

EXHIBIT 10.3

Causes of Pancreatitis in Pregnancy

- Gallstones
- Alcohol
- Idiopathic
- Hyperlipidemia
- Hyperparathyroidism
- Trauma
- Medications
- Acute fatty liver of pregnancy

Source: Adapted from Eddy et al. (2008).

The most common cause of pancreatitis in pregnancy is gallstones (66%; Eddy et al., 2008). Other causes of pancreatitis in pregnancy are listed in Exhibit 10.3.

Risk factors for pancreatitis include a history of gallstones, alcohol use, hyperlipidemia, or tobacco use. Physiologic changes during pregnancy such as smooth muscle relaxation of the gallbladder due to progesterone case induce bile stasis and gallstone formation. In addition, pregnancy is thought to be associated with a two- to four-fold increase in plasma triglyceride levels (Crisan, Steidl, & Rivera-Alsina, 2008). Medications that have been associated with pancreatitis include erythromycin, mesalamine, sulfasalazine, acetaminophen, didanosine, and steroids (Papadakis, Sarigianni, Mikhailidis, Mamopoulos, &, Karagiannis, 2011).

PHYSICAL EXAMINATION

Vital signs of a patient with acute pancreatitis may be notable for fever, tachycardia, or tachypnea. Physical examination findings may include abdominal tenderness especially in the epigastric area, signs of an acute abdomen, or signs of dehydration.

LABORATORY AND IMAGING STUDIES

The diagnosis of acute pancreatitis can be confirmed by increased serum amylase and/or lipase. Amylase and lipase levels in pregnancy are similar to levels in the nonpregnant state (Karsenti et al., 2001). An elevated amylase level can be a nonspecific finding as it can be elevated in other disease states. Typically in acute pancreatitis, the amylase level is three times the normal range. Serum lipase has also been found to be more specific than amylase in the evaluation of acute pancreatitis (Treacy et al., 2011). Other laboratory findings may include elevated liver function tests, leukocytosis, and increased serum cholesterol levels.

An ultrasound of the right upper quadrant may be performed as it is safe in pregnancy and can reliably detect gallstones and biliary duct dilation. Figure 10.1 illustrates gallstones in the gall bladder or ultrasound imaging.

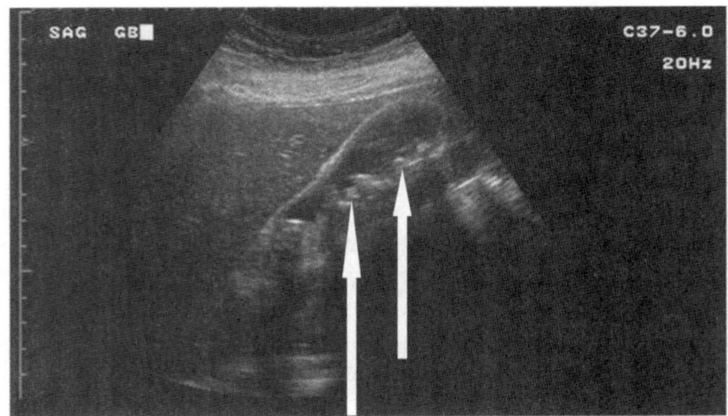

FIGURE 10.1 Gallstones on ultrasound.

Source: Courtesy of Department of Radiology, Women & Infants Hospital, Providence, RI.

However, ultrasound has low-diagnostic value for acute pancreatitis (Koo, Chinogureyi, & Shaw, 2010). Magnetic resonance cholangiopancreatography (MRCP) can allow for visualization of the pancreatic parenchyma and common bile duct with a sensitivity of over 90% (Roumieu et al., 2008). In addition, it avoids exposure to radiation for the patient and her fetus.

DIFFERENTIAL DIAGNOSIS

The differential diagnosis of pancreatitis in pregnancy encompasses diseases from many organ systems. It includes cholecystitis, cholelithiasis, choledocholithiasis, preeclampsia, acute fatty liver of pregnancy, hyperemesis gravidarum, gastroenteritis, gastric ulcer, appendicitis, nephrolithiasis, and pyelonephritis.

CLINICAL MANAGEMENT AND FOLLOW-UP

Pregnant women with presumed acute pancreatitis are most often admitted to the hospital for further workup and clinical management. Clinical and laboratory risk factors or various severity grading systems can be used to access the severity of disease (Geng et al., 2011). If the woman is clinically stable and has a mild form of the disease, it is reasonable to proceed with conservative management including intravenous fluid therapy, bowel rest, and pain control. The mean length of stay in the hospital in a recent study was estimated at approximately 6 days (Hernandez et al., 2007). Once symptoms resolve, the woman can be discharged home with close follow-up. A low-fat diet should be encouraged in all patients with pancreatitis. The rate of recurrence of gallstone pancreatitis during pregnancy is approximately 30% to 50% (Eddy et al., 2008; Hernandez et al., 2007). A cholecystectomy can be performed safely in pregnancy, ideally during the second trimester, and may be considered once symptoms resolve (Date, Kaushal, & Ramesh, 2008).

If symptoms do not improve, enteral or parenteral nutrition may be needed after approximately 7 days. Women who are clinically unstable or have evidence of septic shock will need admission to the intensive care unit.

Consultation with gastroenterology or general surgery to assist with further imaging and management may be considered.

Antibiotic prophylaxis in the setting of acute pancreatitis is controversial and debated in the literature. In cases of suspected sepsis or cholangitis, broad spectrum antibiotics are recommended. However, in mild pancreatitis, antibiotics can be deferred unless the clinical situation changes (Pitchumoni & Yegneswaran, 2009).

Later in gestation, women with acute pancreatitis are at-risk for preterm delivery. The rate of preterm delivery in pregnant women with a history of acute pancreatitis is estimated to be approximately 32% (Eddy et al., 2008). The risk of preterm delivery is thought to be increased in patients with non-gallstone pancreatitis or in severe cases of pancreatitis (Geng et al., 2011).

REFERENCES

Archabald, K. L., Friedman, A., Raker, C. A., & Anderson, B. L. (2009) Impact of trimester on morbidity of acute pyelonephritis in pregnancy. *American Journal of Obstetrics & Gynecology, 201*(4), 406, e1–e4.

Bánhidy, F., Acs, N., Puhó, E. H., & Czeizel, A. E. (2007). Maternal kidney stones during pregnancy and adverse birth outcomes, particularly congenital abnormalities in the offspring. *Archives of Gynecology and Obstetrics, 275*(6), 481–487.

Butler, E. L., Cox, S. M., Eberts, E. G., & Cunningham, F. G. (2000). Symptomatic nephrolithiasis complicating pregnancy. *Obstetrics and Gynecology, 96*, 753–756.

Crisan, L. S., Steidl, E. T., & Rivera-Alsina, M. E. (2008). Acute hyperlipidemic pancreatitis in pregnancy. *American Journal of Obstetrics and Gynecology, 198*, e57–e59.

Date, R. S., Kaushal, M., & Ramesh, A. (2008). A review of the management of gallstone disease and its complications in pregnancy. *American Journal of Surgery, 196*, 599–608.

Eddy, J. J., Gideonsen, M. D., Song, J. Y., Grobman, W. A., O'Halloran, P. (2008). Pancreatitis in pregnancy. *Obstetrics and Gynecology, 112*(5), 1075–1081.

Geng, Y., Li, W., Sun, L., Tong, Z., Li, N., Li, J. (2011). Severe acute pancreatitis during pregnancy: Eleven years experience from a surgical intensive care unit. *Digestive Diseases and Sciences, 56*(12), 3672–3677.

Hernandez, A., Petrov, M. S., Brooks, D. C., Banks, P. A., Ashley, S. W., Tavakkolizadeh, A. (2007). Acute pancreatitis and pregnancy: A 10-year single center experience. *Journal of Gastrointestinal Surgery, 11*(12), 1623–1627.

Hill, J. B., Sheffied, J. S., McIntire, D. D., & Wendel, G. D. (2005). Acute pyelonephritis in pregnancy. *Obstetrics & Gynecology, 105*(1), 18–23.

Jolley, J., & Wing, D. (2010). Pyelonephritis in pregnancy: An update on treatment options for optimal outcomes. *Drugs, 70*(13), 1643–1655.

Karsenti, D., Bacq, Y., Bréchot, J. F., Mariotte, N., Vol, S., & Tichet, J. (2001). Serum amylase and lipase activities in normal pregnancy: A prospective case-control study. *American Journal of Gastroenterology, 96*(3), 697–699.

Koo, B. C., Chinogureyi, A., & Shaw, A. S. (2010). Imaging acute pancreatitis. *British Journal of Radiology, 83*, 104–112.

Le, J., Briggs, G. G., McKeown, A., & Bustillo, G. (2004). Urinary tract infections during pregnancy. *Annals of Pharmacotherapy, 38*(10), 1692–1701.

Lenke, R. R., VanDorsten, J. P., & Schifrin, B. S. (1983). Pyelonephritis in pregnancy: A prospective randomized trial to prevent recurrent disease evaluating suppressive therapy with nitrofurantoin and close surveillance. *American Journal of Obstetrics & Gynecology, 146*(8), 953–957.

Meria, P., Hadjadj, H., Jungers, P., Daudon, M., & Members of the French Urological Association Urolithiasis Committee. (2010). Stone formation and pregnancy: Pathophysiological insights gained from morphoconstitutional stone analysis. *Journal of Urology, 183*(4), 1412–1416.

Papadakis, E. P., Sarigianni, M., Mikhailidis, D. P., Mamopoulos, A., Karagiannis, V. (2011). Acute pancreatitis in pregnancy: An overview. *European Journal of Obstetrics, Gynecology, and Reproductive Biology, 159*(2), 261–266.

Pitchumoni, C., & Yegneswaran, B. (2009). Acute pancreatitis in pregnancy. *World Journal of Gastroenterology, 15*(45), 5641–5646.

Rosenberg, E., Sergienko, R., Abu-Ghanem, S., Wiznitzer, A., Romanowsky, I., Neulander, E. Z., & Sheiner, E. (2011). Nephrolithiasis during pregnancy: Characteristics, complications, and pregnancy outcome. *World Journal of Urology, 29*(6), 743–747.

Srirangam, S. J., Hickerton, B., & Van Cleynenbreugel, B. (2008). Management of urinary calculi in pregnancy: A review. *Journal of Endourology, 22*(5), 867–875.

Swartz, M. A., Lydon-Rochelle, M. T., Simon, D., Wright, J. L., Porter, M. P. (2007). Admission for nephrolithiasis in pregnancy and risk of adverse birth outcomes. *Obstetrics and Gynecology, 109*(5),1099–1104.

Travassos, M., Amselem, I., Filho, N. S., Miguel, M., Sakai, A., Consolmagno, H., Nogueira, M., & Fugita, O. (2009). Ureteroscopy in pregnant women for ureteral stone. *Journal of Endourology, 23*(3), 405–407.

Treacy, J., Williams, A., Bais, R., Willson, K., Worthley, C., Reece, J...., Thomas, D. (2001). Evaluation of amylase and lipase in the diagnosis of acute pancreatitis. *ANZ Journal of Surgery, 71*(10), 577–582.

Wing, D., Park, A. S., DeBuque, L., Millar, L. K. (2000). Limited clinical utility of blood and urine cultures in the treatment of acute pyelonephritis during pregnancy. *American Journal of Obstetrics and Gynecology, 182*(6), 1437–1441.

III: MANAGEMENT OF OBSTETRIC CONDITIONS (GREATER THAN VIABILITY)

Fetal Evaluation and Clinical Applications 11

Edie McConaughey

Electronic fetal heart rate monitoring (EFM) technologies and ultrasound are the primary surveillance tools used for fetal evaluation in an obstetric (OB) triage setting. Approximately 85% of live births in the United States are assessed with EFM, making it one of the most widely used OB tools (Freeman, Garite, & Nageotte, 2003; Tucker, Miller, & Miller, 2009). Technologic advances have produced a machine that provides clinicians with a valuable tool to display fetal heart rate (FHR) patterns accurately. The benefits of EFM include decreased intrapartum death rates, improved Apgar scores, and the determination of well-being in the high-risk fetus. The goals of fetal evaluation are to accurately identify reassuring fetal status, permit expectant management, and recognize the fetus at risk, thus preventing adverse perinatal outcomes (ACOG, 1999; Devoe, 2008; Signore, Freeman, & Spong, 2009). Common maternal and fetal indications for EFM testing in an OB triage setting are presented in Exhibit 11.1.

Despite widespread use of these technologies, there is limited evidence to guide type of test, testing intervals, gestational ages at which to initiate testing, or optimal frequency of testing (Signore et al., 2009). Key measures of the effectiveness of a test include the false negative rate (incidence of fetal death within 1 week of normal antepartum test) and the false positive rate (abnormal test that prompts delivery of a healthy fetus; Tucker et al., 2009). These rates are presented for each of the current testing methods as described in Table 11.1.

FETAL TESTING METHODS AND EVALUATION

Nonstress Test

Nonstress tests (NST) are often the first cardiotocographic test performed in assessing fetal well-being and are initiated for a variety of maternal and fetal conditions. The characteristics of the baseline FHR unrelated to contractions are observed with healthy fetuses displaying normal fluctuations and oscillations in the baseline. In addition, the presence of accelerations correlates with fetal well-being (Freeman et al., 2003) and normal fetal autonomic functioning (ACOG, 1999). Absence of accelerations on a baseline FHR tracing can be associated with a fetal sleep cycle, medication administration, congenital

EXHIBIT 11.1

Common Indications for Electronic Fetal Monitoring Evaluation in OB Triage

- Postterm pregnancy
- Amniotic fluid abnormalities
- Preterm premature rupture of membranes (PPROM)
- Decreased fetal movement (DFM)
- Hypertensive disorders
- Diabetes
- Multiple gestation
- Fetal growth restriction
- History of stillbirth
- Minor trauma

Source: Adapted from ACOG (1999) and Signore et al. (2009).

abnormalities or adverse fetal outcomes (Signore et al., 2009), and acidosis (ACOG, 1999; Freeman et al., 2003).

Both the external tocodynamometer and the ultrasound transducer are secured to the woman's abdomen to record uterine contractions and FHR, respectively. A separate "event marker" button is given to the mother to record perceived fetal movements. The fetal monitor tracing is recorded for 20 minutes during which clinicians can observe FHR baseline, variability, the presence or absence of accelerations, decelerations, and contractions along with maternal perception of fetal movements.

Interpretation and Management

Accelerations of the FHR in response to fetal movements are the basis for interpretation and management of the NST. There is no universal agreement for defining a "reactive" NST, the number of accelerations, or length of testing (Freeman et al., 2003). Generally, for a fetus beyond 32 weeks' gestation, a normal or reactive NST consists of two accelerations of the FHR greater than 15 beats above baseline lasting at least 15 seconds occurring in 20 minutes. When the fetus is less than 32 weeks, the immature central nervous system may not respond as vigorously. In these fetuses, a reactive NST consists of two accelerations of greater than 10 beats above baseline lasting at least 10 seconds (Tucker et al., 2009). The NST may continue for 40 minutes or more to account for a fetal sleep cycle.

Vibroacoustic stimulation, using an artificial larynx, may be used to stimulate fetal movement and shorten the test duration (Tan & Smyth, 2001). FHR accelerations, in response to fetal scalp stimulation or fetal acoustic stimulation, are predictive of a normal fetal scalp pH (Tucker et al., 2009). A reactive NST may occur without maternal perception of fetal movement (ACOG, 1999; Freeman et al., 2003; Tucker et al., 2009).

An NST is considered nonreactive when two accelerations do not meet the gestational age requirements in 40 minutes (ACOG, 1999). Nonreactive NSTs, along with reactive NSTs with decelerations, warrant additional testing including amniotic fluid (AF) assessment, contraction stress test (CST),

TABLE 11.1 Comparison of Fetal Evaluation

NAME	COMPONENTS	RESULTS/SCORING	FALSE NEGATIVE (%)	FALSE POSITIVE (%)	COMMENTS
Nonstress test	Continuous FHR monitoring. FHR accelerations: ≥32 wk: reaching 15 bpm above baseline and lasting ≥15 sec <32 wk: 10 beat amplitude lasting ≥10 sec	**Reactive**: ≥2 accelerations within 20 min (may be extended to 40 min) **Nonreactive**: <2 accelerations in 40 min	0.2–0.65	55–90	Preterm fetus 24–28 wk, up to 50% of NSTs are nonreactive Preterm fetus 28–32 wk, 15% of NSTs may be nonreactive
Modified BPP	NST and AFI	**Normal**: Reactive NST and AFI > 5 cm **Abnormal**: Nonreactive NST and/or AFI ≤5 cm	0.08	60	NST short-term indicator of fetal acid–base status Normal AFI >5 cm—indicator of long-term placental function
BPP	Presence or absence of five components within 30 min: Reactive NST ≥ one episode of fetal breathing movements lasting ≥30 sec ≥ 3 discrete body or limb movements ≥ one episode of extremity extension with return to flexion or opening or closing of a hand Maximum vertical AF pocket > 2 cm or AFI > 5 cm Continuous FHR monitoring	Each component present is assigned a score of 2 points; maximum score is 10/10 **Normal**: ≥8/10 or 8/8 excluding NST **Equivocal**: 6/10 **Abnormal**: ≤4/10	0.07–0.08	40–50	Assesses both acute (NST, breathing, fetal movement) and chronic (AFV/AFI) hypoxia. Correlates with fetal pH
Contraction stress test (Oxytocin challenge test)	At least three contractions of ≥40 sec duration within 10 min that occur spontaneously, with nipple stimulation or with IV oxytocin	**Negative**: no late or significant variable decelerations **Positive**: late decelerations following ≥50% of contractions	0.04	35–65	Relative contraindications: PTL Preterm ROM Classical C/S

Continued

TABLE 11.1 Comparison of Fetal Evaluation *Continued*

NAME	COMPONENTS	RESULTS/SCORING	FALSE NEGATIVE (%)	FALSE POSITIVE (%)	COMMENTS
Contraction stress test (*continued*)		**Equivocal—suspicious**: intermittent late decelerations or significant variable decelerations **Equivocal—hyperstimulatory**: decelerations with contractions occurring more frequently than q 2 min or lasting greater than 90 sec **Unsatisfactory—**Less than 3 contractions in 10 min or uninterpretable FHR tracing			Known placenta Previa Repeat equivocal CSTs within 24°
Doppler indices					
Uterine artery	Evaluation of maternal flow to placenta	Increased resistance to uterine artery blood flow			Associated with development of future preeclampsia, IUGR, and/or perinatal death
Umbilical artery	Evaluation of high-velocity diastolic flow, i.e., systolic-to-diastolic (SD) ratio	Decreased, absent, or reversed diastolic flow in early IUGR fetuses associated with fetal hypoxia			Indicated for early onset IUGR fetuses with uteroplacental insufficiently ACOG currently supports use with IUGR fetuses
Middle cerebral artery	Doppler measurement of flow	Detects blood redistribution from periphery to brain			Brain sparing Limited data available

Source: Adapted from ACOG (1999), Devoe (2008), Signore et al. (2009), and Cunningham et al. (2010).

or biophysical profile (BPP; Tucker et al., 2009). See Figure 11.1 for a sample management algorithm for EFM testing in the OB triage setting.

Amniotic Fluid Assessment

AF is an important assessment of fetal well-being. It provides a protective environment for fetal development by shielding the fetus from trauma and infection, allowing for fetal movement, and preventing compression of the umbilical cord. Its volume is the sum of fluid flowing into and out of the amniotic cavity from fetal urine, fetal swallowing, and intramembranous absorption. As long as there is no rupture of membranes, oligohydramnios is believed to indicate a fetal response to chronic stress. It is associated with increased fetal and neonatal morbidity and mortality including fetal anomalies, growth restriction, postterm pregnancies, and maternal hypertensive disorders (Nabhan & Abdelmoula, 2008).

Ultrasound measurement of AF is used during fetal surveillance by estimating an amniotic fluid volume (AFV) in a single vertical pocket or the amniotic fluid index (AFI). Several AFV measurements have been suggested in the

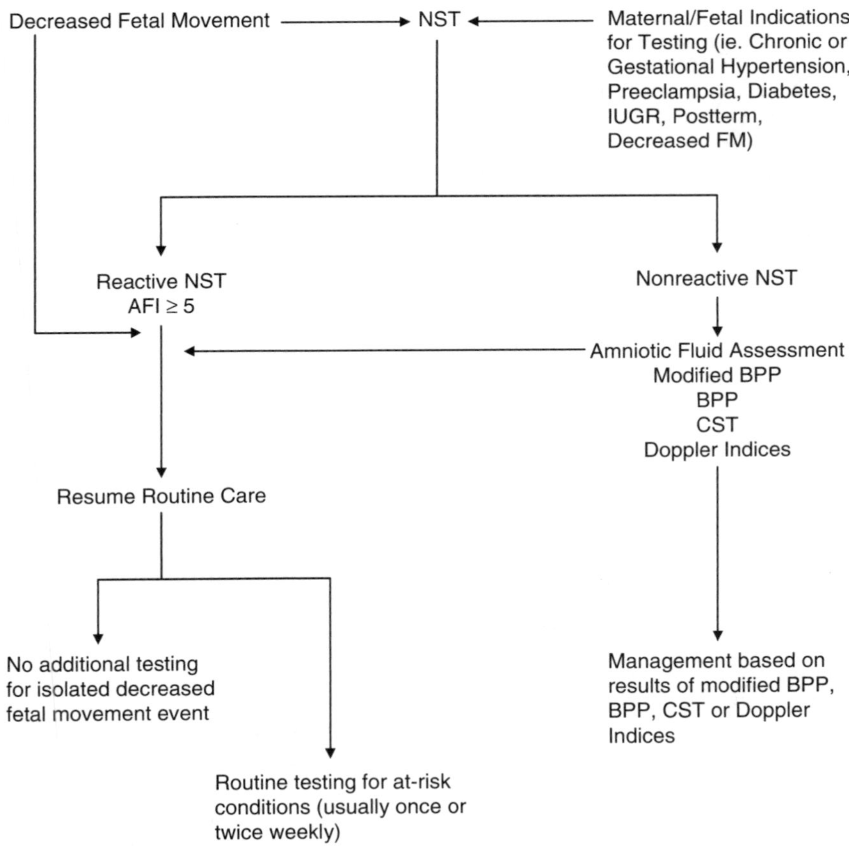

FIGURE 11.1 Algorithm for electronic fetal monitoring testing.

literature, but a 2 cm vertical pocket is the most commonly used lower limit of normal (ACOG, 1999; Nabhan & Abdelmoula, 2008). When calculating the AFI, the clinician divides the uterus into four quadrants. The AFI is the sum of the largest vertical fluid pocket in each of the four quadrants that does not contain umbilical cord (Nabhan & Abdelmoula, 2008).

Interpretation and Management

An AFI of ≤ 5 cm or the absence of a 2 cm vertical pocket identifies oligohydramnios and has been associated with fetal compromise especially with high-risk pregnancies (Nabhan & Abdelmoula, 2008). No consensus exists for the best method of testing or for the ideal cutoff for intervention (ACOG, 1999). Many clinicians will plan delivery for oligohydramnios at term but will also consider maternal and fetal clinical condition as determined by other tests of fetal well-being (ACOG, 1999; Nabhan & Abdelmoula, 2008). Evaluating the pregnant woman for ruptured membranes should be considered based on clinical history. In the preterm pregnancy, expectant management may be the most suitable course of action but follow-up AF and fetal growth assessments are warranted (ACOG, 1999).

Modified Biophysical Profile

Interpretation and Management

The modified biophysical profile (mBPP) uses two biophysical parameters, the NST to reflect current fetal oxygenation and the AFI that reflects chronic oxygenation (Devoe, 2008; Tucker et al., 2009). A normal mBPP consists of a reactive NST and an AFI of greater than 5 cm (Tucker et al., 2009), and the woman may resume routine prenatal care regimen as directed by her risk status. An abnormal test result is obtained when either or both of these components are absent and additional testing is necessary. Further assessment usually consists of the complete BPP or the CST. Management is directed by the results of these additional tests.

Biophysical Profile

The original research for the BPP in 1980, published by Manning and coworkers, endorsed the combined use of multiple biophysical components measured by ultrasound as a more accurate assessment of fetal well-being than the NST alone (Cunningham, Leveno, Bloom, Hauth, Rouse, 2010). The elements of the BPP consist of an NST, fetal movement, fetal tone, and fetal breathing as indicators of acute central nervous system functioning. An ultrasound assessment of AFV indicates long-term placental functioning (Tucker et al., 2009).

Four ultrasound components of the BPP are assessed over a 30-minute time frame with the NST obtained using a fetal monitor. Each of the tests is assigned a score of 0 or 2 according to specific criteria. Two points are assigned for a reactive NST, three distinct fetal movements, 30 continuous seconds of fetal breathing, and an AFV greater than 2 cm in a single vertical pocket. In addition, the presence of at least one episode of flexion and extension of an extremity or opening and closing of a hand provides two points for tone. The absence of any of these five components provides a score of 0 for that assessed parameter. The presence of all five components yields a score of 10/10.

Interpretation and Management

A BPP result of 8 or 10 out of 10 is considered a normal test, and the woman will continue a routine testing schedule if the fetus is felt to be at risk. A score of 6 is equivocal and warrants repeat testing within 6 to 24 hours. The BPP is abnormal if the score is four or less and necessitates evaluation for delivery. Management may be gestational age dependent with later gestations considered for delivery and very early gestations managed with daily, ongoing fetal assessment. The presence of oligohydramnios necessitates additional evaluation (ACOG, 1999; Signore et al., 2009).

Contraction Stress Test

The CST, or oxytocin challenge test (OCT), was originally based on observations of the FHR during labor (Cunningham et al., 2010) when examiners observed periods of heart rate decelerations occurring with contractions as a result of impaired oxygenation. When uteroplacental pathology existed during some at-risk pregnancies, the fetus would exhibit recurrent late decelerations.

The external tocodynamometer and the ultrasound transducer are secured to the woman's abdomen to record uterine contractions and FHR, respectively. Contractions may be spontaneously occurring or they may be induced with oxytocin or with nipple stimulation. When Pitocin or nipple stimulation is used, EFM monitoring is continuous until three contractions in 10 minutes are achieved and the test is completed. Clinicians observe FHR response to uterine contractions.

Interpretation and Management

A negative test occurs with the absence of late decelerations. A positive test exhibits the presence of persistent late decelerations occurring with more than 50% of the contractions. Depending on gestational age, the woman may be evaluated for delivery. Equivocal tests are repeated within 24 hours (Signore et al., 2009).

Doppler Velocimetry

Research is expanding in the field of Doppler assessment and is used as an adjunct to fetal evaluation (Freeman et al., 2003). Doppler measurement of blood flow in the maternal and fetal vessels provides information about the fetal response to diminished uteroplacental blood flow (Signore et al., 2009; Tucker et al., 2009). Abnormal blood flow is characterized by absent or reversed end-diastolic flow, and this abnormal flow has been associated with fetal growth restriction, acidosis, and perinatal morbidity (Tucker et al., 2009). Further assessment and timing of delivery are suggested with abnormal testing results. At present, umbilical artery Doppler velocimetry is recommended in pregnancies complicated by fetal growth restriction (ACOG, 1999), whereas middle cerebral artery (MCA) testing is used for detection and management of fetal anemia (Cunningham et al., 2010).

Overview

A challenge faced by clinicians in OB triage settings is to understand and fulfill the legal requirements for care of the pregnant woman. The Emergency Medical Treatment and Active Labor Act (EMTALA) was enacted so that patients with medical emergencies, including labor, are not denied treatment and are not inappropriately transferred (Angelini & Mahlmeister, 2005). EMTALA requires that OB triage clinicians perform a medical screening exam in a timely fashion to determine if a medical condition exists, provide necessary stabilizing treatments, and, if warranted, provide proper transfer to another hospital (Angelini & Mahlmeister, 2005).

The minimal initial assessment includes maternal vital signs, FHR tracing, and the presence or absence of contractions. The OB triage clinician additionally assesses for the presence or suspicion of vaginal bleeding, acute abdominal pain, fever ≥ 100.4°F, preterm labor, preterm rupture of membranes, hypertension, or abnormal EFM pattern (Simpson, 2009). Concise and complete documentation of screening examinations, stabilizing treatments, and consultation with the referring hospital is necessary to reduce liability and claims of an EMTALA violation (Angelini & Mahlmeister, 2005).

Care of the pregnant woman presenting to OB triage settings must adhere to national, evidence-based standards that are typically derived from recommendations from the American College of Obstetricians and Gynecologists (ACOG) and the American Academy of Pediatrics (AAP; Angelini, 2006). The topics mentioned below have been identified as demonstrating increased liability in the OB triage environment (Angelini, 2006). These include decreased fetal movement (DFM), minor trauma, and liability of assessing fetal status in labor or upon discharge.

Decreased Fetal Movement

Most women perceive fetal movements between 16 and 20 weeks with a woman's perception of fetal movement frequency increasing as gestational age approaches term. Movements decrease in response to fetal hypoxemia (Signore et al., 2009) and have been thought to be associated with impending fetal death (Freeman et al., 2003). Many clinicians have encouraged fetal movement counting but results of clinical trials for routine fetal movement counting are mixed (Signore et al., 2009). One randomized trial in Denmark noted that fetal movement counting had a 73% reduction in stillbirths (relative risk [RR] = 0.27, 95% CI: 0.08–0.93; Signore, et al., 2009). However, a large international study found no difference in avoidable fetal deaths when women were instructed to count movements routinely versus women who were not given specific instructions for counting (Signore et al., 2009).

The diagnosis of DFM is based on the woman's subjective perception of a decline in fetal activity. When a pregnant woman ≥ 24 weeks' gestation presents to OB triage with DFM, an assessment of the woman's prenatal health and risk status along with fetal assessment and risk status is initiated as soon as possible. This woman is prioritized ahead of those with nonemergent problems and not kept waiting (Angelini & Mahlmeister, 2005). The clinical assessment of the woman with DFM includes evaluation of maternal or fetal risk factors with a NST, an ultrasound assessment of AF, and other biophysical parameters if warranted, as well as a review of fetal growth during the pregnancy (Preston et al., 2010). No consensus exists for the optimal management of DFM. However, the NST combined with ultrasound evaluation of AF are the most useful tests for fetal surveillance in DFM (FrØen et al., 2008).

Clinical Management

A nonreactive NST or decreased AF requires additional evaluation of fetal well-being such as with BPP, CST, or Doppler indices if growth restriction is revealed. An isolated episode of DFM requires no additional follow-up.

No trials have defined an agreed-upon method for fetal movement counting or at what threshold decreased movements signifies increased risk. The current definition of DFM recommended by the AAP and the ACOG has the woman count 10 movements. If it takes longer than 2 hours for those movements to occur, the woman is instructed to call the provider or present to the OB triage unit as soon as possible for additional follow-up (AAP & ACOG, 2007). A recent Cochrane review of fetal movement counting for assessing well-being concluded that there is insufficient evidence to recommend routine counting to prevent stillbirth (Signore et al., 2009).

Minor Trauma in Pregnancy

Trauma affects up to 6% to 7% of all pregnancies with the majority accidental and noncatastrophic. Motor vehicle accidents, falls, and assaults are the most common causes. Most trauma is blunt trauma and often without direct fetal injury. However, injury may be noted in minor trauma and complications include not only direct maternal consequences but also pregnancy-related conditions such as placental abruption, preterm labor, fetal-maternal hemorrhage, and fetal demise (Chames & Pearlman, 2008).

Clinical Management

Timely and systematic care must be provided to the minor trauma victim who presents to OB triage. A complete physical examination and trauma clearance of the pregnant woman is necessary, evaluating for maternal injury along with contractions, vaginal bleeding, and fetal movement. Laboratory testing may be obtained for complete blood count, blood type, and antibody screen. The Kleihauer-Betke test may be ordered in the Rh-negative woman for appropriate dosing of Rh immune globulin. Once the woman's condition is considered to be stable, continuous fetal monitoring is recommended if the pregnancy is ≥ 24 weeks. Four hours of continuous EFM is a widely accepted minimum duration of monitoring. Lateral displacement of the uterus is recommended to avoid compression of the vena cava by the gravid uterus. Women with ≤ 6 contractions per hour during this 4-hour period and no evidence of uterine tenderness, bleeding, significant maternal injury, or nonreassuring fetal tracing (i.e., tachycardia, bradycardia, decelerations) may be discharged with instructions and warning signs of abruption. Inpatient observation for 24 hours with continuous EFM has been recommended with ≥ 6 contractions per hour or concern for abruption (Chames & Pearlman, 2008).

Liability in Assessing Fetal Status in Labor or Upon Discharge

Evaluation of the woman presenting to OB triage in labor includes assessment of maternal vital signs, uterine activity, fetal assessment, cervical examination, and membrane status (Simpson, 2009). Labor is established by progressive cervical change with regular contractions. EMTALA specifies that a woman experiencing contractions is in labor unless a qualified clinician certifies that, after a period of observation, the woman is in false labor (Angelini, 2005; Simpson, 2009). Prior to discharging the woman in early or false labor, fetal well-being is established usually by a reactive NST, when gestational age is

TABLE 11.2 Electronic Fetal Monitoring Standardized Definitions

PATTERN	DEFINITION
Baseline	Mean FHR rounded to nearest 5 beats per min (bpm) in 10-min segment excluding accelerations, decelerations, or periods of marked variability Minimum of 2 min of tracing Normal baseline FHR: 110–160 bmp Tachycardia: >160 bmp Bradycardia: <110 bmp
Baseline variability	Fluctuations in baseline FHR in a 10-min window, peak-to-trough amplitude, and frequency quantified in bpm *Absent*—range undetectable *Minimal*—range detectable 5 bpm or less *Moderate (normal)*—range between 6–23 bpm *Marked*—range >25 bmp
Accelerations	*Abrupt* (onset to peak <30 sec) increase in FHR above baseline Peak of acceleration is 15 bpm above baseline and is sustained for ≥15 sec but less than 2 min Before 32 weeks' gestation: 10 bpm amplitude for at least 10 sec but less than 2-min duration Prolonged acceleration: >2 min but <10 min If ≥10 minutes is a baseline change
Early deceleration	*Gradual* (onset to nadir >30 sec) decrease and return of FHR associated with a contraction Nadir of deceleration occurs with peak of contraction and returns to baseline with end of contraction
Late deceleration	*Gradual* (onset to nadir >30 sec) decrease in FHR below baseline occurring with a contraction "Delayed" timing: nadir of deceleration occurs *after* the peak of the contraction and ends after contraction is finished "Repetitive": occurs with >50% of uterine contractions
Variable deceleration	*Abrupt* (onset to nadir <30 sec) decrease in FHR ≥15 bpm drop below the baseline lasting ≥15 sec, but less than 2 min
Prolonged deceleration	FHR decrease ≥15 bpm lasting ≥2 min but <10 min If ≥10 min, it is a baseline change
Sinusoidal pattern	Smooth, sine-like undulating pattern of FHR baseline with a cycle frequency of 3–5/min lasting for ≥20 min
Uterine contractions frequency	The number of contractions in a 10-min window averaged over 30 min ≤5 is "normal" >5 is "tachysystole" Management guided by presence or absence of deceleration

Source: Adapted from ACOG (2009, 2010) and Miller (2010).

appropriate (Simpson, 2009). Fetal assessment in the laboring woman uses nomenclature and interpretation as defined and revised by the National Institute of Child Health and Human Development (NICHD) consensus in 2008 (ACOG, 2009; Miller, 2010). Refer to Table 11.2 for EFM definitions (ACOG, 2010).

If the FHR tracing is considered to be nonreassuring, then additional evaluation methods such as an AFI, BPP, or CST are needed (Angelini & Mahlmeister, 2005). When fetal bradycardia, tachycardia, or repetitive decelerations occur in OB triage settings, intrauterine resuscitative measures including intravenous fluid administration, maternal oxygen therapy, and repositioning are employed to promote fetal well-being (Garite & Simpson, 2011). Recommended interpretation and management of FHR tracings are further delineated into three categories as noted in Exhibit 11.2.

The purpose of the categories is to assist clinicians in identifying EFM tracings that are normal versus those that require additional intrauterine resuscitation or delivery. In addition, the categories are integral to determining necessity of timing of transport to a labor and delivery unit/facility and in alerting an operating room team. For example, Category 1 FHR tracings are considered normal and no specific action is required. Category 2 tracings are

EXHIBIT 11.2

Three-Tiered FHR Classification System

Category I. Includes all of the following:

Baseline: 110–160 bpm
Moderate FHR variability
No late or variable decelerations
Early decelerations may be present or absent
Accelerations may be present or absent

Category II. All FHR tracings not specifically categorized as Category I or III:

Baseline rate: bradycardia without absent variability; tachycardia
Baseline variability: minimal or marked variability; absent variability without decelerations
Absence of accelerations with scalp stimulation
Recurrent variable decelerations with minimal or moderate variability
Prolonged deceleration
Recurrent late decelerations with moderate variability
Variable decelerations with "slow return to baseline" "overshoots" or "shoulders"

Category III. Includes either:

Absent baseline variability with the presence of any of the following:
Recurrent late or variable decelerations
Bradycardia
Or sinusoidal pattern

Source: Adapted from ACOG (2009, 2010) and Miller (2010).

considered indeterminate. This category requires evaluation and surveillance and possibly other tests to ensure fetal well-being. Category 3 tracings are considered abnormal and require prompt evaluation. An abnormal FHR tracing may require intrauterine resuscitation prior to transporting the pregnant woman. (ACOG, 2009, 2010; Miller, 2010).

Many different fetal testing modalities are used prior to discharging the pregnant woman from OB triage. In all situations prior to discharge, clinicians must adequately assess the EFM tracing to obtain evidence of maternal and fetal well-being and have complete documentation that supports management of any non-Category 1 fetal tracing. Any pregnant woman discharged from an OB triage unit or emergency setting must have evidence of fetal well-being. Failure to adequately assess the FHR tracing or failure to respond to a non-Category 1 tracing can affect fetal and maternal outcomes.

REFERENCES

ACOG Practice Bulletin No. 9. (1999; Reaffirmed 2009). Antepartum fetal surveillance. American College of OB/GYN. *Obstetrics and Gynecology, 94*(4), 927–937.

ACOG Practice Bulletin No. 106. (2009). Intrapartum fetal heart rate monitoring: Nomenclature, interpretation, and general management principles. *Obstetrics and Gynecology, 114* (1), 192–202.

ACOG Practice Bulletin No. 116. (2010). Management of intrapartum fetal heart rate tracings. American College of OB/GYN. *Obstetrics and Gynecology, 116*(5), 1232–1240.

American Academy of Pediatrics (AAP) & The American College of Obstetricians and Gynecologists (ACOG). (2007). *Guidelines for perinatal care* (6th ed., pp. 111–117). Washington, DC: AAP and ACOG.

Angelini, D. J. (2006). Obstetric triage: State of the practice. *Journal of Perinatal and Neonatal Nursing, 20*(1), 74–75.

Angelini, D. J., & Mahlmeister, L. R. (2005). Liability in triage: Management of EMTALA regulations and common obstetric risks. *Journal of Midwifery and Women's Health, 50*, 472–478.

Chames, M. C., & Pearlman, M. D. (2008). Trauma during pregnancy: Outcomes and clinical management. *Clinical Obstetrics and Gynecology, 51*(2), 398–408.

Cunningham, F. G., Leveno, K. J., Bloom, S. L., Hauth, J. C., Rouse, D. J. (2010). Antepartum assessment. In F. G. Cunningham, K. J. Leveno, S. L. Bloom, J. C. Hauth, D. J. Rouse (Eds.), *Williams obstetrics* (23rd ed.; pp. 334–348). Columbus, OH: The McGraw-Hill Companies, Inc.

Devoe, L. D. (2008). Antenatal fetal assessment: Contraction stress test, nonstress test, vibroacoustic stimulation, amniotic fluid volume, biophysical profile, and modified biophysical profile—An overview. *Seminars in Perinatology, 32*, 247–252.

Freeman, R. K., Garite, T. J., & Nageotte, M. P. (2003). Antepartum fetal monitoring. In R. K. Freeman, T. J. Garite, & M. P. Nageotte (Eds.), *Fetal heart rate monitoring*. (3rd ed., pp. 181–202). Philadelphia, PA: Lippincott Williams & Wilkins.

FrØen, J. F., Tveit, J. V., Saastad, E., Børdahl, P. E., Stray-Pedersen, B., Heazell, A. E., Flenady, V., & Fretts, R. C. (2008). Management of decreased fetal movements. *Seminars in Perinatology, 32*(4), 307–311.

Garite, T. J., & Simpson, K. R. (2011). Intrauterine resuscitation during labor. *Clinical Obstetrics and Gynecology, 54*(1), 28–39.

Miller, D. A. (2010). Intrapartum fetal monitoring: Maximizing benefits and minimizing risks. *Contemporary OB/GYN, 55*(2), 26–36.

Nabhan, A. F., & Abdelmoula, Y. A. (2008). Amniotic fluid index versus single deepest vertical pocket as a screening test for preventing adverse pregnancy outcome. *Cochrane Database of Systematic Reviews*, (3), CD006593.

Preston, S., Mahomed, K., Chadha, Y., Flenady, V., Gardener, G., MacPhail, J.... Frøen, F. (2010). The Australia and New Zealand Stillbirth Alliance (ANZSA). *Clinical practice guideline for the management of women who report decreased fetal movements*. Retrieved from http://www.stillbirthalliance.org.au/guideline4.htm

Signore, C., Freeman, R. K., & Spong, C. Y. (2009). Antenatal testing—A reevaluation. *Obstetrics and Gynecology, 113*(3), 687–701.

Simpson, K. R. (2009). Obstetrical triage: Stable for discharge. *MCN American Journal of Maternal and Child Nursing, 34*(4), 268.

Tan, K. H., & Smyth, R. (2001). Fetal vibroacoustic stimulation for facilitation of tests of fetal wellbeing. *Cochrane Database of Systematic Reviews*, (1), CD002963. Published Online 20 January 20, 2010.

Tucker, S. M., Miller, L. A., & Miller, D. A. (2009). *Mosby's pocket guide to fetal monitoring a multidisciplinary approach* (6th ed.). St. Louis, MO: Mosby.

Limited or No Prenatal Care at Term

12

Linda Steinhardt

The essential elements of care for the pregnant woman at term who presents to the obstetric triage unit or emergency department with late or no prenatal care (PNC) will be reviewed. The goals of such a visit include establishing maternal and fetal well-being; determining the gestational age of the pregnancy, number of fetuses, fetal presentation, labor status; and addressing immediate needs. If a woman is not admitted to the hospital, enrollment into PNC will need to be expedited. The U.S. Department of Health and Human Services (DHHS) defines late or no PNC as: births that occur to mothers who reported receiving PNC only in the third trimester of their pregnancy, or reported receiving no PNC on the child's birth certificate (DHHS, 2010). This population includes a wide range of women, who for a variety of reasons experience barriers to obtaining PNC.

INCIDENCE

Statistics from 2009 represent the most recent published data regarding this population in the United States. In that year, there were 4,130,665 (Centers for Disease Control and Prevention [CDC], 2012) live births. Four to seven percent of all reported births were to women with late or no PNC (DHHS, 2010). Hispanic women of childbearing age were more than twice as likely as non-Hispanic White women to be uninsured. Younger women were more likely to be uninsured than older women, and impoverished women were more likely than nonimpoverished women to be uninsured (March of Dimes, 2010; DHHS, 2010). These represent a large number of pregnant women who may present to the emergency department for their first and/or only PNC. Infants born to mothers who receive no PNC are three times more likely to be born with low birth weight, five times more likely to die (Vintzileos, Ananth, Smulian, Scorza, & Knuppel, 2002), and have twice the risk of preterm birth (Cunningham et al., 2010) than those whose mothers received PNC.

WHY WOMEN DO NOT SEEK PNC

Pregnant women may not seek PNC for a variety of social, economic, and medical reasons. Analysis of birth certificate data by the CDC found that reasons for inadequate PNC included social and ethnic group, age and method of payment for services (CDC, 2011), undocumented status (Guttmacher Institute, 2000a), or other problems (Guttmacher Institute, 2000b). The most common reasons cited were that a woman did not know she was pregnant, lacked money or insurance, and was unable to secure an appointment for care (Cunningham et al., 2010). Other reasons include social pressures such as denial, undocumented legal status, relocation, drug abuse, fear of interacting with "the system," or difficulty with assessing care.

In 2010, almost 22% of women of childbearing age (ages 15–44) in the United States did not have health insurance (March of Dimes, 2010). Access to care for minors can be a complicating factor (Guttmacher Institute, 2011). National trends toward restrictive access to abortion services can create a situation where a woman does not desire a pregnancy yet cannot terminate it (Guttmacher Institute, 2011). Social services often available in the emergency setting provide vital assistance in identifying/assessing barriers and expediting the process to obtain necessary documentation, insurance, mental health assistance, and referrals to appropriate agencies.

EMERGENCY MEDICAL TREATMENT AND ACTIVE LABOR ACT

The Emergency Medical Treatment and Active Labor Act (EMTALA) mandates a medical screening exam (MSE) for any pregnant woman, regardless of age, who presents to obstetric triage with uterine contractions, or who might be in active labor (EMTALA Guidelines and Review CMS, Center for Medicare and Medicaid Services, 2002). The examination includes, at a minimum, assessment of vital signs, fetal heart tracing (FHT) status, frequency and intensity of uterine contractions, fetal presentation, cervical dilatation, status of membranes, and rapid assessment of the presenting complaint (EMTALA Guidelines and Review CMS, Center for Medicare and Medicaid Services, 2002). The MSE examination must be performed by a "qualified medical examiner" (QME) (EMTALA Guidelines and Review CMS, Center for Medicare and Medicaid Services, 2006). The QME must be someone who is credentialed to perform this function within this setting and who meets hospital credentialing requisites, as well as state rules and regulations for practice (EMTALA Guidelines and Review CMS, Center for Medicare and Medicaid Services, 2006). The QME may include physicians, certified nurse midwives, nurse practitioners, physician assistants, or registered nurses (RN) (EMTALA Guidelines and Review CMS, Center for Medicare and Medicaid Services, 2006). Nurses must be credentialed to perform the MSE within their respective hospitals, and in addition, they must meet individual state rules and regulations for nursing practice (EMTALA Guidelines and Review CMS, Center for Medicare and Medicaid Services, 2006).

CARE OF MINORS

State law is superseded by EMTALA in the case of pregnant minors who are pregnant and contracting (EMTALA Guidelines and Review CMS, Center for Medicare and Medicaid Services, 2002). In the case of a minor who is pregnant but not contracting, regulations differ by state. The great majority of U.S. states and the District of Columbia currently allow a minor to obtain confidential PNC, including regular medical visits and routine services for pregnancy (Guttmacher Institute, 2011). State by state information is available at www.guttmacher.com (Guttmacher Institute, 2011).

EXAMINATION OF THE WOMAN WITH LATE OR NO PNC AT TERM

PRESENTING SYMPTOMATOLOGY

Even when a woman is obviously pregnant, the presenting complaint may not include pregnancy (Givens, Jackson, & Kulick, 1994; Minnerop, Garra, Chohan, Troxell, & Singer, 2011). The history alone has not been shown to be a reliable method of confirming pregnancy (Causey, Seago, Wahl, & Voelker, 1997; Givens et al., 1994; Minnerop et al., 2011). Key questions needed to ascertain a relevant pregnancy history are summarized in Exhibit 12.1. The most frequent presenting symptomology includes the following: gastrointestinal and gynecologic complaints, urinary issues, trauma, psychiatric problems, syncope, chest pain, or respiratory difficulty. Pregnancy or a missed period may not be mentioned (Givens, 1992). In addition to determining the chief complaint, it is crucial to obtain as much information as possible about the pregnancy to date.

PHYSICAL EXAMINATION

Vital signs are performed at the point of care to evaluate maternal status and confirm a viable, intrauterine pregnancy. Establishing gestational age is crucial at this time. Ideally, this is performed and confirmed by ultrasound

EXHIBIT 12.1

Key Questions to Ascertain Relevant Pregnancy History

1. When was your last menstrual period?
2. Do you know when your due date is?
3. Were you using contraception?
4. What number pregnancy is this for you?
5. What happened with your previous pregnancies?
   a. Were they term?
   b. Were they normal vaginal deliveries or cesarean sections?
6. Have you received any prenatal care anywhere? If so, where?
7. Do you have any medical problems
8. Do you take any medications? Any drug usage?
9. Do you have any allergies?
10. Do you feel fetal movement?
11. Do you have vaginal bleeding?
12. Are you having contractions, if so, how frequently?
13. Have you noticed leaking of fluid?
14. Domestic violence screening questions

identifying the following: fetal presenting part, number of fetuses, placental location, amniotic fluid index, and biometry. Biometry is the measurement of fetal head circumference, abdominal circumference, and femur bone length that are used to calculate an estimated fetal weight (EFW). Fetal weight loosely corresponds to gestational age although the accuracy of ultrasound for estimation of EFW decreases as pregnancy advances (Cunningham et al., 2010). Figure 12.1 shows a near-term fetus with cephalic presentation.

The abdominal examination consists of observing for any scars suggestive of previous cesarean section or other uterine surgeries, palpation of fundal height for an estimation of gestational age and evaluation for uterine contractions. Leopold's maneuvers are performed, which are a series of gentle and deliberate palpations of the abdomen that can help to establish fetal position, lie, presentation, and EFW of the fetus (Fraser & Cooper, 2009).

An external fetal monitor is applied to assess the fetal heart rate and frequency/intensity of uterine contractions. Establishing fetal well-being is a vital part of the evaluation. A normal fetal heart rate baseline is between 110 to 160 beats per minute. Fetal Doppler or external fetal monitor is used to ascertain the fetal heart rate and assess for baseline, variability and presence or absence of accelerations and decelerations.

An abdominal ultrasound is performed to eliminate the finding of placenta previa. A vaginal examination performed in the presence of placenta previa can cause a life-threatening hemorrhage to mother and fetus. A speculum examination is performed to observe for the following: lesions, bleeding, fluid pool, vaginal discharge, signs of infection, cervical dilation, presenting part, or prolapsing umbilical cord. A vaginal examination is performed to assess cervical dilation, effacement, station, and fetal presentation.

LABORATORY AND IMAGING STUDIES

Specimens collected during the sterile speculum examination might include amniotic fluid testing for nitrazine and ferning, as well as a wet mount. An Affirm test might also be taken. This is a vaginal culture to assess for varying types of vaginitis. Cultures for gonorrhea and chlamydia as well as a Group

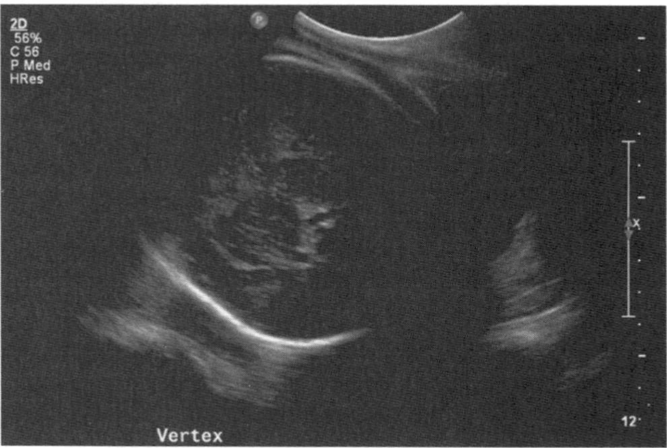

FIGURE 12.1 Ultrasound image of cephalic presentation, at term.

Source: Courtesy of Women & Infants Hospital, Department of Radiology, Providence, RI.

B Strep (GBS) culture need to be obtained. A urine drug screen may be warranted, and the woman's consent is usually necessary before this can be collected and sent for analysis.

GBS is a bacterium associated with neonatal infection and sepsis. It is transmitted from mother to fetus during the birth process. In order to minimize this complication, women with unknown GBS status are treated based on risk factors; however, a confirming culture may prove useful in care of the neonate. Treatment is comprised of appropriate antibiotics administered during labor and until the infant is born. Exhibit 12.2 summarizes risk factors for GBS when a woman's status is unknown.

In addition to the routine prenatal laboratory panel, which is listed in Table 12.1, additional labs may be necessary based on individual cases. For instance, if a woman has recently been out of the country or is a recent immigrant, she might have been exposed to a variety of infectious or communicable diseases. These can include a wide range of possibilities including parasitic infections. Measles, mumps, diphtheria, and other infections, such as malaria, not commonly seen in the United States, may also present and will need to be considered in the emergency setting. In addition, women may present with previously undiagnosed conditions such as tuberculosis and will need appropriate precautions and isolation as indicated. In some areas of the United States, testing for tuberculosis or malaria may be considered in women from areas where these diseases are endemic.

DIFFERENTIAL DIAGNOSIS

The differential diagnoses often include assessment of labor, evaluation of ruptured membranes, and monitoring of other pregnancy or medical conditions. Other conditions such as placental abruption, umbilical cord prolapse, and chorioamnionitis need to be addressed accordingly.

CLINICAL MANAGEMENT AND FOLLOW-UP

Clinical management and follow up care can take several pathways. Some pregnant women presenting to obstetric triage at term with scant or no previous PNC may be in active labor or could be close to delivery when they present for

EXHIBIT 12.2

GBS Risk Factors

If GBS status is unknown, the recommendation is to give intrapartum prophylaxis by risk factors

1. Preterm labor less than 37 weeks
2. Preterm premature rupture of membranes less than 37 weeks
3. Rupture of membranes greater than 18 hours
4. Maternal fever during labor greater than 38°C or 100.4°F
5. Previous infant with GBS sepsis
6. GBS bacteriuria during current pregnancy

Source: ACOG Committee Opinion, No. 279, December (2002).

TABLE 12.1 Prenatal Laboratory Panel for Women with No Prenatal Care at Term

	INFORMATION YIELDED
Blood	
CBC	Anemia, inherited anemias, thrombocytopenia
Blood type and Rh	Need for Rhogam
Blood antibody screen	Hemeglobinopathies
HBsAg	Screen for hepatitis B
HCV	Screen for hepatitis C
RPR or VDRL	Syphilis status
HIV	Special care plan and medications
Rubella titer	Screen need for PP vaccination
Hemoglobin electrophoresis	Sickle cell syndromes or thalassemias
Vaginal	
Chlamydia, gonorrhea cultures	Sexually transmitted infections (STI) testing
Group beta strep culture	Screen for prophylaxis in labor if greater than or equal to 35–37 weeks' gestation
Nitrazine	Vaginal pH and screen for ruptured membranes
Dry slide of vaginal discharge	Ferning for ruptured membranes
Wet prep slide	Screen for infections (*Candida*, bacterial vaginosis, *Trichomonas*)
Urine	
Urinalysis (UA)	Screen for infection, ketones, proteinuria, blood
Urine culture and sensitivity	Rule out infection if you suspect based on symptoms or UA
Urine drug screen (consent needed)	Screen for substance abuse

Source: Adapted from Cunningham et al., (2010).

care. In the case of those women not in active labor but with reassuring fetal status, referral for a prompt formal ultrasound and access to PNC are critical. Some women may simply have been unaware of services available to them. Social services can help to identify needed supports and establish access to services and/or insurance. Still other women require substantial social services to address homelessness, abusive situations, drug use, or mental health problems.

The key factors in the assessment of the woman with little or no PNC at term include identifying labor and addressing immediate needs. Appropriate follow up care include admission to the hospital or referral for appropriate services.

REFERENCES

ACOG Committee Opinion No. 279. (2002). Prevention of early-onset group B streptococcal disease in newborns. *American College of Obstetricians and Gynecologists.*

Causey, A. L., Seago, K., Wahl, N. G., & Voelker, C. L. (1997). Pregnant adolescents in the emergency department: Diagnosed and not diagnosed. *American Journal of Emergency Medicine, 15*(2), 125–129.

Centers for Disease Control and Prevention (CDC). (2011). *National Vital Statistics Report*. Volume 59, No. 7; July 27, 2011. Hayattsville, MD. Retrieved on September 14, 2011, from http://www.cdc.gov/nchs/data/nvsr/nvsr59/nvsr59_07.pdf

Centers for Disease Control and Prevention (CDC). (2012). *National Vital Statistics System*. Retrieved April 25, 2012 from http://www.cdc.gov/nchs/births.htm

Cunningham, F. G., Leveno, K. J., Bloom, S. L., Hauth, J. C., Rouse, D. J., & Spong, C. Y. (2010). *Williams Obstetrics* (23rd ed.). Columbus, OH: The McGraw-Hill Companies, Inc.

EMTALA Guidelines and Review CMS, Center for Medicare and Medicaid Services. (2002). Certification of False Labor. January 16, 2002. Retrieved on October 3, 2011, from http://www.cms.gov/SurveyCertificationGenInfo/downloads/SCLetter02–14.pdf

EMTALA Guidelines and Review CMS, Center for Medicare and Medicaid Services. (2006). Revisions to Special Responsibilities of Hospital under EMTALA (The definition of "Labor" is revised to expand types of health care practitioners who may certify false labor.) September 30, 2006. Retrieved on October 3, 2011, from http://www.cms.gov/SurveyCertificationGenInfo/downloads/SCLetter06–32.pdf

Fraser, D. M. & Cooper, M. A. (2009). *Myles textbook for midwives* (15th ed.). New York, NY: Churchill Livingstone.

Givens, T. G., Jackson, C. L., & Kulick, R. M. (1994). Recognition and management of pregnant adolescents in the pediatric emergency department. *Pediatric Emergency Care, 10*(5), 253–255.

Guttmacher Institute. (2000a). Cutting public funding for undocumented immigrants' prenatal care would raise the cost of neonatal care. Family Planning Perspectives; Vol. 32, No. 3, May/June 2000. Retrieved on August 2, 2011, from www.guttmacher.org

Guttmacher Institute. (2000b). Preexisting factors, but not logistical barriers, inhibit timely use of prenatal care. Family planning perspectives. Vol. 32, No. 5. September/October 2000. Retrieved on August 2, 2011, from www.guttmacher.org

Guttmacher Institute. (2011). State policies in brief. Minors' access to prenatal care. As of August 1, 2011. Retrieved on August 2, 2011, from www.guttma cher.org

March of Dimes (2010). Prenatal care, health insurance overview. US, 2010. Retrieved on December 12, 2011, from www.marchofdimes.com/peristats

Minnerop, M. H., Garra, G., Chohan, J. K., Troxell, R. M., & Singer, A. J. (2011). Patient history and physician suspicion accurately exclude pregnancy. *American Journal of Emergency Medicine, 29*, 212–215.

U.S. Department of Health and Human Services. (2010). Health resources and services administration, maternal and child health bureau. *Child Health USA 2010*, Rockville, MD: Author. Retrieved on December 12, 2011, from www.hrsa.gov

Vintzileos, A. M., Ananth, C. V., Smulian, J. C., Scorza, W. E., & Knuppel, R. A. (2002). The impact of prenatal care on neonatal deaths in the presence and absence of antenatal high-risk conditions. *American Journal of Obstetrics and Gynecology, 186*(5), 1011–1016.

Preterm Labor

13

Linda A. Hunter

Defined as a delivery that occurs prior to 37 weeks' gestation, preterm birth is the leading cause of perinatal mortality and long-term infant morbidity worldwide (Muglia & Katz, 2010). Although the National Center for Health Statistics recently reported a drop from 12.8% in 2006 to 12.3% in 2008, the preterm birth rate in the United States remains one of the highest among industrialized nations (Martin, Osterman, & Sutton, 2010). Unfortunately, research has yet to produce reliable methods of accurately predicting or preventing spontaneous preterm births from occurring. While advances in perinatal and neonatal medicine have improved the survival rates for these infants, the consequences of prematurity still pose lifelong disability and economic burden (Muglia & Katz, 2010). Diagnosis and management of spontaneous preterm labor occurring between 24 and 34 weeks' gestation will be presented.

PRESENTING SYMPTOMATOLOGY

Etiology and Risk Factors

Regular and painful uterine contractions that result in cervical change have been the long-accepted definition of labor. Until recently, this "common pathway of parturition" was thought to occur similarly in both full-term and preterm labor (Romero et al., 2006). Muglia and Katz (2010), for example, surmise that unlike labor at full-term gestations, spontaneous preterm labor is an enigmatic process that occurs when the normal labor pathway is triggered through pathological mechanisms. Intrauterine infection or inflammation, immunologic reactions, hormonal disorders, cervical insufficiency, and uterine ischemia, hemorrhage or overdistension have all been implicated in what Romero and his colleagues (2006) refer to as "the preterm parturition syndrome."

Consequently, a number of contributing factors have been identified that increase a woman's chances of giving birth before 37 weeks. This comprehensive list represents years of epidemiological investigation that has yet to establish a clear chain of causality (Goldenberg, Culhane, Iams, & Romero, 2008). A summary of preterm birth risk factors can be found in Exhibit 13.1.

EXHIBIT 13.1

Risk Factors Associated With Spontaneous Preterm Birth

Major Risk Factors

- Previous preterm birth[a]
- Non-White race[b]
- Infection/inflammation[c]
- Cervical insufficiency[d]
- Multiple gestation
- Bleeding in second trimester
- Mullerian uterine anomalies

Associated Risk Factors

- Low socioeconomic status
- Maternal age less than 18 or greater than 40
- Limited maternal education
- Unmarried
- Poor nutrition/underweight
- Short inter-conception period (<6 months)
- Smoker
- Drug abuse
- Life stressors
- Occupational fatigue
- Family history of preterm birth
- Periodontal disease
- Sexually transmitted infections
- Shifts in vaginal ecosystem

[a]Induced or spontaneous.
[b]Black, African American, Afro Caribbean.
[c]Chorioamnionitis or systemic infections (pneumonia, pyelonephritis, appendicitis).
[d]Shortened cervix less than or equal to 2.5 mm on transvaginal ultrasound in second trimester.

Source: Adapted from Goldenberg, R. L., Culhane, J. F., Iams, J. D., & Romero, R. (2008).

HISTORY AND DATA COLLECTION

Subjective Assessment

Women with threatened preterm labor often present with a myriad of nonspecific symptoms such as constant low backache, pelvic pressure, mild irregular uterine cramping, and increased watery vaginal discharge. Overdiagnosis is common and approximately half of the women admitted to the hospital for treatment of presumed preterm labor will go on to deliver at full-term gestations (McPheeters et al., 2005). Regardless, any persistent abdominal, pelvic, or vaginal symptoms could be signs of impending preterm birth and warrant a full obstetric evaluation.

A higher predictive value for the diagnosis of true preterm labor is seen when women present with more than six contractions per hour with cervical dilation of at least 3 cm and/or effacement of at least 80% (Wax, Cartin, &

Pinette, 2010). The presence of any vaginal bleeding or premature rupture of membranes greatly adds to the likelihood of impending birth. More importantly, in many cases of overt preterm labor, the transition from subclinical parturition has been gradual and often triggered by some underlying pathology (Romero et al., 2006). Consequently, the presence of past or current risk factors for preterm birth is important to ascertain, as well as any recent associated symptoms such as fever, malaise, nausea, vomiting, diarrhea, urine symptoms, drug use, and trauma. Previous cervical assessments (digital or ultrasound) or recent sexual intercourse are also noted.

Gestational Age Assessment

A crucial next step in data collection is a thorough review of the dating criteria used to determine gestational age. Women who conceive with assisted reproductive technologies will have the most accurate pregnancy dating, followed by first trimester ultrasound assessment (Beydoun, Ugwu, & Oehninger, 2011). Menstrual dating is still considered to be reliable, especially when corroborated by an ultrasound performed prior to 20 weeks' gestation (Beydoun, Ugwu, & Oehninger, 2011). On the other hand, women who present with no prenatal care, unsure menstrual history, or third trimester ultrasound dating could have a gestational age discrepancy of up to 2 weeks (ACOG, 2002). No matter how the gestational age was determined, some margin of error exists and clinicians must use the best evidence-based criteria to discern the boundaries for preterm labor treatment.

PHYSICAL EXAMINATION

Pregnant women with a gestational age of greater than 24 weeks who present with any symptoms suggestive of preterm labor require continuous external fetal monitoring for contractions and assessment of fetal well-being. Observation of the woman's demeanor and response to contractions is ongoing while the remainder of the physical examination is completed. Constitutional assessment includes temperature, pulse, respirations, and blood pressure paying careful attention for the presence of any fever, tachycardia, or tachypnea. Auscultation of the heart and lungs is performed, as well as thorough palpation of the abdomen and uterine fundus for any signs of tenderness, rebound, or guarding. Percussion of the flank area for costovertebral angle tenderness is another requisite component of this evaluation to assess for signs of renal etiologies.

Lastly, a complete pelvic exam is performed. It is imperative that a digital examination is *not* performed until the vagina and cervix are first visually inspected using a sterile speculum. This enables the clinician to initially exclude the possibility of preterm premature of membranes (PPROM); inspect the cervix and vagina for any bleeding, discharge, or dilation; and obtain any necessary specimens for further evaluation. Regardless of the appearance of the cervix, once PPROM is ruled out and the possibility of placenta previa also excluded, a digital examination can be safely performed to more thoroughly assess cervical dilation, effacement, consistency, and position.

LABORATORY AND IMAGING STUDIES

Since there are a number of pathological processes that could lead to preterm labor, the physical examination must be accompanied by laboratory studies that will facilitate accurate diagnosis of etiologies such as intrauterine and extrauterine infections. A complete blood count and clean catch urinalysis (with micro) are basic first steps of this evaluation. During the pelvic examination, cultures for gonorrhea, chlamydia, and a vaginal swab for wet mount assessment are collected. Specifically a wet mount is obtained to identify the presence of either bacterial vaginosis or trichomoniasis. These infections have been implicated as risk factors for preterm labor and should be treated when encountered, but absolute causality has not been established (Iams, Romero, & Creasy 2009).

Fetal Fibronectin

Fetal fibronectin (fFN) is an extracellular glycoprotein normally found in the amniochorionic membrane prior to 20 weeks' gestation and again as labor approaches in full-term gestations due to physiologic cervical remodeling and effacement (Iams et al., 2009). For women presenting with threatened preterm labor between 24 and 34 weeks' gestation, the presence or absence of fFN might therefore enhance the diagnostic accuracy in predicting impending delivery. In a large meta-analysis, however, Sanchez-Romero and his colleagues (2009) reported fFN had only a 25.9% positive predictive value but more importantly a negative predictive value of 97.6%. Although fFN assessment is not recommended as a screening test, its negative predictive value may still provide improved triaging in less clear clinical scenarios (Iams et al., 2009; Wax et al., 2010).

Regardless, the fFN sample must be collected prior to any other vaginal or cervical examination and its validity is greatly hampered by the presence of lubricants, bleeding, amniotic fluid, and sexual intercourse within 24 hours (Wax et al., 2010). Proper technique requires that the swab is placed in the posterior vaginal fornix (avoiding the cervical os) during the speculum examination but can also be inserted blindly into the vagina (Wax et al., 2010). In either case, the swab is left in position for a minimum of 10 seconds and placed in the appropriate culture medium according to manufacturer's instructions. The specimen can then be set aside and either sent or discarded as the clinical situation dictates.

Cervical Length Assessment

Initially, real time abdominal ultrasound is performed to confirm the presenting part, identify placental location, or gauge an approximate gestational age, if needed. Ultrasound can also be utilized to provide a transvaginal measurement of cervical length (CL). When compared to digital assessments performed in early labor, transvaginal cervical sonography imparts a more consistent and objective measurement of the cervix (Iams et al., 2009). Moreover, decreasing CL has been associated with increased risks of spontaneous preterm birth (Iams et al., 2009; Owen et al., 2010; Wax et al., 2010). As a screening tool in selected asymptomatic high-risk women (those with a history of prior preterm birth), a second trimester CL measurement of 25 mm is considered the threshold discriminator for predicting future recurrence risk of preterm delivery and may indicate cervical insufficiency (Owen et al., 2010).

For women presenting with preterm contractions at 24 weeks or beyond, a transvaginal CL measurement of 30 mm or greater is considered normal and precludes the likelihood of preterm birth (Iams et al., 2009; Rose et al., 2010;

Wax et al., 2010). In fact, when combined with a negative fFN assay, a normal CL measurement can greatly reduce false positive diagnoses and provide a more cost-effective alternative to hospital admission (Rose et al., 2010). Some authors now advocate standardized algorithms for preterm labor triage that incorporate ultrasound assessment of the CL as a predeterminant for sending the fFN specimen (Rose et al., 2010; Wax et al., 2010). See Figure 13.1 for a transvaginal measurement of shortened CL with funneling.

DIFFERENTIAL DIAGNOSIS

Women experiencing the wide array of symptoms associated with threatened spontaneous preterm labor will generate a broad list of differential diagnoses. This inventory includes fairly straightforward etiologies such as Braxton Hicks contractions and round ligament pain. More serious causes such as pyelonephritis or chorioamnionitis must be conclusively ruled out. Regardless of the presumed cause(s), overt preterm labor calls for expeditious treatment, especially in cases where birth seems imminent. A comprehensive list of differential diagnoses is noted in Exhibit 13.2.

CLINICAL MANAGEMENT

Once the diagnosis of spontaneous preterm labor is made, clinical management is focused on strategies that have been shown to improve neonatal outcomes such as expeditious transfer to a neonatal intensive care facility (Iams et al., 2009). Other key interventions include antenatal corticosteroids, delay of delivery, administration of antibiotics, and fetal neuroprotection.

Antenatal Corticosteroids

Numerous studies coalesced into a recent Cochrane review conclusively uphold that a single course of antenatal corticosteroids administered to women

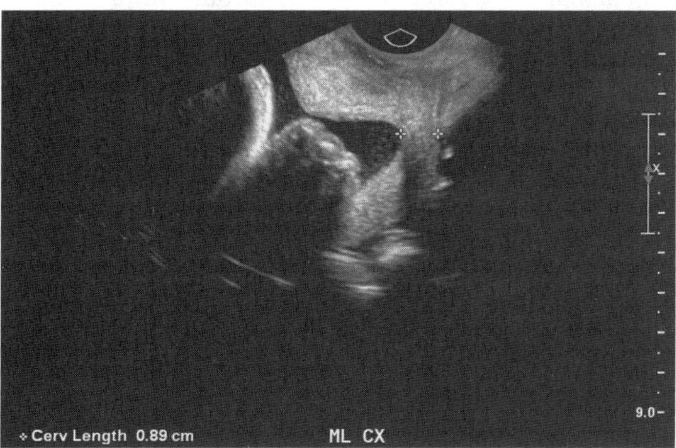

FIGURE 13.1 Sonographic image of shortened cervix with funneling.
Source: Courtesy of Department of Radiology, Women & Infants Hospital, Providence, RI.

EXHIBIT 13.2

Differential Diagnoses for Spontaneous Preterm Labor

Physiologic

- Braxton Hicks contractions
- Uterine irritability
- Dehydration
- Lax vaginal tone
- Round ligament pain
- Sacroiliac joint instability
- Unknown cause

Pathologic

- Intrauterine infections
  - Chorioamnionitis
  - Decidual inflammation
- Extrauterine infections
  - Urinary tract infection
  - Kidney stone
  - Pyelonephritis
  - Appendicitis
- Genital tract infections
  - Gonorrhea/chlamydia
  - Bacterial vaginosis
  - Trichomoniasis
- Placental abruption
- Trauma

This list is not all inclusive and does not imply causality.

Source: Adapted from Goldenberg, R. L., Culhane, J. F., Iams, J. D., Romero, R. (2008).

in preterm labor between 24 and 34 weeks' gestation significantly reduces the incidence of neonatal respiratory distress syndrome, intraventricular hemorrhage, and other morbidities associated with prematurity (Neilson, 2007). This review has also shown antenatal corticosteroids are most effective when given within a week of actual delivery; however, even one dose given within 24 hours of birth will convey some neonatal benefit (Neilson, 2007). Currently, the American College of Obstetricians and Gynecologists (ACOG) advocates the use of either betamethasone or dexamethasone to hasten neonatal lung maturity for women between 24 and 34 weeks' gestation at risk for delivery within 7 days (ACOG, 2011). For women who do not deliver, these guidelines also state that an additional dose of "rescue steroids" can be given if a) more than 2 weeks have passed, b) the gestational age is less than 32 6/7 weeks, and c) the risk of delivery is within 7 days (ACOG, 2011). See Table 13.1 for current corticosteroid options and dosing recommendations.

Intrapartum Antibiotics

Infants born prior to 34 weeks are particularly susceptible to early-onset Group B Streptococcus (GBS) disease with a reported neonatal mortality

TABLE 13.1 Current Guidelines for Antenatal Corticosteroids[a]

BETAMETHASONE	DEXAMETHASONE
12 mg IM 2 doses given 24 hours apart	6 mg IM 4 doses given 12 hours apart

IM = intramuscular.
[a]Recommended for preterm labor 24 to 34 weeks' gestation and birth likely within 1 week

Source: ACOG Committee Opinion No. 475, (2011).

rate of 20% to 30% (Centers for Disease Control and Prevention [CDC], 2010). Since routine GBS screening does not occur until 35 to 37 weeks' gestation, most women presenting in preterm labor prior to this gestational age will have unknown colonization status. Consequently, if preterm delivery seems likely, a culture for GBS colonization should be obtained and prophylactic treatment with either intravenous penicillin or ampicillin initiated (CDC, 2010). Other antibiotics can be used when a penicillin allergy exists; however, if GBS colonization or sensitivities are unknown, vancomycin is the recommended alternative (CDC, 2010).

Delay of Delivery

One of the more controversial aspects of preterm labor management has continued to revolve around the utility, efficacy, safety, and side effects of tocolytic medications. Many different pharmacological agents have been utilized over the past 50 years as researchers have fervently sought to prolong pregnancy in hopes of reducing the preterm birth rates. All of these medications have certainly demonstrated the ability to produce some degree of uterine quiescence which in theory, should have achieved this goal. Unfortunately, many of these drugs cause untoward side effects and increased risks of toxcicity (Haas et al., 2009). More importantly, tocolysis has not been shown to prevent preterm births from occurring or reduce neonatal morbidity or mortality (Conde-Agudelo, Romero, & Kusanovic, 2011; Haas et al., 2009; Iams et al., 2009). At best, tocolytic medications will delay preterm delivery from 2 to 7 days, allowing time for a full course of antenatal corticosteroids and transfer to a tertiary center if needed (Haas et al., 2009).

Until recently, the most commonly used tocolytic medications in the United States included calcium channel blockers (nifedipine), prostaglandin synthetase inhibitors (indomethacin), beta-mimetics (terbutaline), and magnesium sulfate (ACOG, 2003; Haas et al., 2009; Mercer & Merlino, 2009). Due to a higher incidence of maternal side effects, potential toxicity, and lowered comparative efficacy; magnesium sulfate and terbutaline have fallen out of favor and are no longer recommended for acute tocolysis by many authors (Blumenfeld & Lyell, 2009; Haas et al., 2009; Iams et al., 2009).

Despite ample evidence discouraging its continued use, magnesium sulfate is still an a priori tocolytic option in the United States, although some reserve it solely for clinical situations in which other agents are contraindicated (Blumenfeld & Lyell, 2009; Haas et al., 2009; Iams et al., 2009). Most sources now recommend using either nifedipine or indomethacin as first-line therapies although indomethacin is recommended for gestations less than 32 weeks due to potential constriction of the fetal ductus arteriosis (Blemenfeld, 2009; Conde-Agudelo, Romero, & Kusanovic, 2011; Haas et al., 2009). Regardless, there is consensus agreement that tocolysis is discontinued after a full course of corticosteroids have been completely administered (Blumenfeld & Lyell, 2009; Iams et al., 2009; Mercer & Merlino, 2009). See Table 13.2 for tocolytic dosing guidelines.

Fetal Neuroprophylaxis

One of the most promising perinatal discoveries in recent years has been the potential benefit of magnesium sulfate therapy in improving neurologic disability for infants born preterm. This neuroprotective role was first described in the 1990s by researchers who reported a decreased incidence of cerebral palsy in preterm infants exposed to antenatal magnesium sulfate (Nelson & Grether, 1995). Numerous studies including 5 randomized controlled trials have since been aggregated into a Cochrane review indisputably confirming this hypothesis (Doyle et al., 2009). Although there has been criticism raised regarding the appropriate use of meta-analysis, this evidence suggests that administration of magnesium sulfate to women in spontaneous preterm labor prior to 32 weeks'

TABLE 13.2 Guidelines for Tocolytic Medication Use

DRUG NAME	DOSING GUIDELINES	CONTRAINDICATIONS	MATERNAL SIDE EFFECTS	FETAL SIDE EFFECTS
Nifedipine	Loading dose: 30 mg orally[a] Maintenance: 10 to 20 mg orally every 4 to 6 hrs for 48 hrs	Cardiac disease, hypotension less than 90/50 **Do not give with magnesium sulfate**	Flushing, headache, dizziness, nausea, transient hypotension	None identified
Indomethacin[b]	Loading dose: 50 to 100 mg orally Maintenance: 25 to 50 mg orally every 6 hrs for 48 hrs	Significant renal or hepatic impairment	Nausea, heartburn	Constriction of ductus arteriosis, pulmonary hypertension, IVH oligohydramnios
Magnesium Sulfate[c]	Loading dose: 4 to 6 g IV Maintenance: 2 to 3 g/hr IV [d] for 48 hrs (discontinue sooner if possible)	Myasthenia gravis **Do not give with Nifedipine**	Flushing, lethargy, muscle weakness, cardiac or respiratory arrest	Lethargy, hypotonia, respiratory depression

[a] Alternative regime: 10 to 20 mg loading dose repeated every 3 to 6 hrs until contractions slow, then 30 to 60 mg every 8 to 12 hrs for 48 hrs.

[b] Recommended only for gestations less than 32 weeks.

[c] Not recommended for acute tocolysis unless Nifedipine or Indomethacin are contraindicated

[d] Must be administered via infusion pump with frequent monitoring of maternal respiratory rate and patellar reflexes.

mg = milligram, hr = hour, IVH = intraventricular hemorrhage, IV = intravenous.

Source: Adapted from ACOG Practice Bulletin No. 43, (2003).

gestation could potentially prevent 1,000 cases of cerebral palsy per year in the United States alone (Rouse, 2009).

Per the current ACOG Committee Opinion (2010) on fetal neuroprotection, clinicians who elect to use magnesium sulfate for this indication must develop their own specific guidelines in accordance with one of the larger randomized controlled trials. Considered by some to be "the best single piece of scientific evidence available," the Beneficial Effects of Antenatal Magnesium Sulfate (BEAM) trial published in 2008 has subsequently become a favored option (Cahill, Stout, & Caughey, 2010). In this regime, intravenous magnesium sulfate is offered to pregnant women between 24 0/7 to 31 6/7 weeks' gestation at high risk for impending delivery within 24 hours (Rouse et al., 2008). Using a shared decision-making approach, pregnant women and their families are also thoroughly informed of all risks and potential fetal benefits of this therapy (Cahill, Stout, & Caughey, 2010). As modeled in the BEAM trial (Rouse et al., 2008), magnesium sulfate is then administered intravenously first as a loading dose of 6 grams/hour over 20 to 30 minutes. This bolus is followed immediately by a continuous intravenous infusion of 2 grams/hour (via an infusion pump) for 12 hours. The full dosing protocol can be repeated after 6 to 12 hours if delivery again seems imminent and/or discontinued once delivery occurs.

FOLLOW-UP

Inpatient observation for advancing cervical dilation is often continued for at least 24 hours following acute tocolysis or for as long as deemed clinically necessary (Blumenfeld & Lyell, 2009; Iams et al., 2009). Continuing to prolong pregnancy beyond this point has not been shown to reduce preterm birth rates nor have interventions such as home contraction monitoring, sedation, or bedrest (Iams et al., 2009). Prior to discharge from the hospital, any potential infectious causes of preterm labor are treated and strategies to reduce preterm birth risks addressed. For those women who re-present at a later date with threatened preterm labor, the clinical appropriateness of rescue steroids, fetal neuroprophylaxis, and GBS prevention must all be reassessed.

REFERENCES

ACOG Committee Opinion No. 455. (2010). Magnesium sulfate before anticipated preterm birth. American College of Obstetricians and Gynecologists. *Obstetrics and Gynecology, 115,* 669–671.

ACOG Committee Opinion No. 475. (2011) Antenatal corticosteroid therapy for fetal maturation. American College of Obstetricians and Gynecologists. *Obstetrics and Gynecology, 117,* 422–424.

ACOG Practice Bulletin No. 38. (2002). Perinatal care at the threshold of viability. American College of Obstetricians and Gynecologists. *Obstetrics and Gynecology. 100,* 617–624.

ACOG Practice Bulletin No. 43. (2003). Management of preterm labor. American College of Obstetricians and Gynecologists. *Obstetrics and Gynecology, 101,* 1039–1047.

Beydoun, H., Ugwu, B., & Oehninger, S. (2011). Assisted reproduction for the validation of gestational age assessment methods. *Reproductive BioMedicine Online. 22*(4), 321–326.

Blumenfeld, Y. J., & Lyell, D. J. (2009). Prematurity prevention: The role of acute tocolysis. *Current Opinion in Obstetrics and Gynecology, 21,* 136–141.

Cahill, A. G., Stout, M. J., & Caughey, A. B. (2010). Intrapartum magnesium for prevention of cerebral palsy: Continuing controversy? *Current Opinion of Obstetrics and Gynecology, 22*, 122–127.

Centers for Disease Control and Prevention. (2010). Prevention of perinatal group B streptococcal disease, revised guidelines from CDC, 2010. *MMWR, 59, No. RR-10*, Retrieved from www.cdc.gov/mmwr/pdf/rr/rr5910.pdf

Conde-Agudelo, A., Romero, R., & Kusanovic, J. P. (2011). Nifedipine in the management of preterm labor: A systematic review and meta-analysis. *American Journal of Obstetrics and Gynecology, 204*, 134.e1–134.e20.

Doyle, L. W., Crowther, C. A., Middleton, P., Maret, S., & Rouse, D. (2009). Magnesium sulfate for women at risk of preterm birth for neuroprotection of the fetus. *Cochrane Database of Systemic Reviews*, Issue 1. Art.No.: CD004661. doi:10.1002/14651858.CD004661.pub3

Goldenberg, R. L., Culhane, J. F., Iams, J. D., & Romero, R. (2008). Epidemiology and causes of preterm birth. *The Lancet, 371*(9606), 75–84.

Haas, D. M., Imperiale, T. F., Kirkpatrick, P. R., Klein, R. W., Zollinger, T. W., & Golichowski, A. M. (2009). Tocolytic therapy: A meta-analysis and decision analysis. *Obstetrics and Gynecology, 113*(3), 585–594.

Iams, J D., Romero, R., & Creasy, R. K. (2009). Preterm labor and birth. In R. K. Creasy, R. Resnik and J. D. Iams (Eds.), *Creasy and Resnick's maternal-fetal medicine: Principles and practice* (6th ed., pp. 545–582). Philadelphia, PA: Saunders Elsevier.

Martin, J. A., Osterman, M. J. K., & Sutton, P. D. (2010). *NCHS Data Brief No. 39, Are preterm births on the decline in the United States? Recent data from the National Vital Statistics System*. Retrieved from www.cdc.gov/nchs/data/databriefs/db39.pdf

McPheeters, M. L., Miller, W. C., Hartmann, K. E., Savitz, D. A., Kaufman, J. S., Garrett, J. M., & Thorp, J. M. (2005). The epidemiology of threatened preterm labor: A prospective cohort study. *American Journal of Obstetrics and Gynecology, 192*(4),1325–1330.

Mercer, B. M., & Merlino, A. A. (2009). Magnesium sulfate for preterm labor and preterm birth. *Obstetrics and Gynecology, 114*(3), 650–668.

Muglia, L. J., & Katz, M. (2010). The enigma of spontaneous preterm birth. *New England Journal of Medicine, 326*(6), 529–535.

Neilson, J. P. (2007). Cochrane update: Antenatal corticosteroids for accelerating fetal lung maturation for women at risk of preterm birth. *Obstetrics and Gynecology, 109*(1), 189–190.

Nelson, K. B., & Grether, J. K. (1995). Can magnesium sulfate reduce the risk of cerebral palsy in very low birth weight infants? *Pediatrics, 95*, 263–269.

Owen, J., Szychowski, J. M., Hankins, G., Iams, J., Sheffield, J. S., Perez-Delboy, A., et al. (2010). Does midtrimester cervical length ≥25mm predict preterm birth in high risk women? *American Journal of Obstetrics and Gynecology, 203*, 393.e1–e5.

Romero, R., Espiniza, J., Kusanovic, J. P., Gotsch, F., Hassan, S., Erez, O., Chaiworapongsa, T., & Mazor, M. (2006). The preterm parturition syndrome. *BJOG. An International Journal of Obstetrics and Gynecology, 113*(Suppl. 3), 17–42.

Rose, C. H., McWeeney, D. T., Brost, B. C., Davies, N. P., & Watson, W. J. (2010). Cost-effective standardization of preterm labor evaluation. *American Journal of Obstetrics and Gynecology, 203*(3), e1–e5.

Rouse, D. J. (2009). Magnesium sulfate for the prevention of cerebral palsy. *American Journal of Obstetrics and Gynecology, 200*(6), 610–612.

Rouse, D. J., Hirtz, D. G., Thom, E., Varner, M. W., Spong, C. Y., Mercer, B. M., et al. (2008). A randomized controlled trial of magnesium sulfate for the prevention of cerebral palsy. *New England Journal of Medicine, 359*(9), 895–905.

Sanchez-Ramos, R., Delke, I., Zamora, J., & Kaunitz, A. M. (2009). Fetal fibronectin as a short-term predictor of preterm birth in symptomatic patients. *Obstetrics and Gynecology, 114*(3), 631–640.

Wax, J. R., Cartin, A., & Pinette, M. G. (2010). Biophysical and biochemical screening for the risk of preterm labor. *Clinics in Laboratory Medicine, 30*(3), 693–707.

Preterm Premature Rupture of Membranes

14

Alex Friedman

Premature rupture of membranes (PROM) is defined as spontaneous rupture of the membranes prior to labor. When PROM occurs at less than 37 weeks' gestational age, it is defined as preterm premature rupture of membranes (PPROM). Suspicion for PPROM is a commonly encountered clinical scenario in obstetric triage. PPROM occurs in 3% of pregnancies and causes one-third of preterm births and is associated with brief latency from rupture of membranes to delivery (Mercer, 2003). Risk factors associated with PPROM include subclinical intrauterine infection, placental abruption, and uterine overdistension (Simhan & Canavan, 2005). However, most women who develop PPROM have no identifiable risk factors (Waters & Mercer 2011). Timely diagnosis and treatment are necessary to optimize care. Even with conservative management, 50% to 60% of pregnant women will deliver within 1 week of rupture (Mercer, 2003). While several interventions have been shown to improve neonatal and maternal outcomes after PPROM, early preterm infants delivered after PPROM commonly face significant complications such as respiratory distress syndrome (RDS), necrotizing enterocolitis (NEC), intraventricular hemorrhage (IVH), and sepsis (Mercer, 2003).

PRESENTING SYMPTOMATOLOGY

The most common presenting symptom for PPROM is a gush of vaginal fluid. However, women may complain of increased discharge, urinary incontinence, perineal moisture, or leakage of small amounts of fluid (Simhan & Canavan, 2005). The differential diagnoses for leakage of fluid or increased perineal dampness include PPROM, urinary incontinence (which increases during pregnancy), increased vaginal discharge (physiologic secondary to pregnancy), and expression of cervical mucus.

HISTORY AND PHYSICAL EXAMINATION

A standard obstetric history in the setting of suspected PPROM includes a past medical, surgical, social, obstetric, gynecologic, and social history. Medications and allergies are included in the history. Careful review of the prenatal chart is important. Clinical risk factors for spontaneous preterm birth such as prior preterm delivery, prior cervical surgery, or shortened cervix on transvaginal ultrasound are included in the history. Frequently, the gestational age is critical in decision making so medical records must be carefully reviewed to determine exact pregnancy dating. The history includes duration and amount of leakage of fluid, and whether fetal movement, contractions, and vaginal bleeding are present. Reports of the color of the fluid and odor need to be noted by the provider.

A physical exam in a pregnant woman with suspicion for PPROM is performed to confirm the diagnosis and assess maternal and fetal status. The physical exam includes all the components of a basic physical exam including vital signs, general appearance, and a cardiac and lung exam. The abdominal exam, noting whether or not fundal tenderness is present, is critical because this finding may represent a diagnosis of chorioamnionitis.

Diagnosis of PPROM is made by sterile speculum exam. On speculum exam, the dilatation and effacement of the cervix are only visually inspected. Prolapsed umbilical cord needs to be ruled out. Fluid seen coming directly from the cervical os confirms the diagnosis. The finding of pooling of vaginal fluid in the posterior fornix increases the likelihood of PPROM having occurred. If present, cervical fluid is analyzed to confirm the diagnosis. However, small amounts of vaginal pooling can occur with urinary incontinence or severe vaginal infections such as herpes simplex virus (HSV). A second clue may be vaginal pH. The vaginal pH is usually acidic with a pH of 4.5 to 6.0, and amniotic fluid is slightly alkaline with a pH of 7.1 to 7.2. Amniotic fluid in the vagina will usually change the color of nitrazine paper from yellow to blue–green as the pH increases beyond 6.4 to 6.8. Blood, semen, bacterial vaginosis, and alkaline urine may all decrease the pH of the vagina and result in a false positive nitrazine test (Simhan & Canavan, 2005).

A final test of vaginal fluid is assessment for "ferning" or "arborization." Amniotic fluid obtained with a sterile swab from the posterior fornix of the vagina and placed on a clean slide and allowed to dry will produce fern-like crystals (secondary to salt content) when viewed with microscope magnification. The slide is allowed to dry for 10 minutes, and the false negative rate increases the less time left to dry. Cervical mucus may also cause ferning, although these crystals tend to be thicker and darker. Because of this risk for false positive results, care should be taken to avoid swabbing cervical mucus (Simhan & Canavan, 2005).

If a pregnant woman provides a clinical history highly suspicious for PPROM, but the diagnosis is not confirmed by initial speculum exam, the woman can be placed in a semi-upright position and reexamined after 1 hour to allow for vaginal pooling. As a last resort, if results are still equivocal, amniocentesis with injection of indigo carmine dye may be performed. A tampon is placed and if any dye leaked from the cervix, a blue staining would be noted on the tampon, confirming the diagnosis of PPROM.

The physical exam includes assessment of fetal well-being with continuous fetal heart rate monitoring. Contractions are assessed by palpation and/or tocometry. Since women with PPROM are at risk for chorioamnionitis, presence or absence of pertinent physical exam findings consistent with infection are noted. Exhibit 14.1 lists the clinical criteria for chorioamniotitis (Gibbs, Blanco, Clair, Castaneda, 1982).

LABORATORY AND IMAGING STUDIES

The AmniSure test for rupture of membranes is another test that may be utilized to confirm rupture of membrane status. The test is an immunoassay for

EXHIBIT 14.1

Clinical Criteria for Chorioamnionitis

Maternal temperature 100°F or higher with no other explanation for fever and any two of the following:

Maternal heart rate over 120 beats per minute
Fetal heart rate over 160 beats per minute
Foul smelling amniotic fluid
Fundal tenderness
Maternal WBC greater than 14K

Source: Adapted from Gibbs et al., (1982).

PAMG-1 (placental alpha microglobulin). There are low levels of PAMG-1 in vaginal secretions and blood, but very high levels in amniotic fluid. AmniSure has been shown to be highly sensitive and specific compared to fern, pool, and nitrazine assessment. An early study demonstrated AmniSure to be 99% sensitive and 100% specific (Cousins, Smok, Lovett, & Poeltler, 2005) in detecting rupture of membranes. Subsequent research has confirmed these results (Birkenmaier, Ries, Kuhle, Burki, Lapaire, Hosli, 2011). Because of the test's cost, Amnisure is primarily used either for women with unclear rupture of membrane status or if providers with appropriate clinical training are unavailable to assess for pooling, ferning, and nitrazine changes.

If a pregnant woman has unknown Group B Streptococcus (GBS) status, vaginal and rectal cultures will be collected during the pelvic exam. If sexually transmitted infections are suspected, appropriate cultures are also collected and sent. A digital cervical exam is contraindicated if the woman is less than 34 weeks' gestation, unless active labor or imminent delivery is suspected. Research demonstrates that latency (time from rupture to delivery) is decreased when serial examinations are performed (Alexander et al., 2000).

If the woman is between 32 and 34 weeks' gestational age and has significant vaginal pooling, amniotic fluid may be obtained for lung maturity testing. Fluid can be collected using a 5 or 10 cc syringe attached to an intravenous catheter (with the needle removed). As much fluid as possible is obtained from the vaginal pool to maximize the probability that the sample is adequate for laboratory analysis for any lung maturity studies.

Ultrasound examination is a critical part of the evaluation for PPROM. Oligohydramnios offers supporting evidence for PPROM having occurred but is not the gold standard for the diagnosis. Normal or increased fluid volume does not preclude the diagnosis. Fetal presentation and placentation are noted additionally. An estimated fetal weight determined by biometry is obtained. In terms of laboratory work, a complete blood count is performed, as well a GBS culture if the woman's status is unknown.

CLINICAL MANAGEMENT

Viability to 34 Weeks' Gestational Age

At most centers, viability is defined as 24 weeks' gestational age. However, many neonates delivered between 23 and 24 weeks are resuscitated, and some fetuses 24 to 26 weeks' gestational age may not be considered viable because of associated conditions (severe intrauterine growth restriction, major congenital anomalies, genetic syndromes, or other conditions predisposing to poor prognoses). Care must be individualized, and determination of viability includes the entire clinical picture, as well as input from neonatologists and the family's goals for care.

The mainstays of management for viable PPROM until 34 weeks include hospital admission, administration of betamethasone, latency antibiotics, and close evaluation of maternal and fetal status. Women who present with PPROM are at risk for chorioamnionitis and abruption, both contraindications to expectant management. The patient is assessed on a daily basis for chorioamnionitis, abruption, preterm labor, and nonreassuring fetal status (either with a nonstress test or biophysical profile).

Evidence supports the administration of betamethasone or dexamethasone in the setting of PPROM from 24 to 34 weeks' gestational age. Steroids reduce the risk of RDS, NEC, and IVH. There appears to be no increased risk of maternal infectious morbidity from steroid administration (Roberts & Dalziel, 2006). Leukocytosis occurs after steroid administration and may not be representative of infection.

Administration of latency antibiotics improves neonatal outcomes. Level 1 evidence demonstrates that antibiotic administration reduces RDS, NEC, neonatal sepsis, bronchopulmonary dysplasia, and pneumonia, while increasing latency (Mercer et al., 1997; Hutzal et al., 2008). Latency antibiotics along with antepartum steroids likely reduce perinatal mortality. A typical antibiotic regimen includes 48 hours of intravenous ampicillin and erythromycin, followed by 5 days of oral ampicillin and erythromycin (Mercer et al., 1997). Ampicillin and amoxicillin cover Group B Streptoccoocus and provide gram negative and some anaerobic coverage. Erythromycin offers coverage of genital mycoplasma along with some coverage of gram positive cocci. Azithromycin, which has a better side effect profile than erythromycin, may be used as an alternate macrolide. Amoxicillin-clavulanic acid should be avoided because of a possible increased risk of NEC. Exhibit 14.2 offers proposed antibiotic regimens, which may vary by medical center.

Many women who present with PPROM at less than 34 weeks may have a prior history of prior preterm birth and may be receiving 17-hydroxyprogesterone (17P). While researchers have hypothesized that 17P may work by an anti-inflammatory mechanism, no evidence exists that receiving 17P in the setting of PPROM increases maternal or neonatal infectious morbidity. No benefit to continuing 17P in the setting of PPROM has been established. Currently there is insufficient evidence to recommend for or against continuing 17P in the setting of PPROM in women less than or equal to 34 weeks' gestational age.

34 to 37 Weeks' Gestational Age

At most clinical centers, the fetal and maternal risks of prolonging pregnancy in the setting of PPROM greater than or equal to 34 weeks outweigh fetal benefits of expectant management and delivery is recommended. However, in remote locations without intensive neonatal care, expectant management may be warranted up until 36 weeks. Alternately, if fetal lung maturity is demonstrated at 32 to 33 weeks, the risks of prolonging the pregnancy may outweigh

EXHIBIT 14.2

Antibiotic Regimens for PPROM

Sample Antibiotic Regimens

Ampicillin 2 g IV every 6 hours for 48 hours followed by amoxicillin 500 mg PO three times daily for 5 days

PLUS EITHER

Erythromycin 250 mg IV every 6 hours for 48 hours followed by erythromycin 333 mg PO every 8 hours for 5 days

OR

Azithromycin 1g PO once

OR

Azithromycin 500 mg IV every 24 hours for 48 hours days followed by azithromycin 250 mg PO daily for 5 days

Sample Antibiotic Regimens for True Penicillin Allergy

Clindamycin 900 mg IV every 8 hours for 48 hours

PLUS

Azithromycin 1 g PO once

OR

Azithromycin 500 mg IV every 24 hours for 48 hours days followed by azithromycin 250 mg PO daily for 5 days

Source: Adapted from Mercer (1997); Personal Communication Brenna Anderson, MD (2011).

the benefits gained from an extra week to 2 weeks of latency and delivery may be indicated prior to 34 weeks.

CONTROVERSIES IN PPROM MANAGEMENT

Cerclage and PPROM

Management of women who present with PPROM with a cerclage is controversial, and data to guide management are limited. One review found that in the setting of PPROM and cerclage, women who did not have cerclage removed were significantly more likely to have at least 48 hours of latency but were at significantly higher risk for maternal chorioamnionitis and neonatal death from sepsis. This led the authors to conclude that for PPROM at less than 23 weeks or greater than or equal to 32 weeks cerclage should be removed immediately. For patients greater than or equal to 23 to less than 32 weeks, the authors recommend cerclage should either be removed immediately or after a 48 hour course of steroids (Giraldo-Isaza and Berghella, 2011). Another review on the same subject found the quality of data to be poor and not useful in guiding management. The review article demonstrated that studies were retrospective, used varying outcome measures, did not perform adjusted analyses, and were mostly performed before the current era of standard PPROM management (steroids and antibiotic administration) (Walsh, Allen, Colford, & Allen, 2010).

Herpes Simplex Virus and PPROM

Management of PPROM in the setting of active HSV infection is controversial. Increased risk of fetal HSV infection with expectant management must be weighed against risks of prematurity from earlier delivery. Because the viral load and risk of neonatal HSV is lower with recurrent infections, expectant management may be warranted in these patients. Data are limited in women with primary HSV outbreaks and PPROM (Ehsanipoor and Major, 2011). There are no clear recommendations for timing of delivery with either recurrent or primary HSV infections.

Magnesium Sulfate for Cerebral Palsy Prevention

The BEAM (beneficial effects of antenatal magnesium sulfate) trial demonstrated that pregnant women at risk for preterm delivery between 24 and 31 weeks because of PPROM or advanced preterm labor who were randomized to magnesium sulfate had a significantly lower risk of a child born with cerebral palsy. However, the primary outcome of this study—stillbirth or infant death by 1 year of age or moderate or severe cerebral palsy—was not different between the two groups (Rouse et al., 2008).

The results of the BEAM trial, as well as findings from previous trials have led some experts to recommend magnesium routinely for cerebral palsy prophylaxis for fetuses at risk for imminent delivery less than or equal to 31 weeks' gestational age (Rouse, 2011). Other authors have expressed concern that findings from the BEAM trial and other studies may be inadequate to routinely recommend magnesium sulfate prophylaxis (Cahill & Caughey, 2009; Sibai, 2011).

Tocolytics in the Setting of PPROM

The use of tocolytics in the setting of PPROM is also controversial. A Cochrane meta-analysis demonstrated an increased risk of chorioamnionitis with tocolysis in the setting of PPROM. Latency was extended in this analysis with tocolysis; however, neonatal outcomes were not improved. These studies were performed prior to universal administration of corticosteroids and antibiotics. The authors concluded that there is insufficient evidence to support tocolytic therapy for women with PPROM (Mackeen, Seibel-Seamon, Grimes-Dennis, Baxter, & Berghella, 2011). In a survey study of maternal-fetal medicine specialists, the majority of respondents reported using tocolytics in PPROM to gain time for antenatal steroid administration (Ramsey et al., 2004). Tocolysis for greater antenatal steroid administration only is not recommended.

REFERENCES

ACOG Practice Bulletin No. 80. (2007). Premature rupture of membranes. Clinical management guidelines for obstetrician-gynecologists. *Obstetrics and Gynecology, 109*(4), 1007–1019.

Alexander, J.M., Mercer, B.M., Miodovnik, M., Thurneau, G. R., Goldenberg, R. L., Das, A. F., Meis, P. J., et al. (2000). The impact of digital cervical examination on expectantly managed preterm rupture of membranes. *American Journal of Obstetrics and Gynecology, 183*(4), 1003–1007.

Birkenmaier, A., Ries, J. J., Kuhle, J., Burki, N., Lapaire, O., & Hosli, I. (2011). Placental alpha-microglobulin-1 to detect uncertain rupture of membranes in a European cohort of pregnancies. *Archives of Gynecology and Obstetrics, 285*(1), 21–25.

Cahill, A. G. & Caughey, A. B. (2009). Magnesium for neuroprophylaxis: Fact or fiction? *American Journal of Obstetrics and Gynecology, 200*(6), 590–594.

Cousins, L. M., Smok, D. P., Lovett, S. M., & Poeltler, D. M. (2005). AmniSure placental alpha microglobulin-1 rapid immunoassay versus standard diagnostic methods for detection of rupture of membranes. *American Journal of Perinatology, 22*(6), 317–320.

Ehsanipoor, R. M., & Major, C. A. (2011). Herpes simplex and HIV infections and preterm PROM. *Clinical Obstetetrics and Gynecology, 54*(2), 330–336.

Gibbs, R. S., Blanco, J. D., St. Clair, P. J., & Castaneda, Y. S. (1982). Quantitative bacteriology of amniotic fluid from women with clinical intraamniotic infection at term. *Journal of Infectious Diseases, 145*(1), 1–8.

Giraldo-Isaza, M. A., & Berghella, V. (2011). Cervical cerclage and preterm PROM. *Clinical Obsterics and Gynecology, 54*(2), 313–320.

Hutzal, C. E., Boyle, E. M., Kenyon, S. L., Nash, J. V., Winsor, S., Taylor, D. J., & Kirpalani, H. (2008). Use of antibiotics for the treatment of preterm parturition and prevention of neonatal morbidity: A meta-analysis. *American Journal of Obstetrics and Gynecology, 199*(6), 620 e621–628.

Mackeen, A. D., Seibel-Seamon, J., Grimes-Dennis, J., Baxter, J. K., & Berghella, V. (2011). Tocolytics for preterm premature rupture of membranes. *Cochrane Database of Systematic Reviews,* (10): CD007062.

Mercer, B. M. (2003). Preterm premature rupture of the membranes. *Obstetrics and Gynecology, 101*(1), 178–193.

Mercer, B. M., Miodovnik, M., Thurnau, G. R., Goldenberg, R. L., Das, A. F., Ramsey, R. D., et al. (1997). Antibiotic therapy for reduction of infant morbidity after preterm premature rupture of the membranes. A randomized controlled trial. National Institute of Child Health and Human Development Maternal-Fetal Medicine Units Network. *JAMA: The Journal of the American Medical Association, 278*(12), 989–995.

Ramsey, P. S., Nuthalapaty, F. S., Lu, G., Ramin, S., Nuthalapaty, E. S., Ramin, K. D., et al. (2004). Contemporary management of preterm premature rupture of membranes (PPROM): A survey of maternal-fetal medicine providers. *American Journal of Obstetrics and Gynecology, 191*(4), 1497–1502.

Roberts, D., & Dalziel, S. (2006). Antenatal corticosteroids for accelerating fetal lung maturation for women at risk of preterm birth. *Cochrane Database of Systematic Reviews,* 3, CD004454.

Rouse, D. J. (2011). Magnesium sulfate for fetal neuroprotection. *American Journal of Obstetrics and Gynecology, 205*(4), 296–297.

Rouse, D. J., Hirtz, D. G., Thom, E., Varner, M. W., Spong, G. Y., Mercer, B. M., Iams, J. D., et al. (2008). A randomized, controlled trial of magnesium sulfate for the prevention of cerebral palsy. *New England Journal of Medicine, 359*(9), 895–905.

Sibai, B. M. (2011). Magnesium sulfate for neuroprotection in patients at risk for early preterm delivery: Not yet. *American Journal of Obstetrics and Gynecology, 205*(4), 296–297.

Simhan, H. N., & Canavan, T. P. (2005). Preterm premature rupture of membranes: Diagnosis, evaluation and management strategies. *BJOG, 112*(Suppl 1), 32–37.

Walsh, J., Allen, V. M., Colford, D., & Allen, A. C. (2010). Preterm prelabour rupture of membranes with cervical cerclage: A review of perinatal outcomes with cerclage retention. *Journal of Obstetric and Gynecology Canada, 32*(5), 448–452.

Waters, T. P. & Mercer, B. (2011). Preterm PROM: Prediction, prevention, principles. *Clinics of Obstetrics and Gynecology, 54*(2), 307–312.

Trauma in Pregnancy

15

Roxanne A. Vrees and Alyson J. McGregor

The focus in the first section of this chapter will be noncatastrophic trauma in viable pregnancies, whereas the latter half discusses pelvic fractures, penetrating trauma, burns, and electrical injuries. A complete review of catastrophic trauma is beyond the scope of this section.

NONCATASTROPHIC TRAUMA

PRESENTING SYMPTOMATOLOGY

Blunt trauma is a common denominator to many injuries during pregnancy. The most common causes include motor vehicle accidents, falls, and direct assaults. The incidence and occurrence for most mechanisms of injury are distributed equally throughout pregnancy. However, falls are far more common during winter and beyond 20 weeks' gestation due to pelvic laxity and imbalance. The gestational age at the time of injury, the type and severity of the injury, and the injury mechanism are all important considerations.

Following trauma in a pregnant woman who is stable, key initial questions to elicit following a motor vehicle accident or fall are listed in Exhibit 15.1. Of note, the responses to these questions are as important as noting whether symptoms were present before or following the injury.

Overall, the management of domestic and sexual violence is similar to that of blunt trauma unless gunshot and/or stab wounds are involved. Sexual assault is often an underreported yet critical component of trauma during pregnancy. Acute traumatic injuries following assault range from minor trauma to more significant injuries, including maternal and fetal death. Pregnant women who are verbally abused are more likely to deliver low-birth weight infants, while those who are physically abused have higher rates of neonatal deaths (Yost, Bloom, McIntire & Leveno, 2005). In addition, the overall risk of injury increases for women who are rape victims by a known assailant, if a weapon is involved, the perpetrator is under the influence of drugs or alcohol, or the assault occurs in the victim's or perpetrator's home (ACOG, 2011).

Maternal death is most often due to either head injury or hemorrhagic shock. Conversely, the most common causes of fetal death are maternal shock

EXHIBIT 15.1

Key Questions to Elicit Following Motor Vehicle Accidents or Falls

Primary

Was there any head or direct abdominal trauma?
Did you have loss of consciousness?
How fast were you traveling?
Were you restrained, driver or passenger?
Any air bag deployment?

Secondary

When is your due date?
Do you have any contractions, vaginal bleeding, or leakage of fluid?
Can you feel the baby move?

and/or death followed by abruptio placentae and direct fetal injury. The risk of fetal, neonatal, and infant death is largely dependent on the gestational age at the time of delivery (El-Kady, Gilbert, Towner, & Smith, 2004). Abruptio placentae complicates up to 40% of pregnancies with major injuries and 3% of minor trauma with direct uterine force (Brown, 2009). The premature separation of the placenta from the uterine wall results in decreased uterine blood flow, which can lead to significant fetal hypoxia and acidemia. In the most severe cases, fetal death can occur.

Uterine rupture, depicted in Figure 15.1, although a rare event, complicates less than 1% of all trauma-related injuries. Although there is a higher incidence of rupture in the presence of pelvic fractures or a prior cesarean section (Aghababian, 2006), uterine rupture can also occur in the absence of obvious risk factors. Of note, findings of both uterine rupture and abruptio placentae are quite similar and often include abdominal pain and tenderness, signs of hypovolemia, and nonreassuring fetal status.

PHYSICAL EXAMINATION

There are a variety of both anatomic and physiologic changes that occur in normal pregnancy as shown in Table 15.1. These changes can both mask and mimic injury in the setting of trauma. A clear understanding of these changes is imperative to both appropriate and optimal management of a pregnant trauma victim.

The physical examination following noncatastrophic trauma includes an assessment of the mother's general appearance; heart, lung, and abdominal examination; assessment of extremities; and a targeted pelvic examination. The pelvic examination is of particular importance because it facilitates differentiation of other potential diagnoses such as preterm labor and placental abruption. Fetal assessment is also a crucial component of the physical examination, as the fetus is an additional patient.

Laboratory and Imaging Studies

Although seemingly obvious, it is imperative to confirm pregnancy status at the forefront of any trauma evaluation. In addition to pregnancy confirmation,

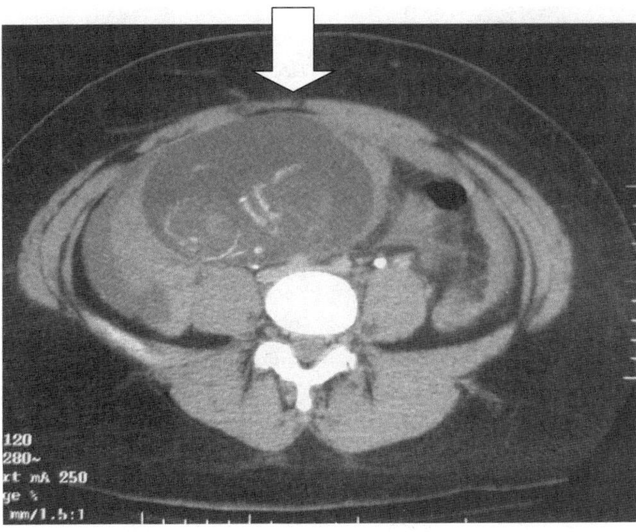

FIGURE 15.1 Uterine rupture post trauma.

Source: Courtesy of the Department of Radiology, Women & Infants Hospital, Providence, RI.

a type and screen is obtained to determine maternal blood type. In an asymptomatic mother with reassuring fetal status, no further laboratory evaluation is necessary.

Fetomaternal hemorrhage (FMH) is the transplacental hemorrhage of fetal blood into the maternal circulation and is a potential complication following trauma. Although the true incidence is largely unknown, it is believed to increase in 8% to 30% of pregnant women involved in trauma (Pearlman, Tintinallli, & Lorenz, 1990). There is no real correlation between the severity of trauma, gestational age and frequency, and/or volume of FMH. Complications include maternal isoimmunization, fetal and neonatal anemia, fetal cardiac arrhythmias, or even fetal death.

FMH is detected by the Kleihauer-Betke (KB) acid elution technique performed on maternal blood. Unfortunately, the sensitivity of the KB test is relatively low, and there is no direct correlation between KB testing and prediction of adverse hemorrhagic sequelae. Thus, routine KB testing is not a standard component in the evaluation of all trauma victims. However, all Rh-negative mothers who present with a history of abdominal trauma should receive one 300 mcg prophylactic dose of Rh immune globulin within 72 hours of the traumatic event. For women in the first trimester, a 50-mcg dose is sufficient when available. Routine KB testing can be advantageous in all pregnant trauma victims regardless of Rh status given its utility in predicting preterm labor (Muench et al., 2004). Presently, the main clinical utility of the KB test in the Rh-negative population is to determine the appropriate dose of Rh immune globulin needed to prevent Rh sensitization.

In conjunction with fetal monitoring, obstetric ultrasound is a critical tool in both maternal and fetal evaluation following trauma. Ultrasound provides invaluable information such as gestational age, placental location, amniotic fluid indices, and fetal well-being via biophysical testing. In addition, ultrasound can provide useful information regarding potential fetal

TABLE 15.1 Changes in Normal Pregnancy That May Affect Trauma Management

AFFECTED VALUE OR SYSTEM	CHANGE DURING NORMAL PREGNANCY
Systolic blood pressure	Decreased by an average of 5–15 mmHg
Diastolic blood pressure	Decreased by 5–15 mmHg
Electrocardiogram	Flat or inverted T waves in leads III, V1, and V2; Q waves in leads III and AVF
Blood volume	Increased by 3%–50%
White blood cell count	May be increased; range: 5,000–25,000/mm^3
Fibrinogen	Increased; range: 264–615/dL
D-dimer	Frequently positive
Respiratory rate	Increased by 40%–50%
Oxygen consumption	Increased by 15%–20% at rest
Partial pressure of oxygen	Increased; range 100–108 mmHg
Partial pressure of carbon dioxide	Decreased; range 27–32 mmHg
Bicarbonate	Decreased; range: 19–25 mEq/L
Base excess	Present; range: 3–4 mEq/L
Blood urea nitrogen	Decreased; range: 3–3.5 mg/dL
Serum creatinine	Decreased; range: 0.6–0.7 mg/dL
Alkaline phosphatase	Increased because of placental production; range: 60–140 IU/L
Kidneys	Mild hydronephrosis
Gastrointestinal tract	Decreased gastric emptying, decreased motility, and increased risk of aspiration
Musculoskeletal system	Widened symphysis pubis and sacroiliac joints, which may lead to misleading of radiologic studies
Diaphragm	Higher position in pregnancy; consequently, chest tubes would need to be placed in one or two interspaces higher
Peritoneum	Small amounts of intraperitoneal fluid are normally present

Source: Adapted from Grossman (2004).

injuries and demise. However, ultrasound has poor sensitivity for detecting placental abruption.

Clinical Management and Follow-Up

Both the impact and management of blunt abdominal trauma on a developing fetus are largely dependent on gestational age at the time of injury. For example, in pregnancies during the first trimester, direct fetal or placental injury is unlikely given the protection from the maternal bony pelvis (ACOG, 1998). Furthermore, in any nonviable fetus, prolonged fetal monitoring is not indicated as the only appropriate fetal intervention is expectant management. In addition to gestational age, critical factors to consider include the degree of maternal injury and mechanism of injury. Table 15.2 provides guidelines for clinical management of noncatastrophic blunt abdominal trauma.

Although the ideal duration of fetal monitoring remains unclear, prolonged and continuous fetal monitoring in conjunction with tocodynamometry is the current standard for fetal assessment following maternal trauma in a viable pregnancy. Recommendations for the duration of fetal monitoring range from 4 to 48 hours (Mirza, Devine, & Gaddipati, 2010).

Placental abruption and preterm labor are the most common and feared complications following maternal blunt abdominal trauma. It can occur up to 24 hours following trauma but has not been seen in women with contractions occurring at a frequency of less than 1 per 10-minute interval, over a 4-hour period (Dahmus & Sibai 1993). The most commonly used fetal monitoring algorithm is continuous monitoring for a total of 4 hours following any maternal trauma even in the absence of obvious signs or symptoms of abdominal injury. At the completion of 4 hours, fetal monitoring can be discontinued if uterine contractions are less frequent than 1 in 10 minutes, the fetal heart tracing is overall reassuring and there is no maternal abdominal pain or vaginal bleeding. If contractions persist at a frequency of greater than or equal to 6 per hour during any portion of the 4 hours, then admission to an obstetric facility for a full 24 hours of monitoring is indicated. Additional indications for prolonged fetal monitoring include fetal tachycardia, significant uterine tenderness, nonreassuring fetal heart tracing, spontaneous rupture of membranes following trauma, significant maternal injuries, or a high risk mechanism of injury (e.g., high-speed collision with air bag deployment). Interestingly, despite the current standard for extensive fetal evaluation following minor trauma in pregnancy, none of the commonly used objective measures adequately predict adverse outcomes (Cahill et al., 2008). This suggests that perhaps shorter durations for fetal monitoring and fewer laboratory studies are indicated.

In viable pregnancies, it is recommended that fetal monitoring be initiated as soon as possible following maternal trauma but not until the mother's condition has been stabilized. Overall, fetal monitoring is most useful for determining reassuring fetal status and for guiding appropriate discharge home. Urgent cesarean delivery is an appropriate intervention in pregnancies at or beyond 24 weeks' gestation, if signs of nonreassuring fetal status such as bradycardia or repetitive decelerations persist in an otherwise adequately resuscitated mother.

CATASTROPHIC TRAUMA

PRESENTING SYMPTOMATOLOGY

Pregnant women who are involved in catastrophic trauma may have no initial symptoms or altered vital signs due to the previously mentioned physiologic changes in pregnancy. However, an investigation for possible intraperitoneal bleeding is indicated in the setting of certain factors. These include altered level of consciousness, unexplained shock, significant thoracic injuries, and multiple major orthopedic injuries.

TABLE 15.2 Guidelines for Clinical Management of Noncatastrophic Blunt Abdominal Trauma

1. Assess maternal vital signs and triage according to emergency severity index
2. Document fetal heart tones
3. Basic blood work—CBC, type and screen, hold tube, KB at provider discretion if Rh negative
4. Obtain targeted history (Include date and time of event, last menstrual period, due date)
5. External fetal monitoring for minimum of 4 hours
   a. Gestational age greater than 24 weeks by estimated date of delivery or fetal biometry
      - 4 hours of continuous fetal monitoring with tocodynamometry
      - Recommend prolonged evaluation if greater than six contractions in any given hour
      - Recommend further evaluation for nonreactive fetal heart tracing (biophysical profile or prolonged continuous monitoring at provider discretion)
   b. Gestational age less than 24 weeks by estimated date of delivery or fetal biometry
      - Fetal heart rate documented by Doppler or real time ultrasound
      - Tocometer if high concern for abruption by history or physical examination
      - Fetal monitoring for periviable gestational age 23–23.6 weeks at institution/provider discretion
6. Administer Rh immune globulin if Rh negative
7. Discharge to home if stable maternal and fetal status
8. Admission for 24 hours of monitoring if greater than six contractions/hour or nonreassuring fetal heart tracing as above
9. Admission labs: coagulation studies, type, and cross if active bleeding and maintain large bore IV access
10. Consider steroids for fetal lung maturity if delivery possible and gestational age less than 34 weeks

Source: Adapted from ACOG (1998); Brown (2009); Dahmus & Sibai (1993); and Muench et al. (2004).

Fetal vasculature is particularly sensitive to catecholamines and the survival of the fetus following trauma is largely dependent on maintenance of adequate uterine perfusion and delivery of oxygen. Once hypovolemic shock ensues, the fetus has likely suffered significant compromise and the possibility of preserving the pregnancy at that point is merely 20% (Desjardins, 2003).

PHYSICAL EXAMINATION

Primary Survey

The primary survey focuses on establishing maternal cardiopulmonary stability: airway, breathing, and circulation. Maternal blood pressure and heart rate are not reliable predictors of blood volume. Thus, with the exception of minor injury cases, early and aggressive intravenous fluid resuscitation with consideration of red blood cell transfusion is critical. It is recommended that vasopressors be avoided unless absolutely necessary as these medications are associated with fetal compromise resulting from diminished uterine blood flow. Physiologic changes in the respiratory system such as a decreased functional residual capacity in conjunction with increased oxygen consumption renders the pregnant trauma victim more vulnerable to hypoxia. Supplemental oxygen and consideration for early intubation in the absence of adequate ventilation is essential. In addition, the elevated level of the diaphragm during pregnancy has implications for chest tube placement and emergency thoracotomy. These procedures are generally performed in one to two intercostals spaces higher than in the nonpregnant patient (Rudloff, 2007).

Secondary Survey

After initial stabilization, it is appropriate to evaluate other maternal injuries. This consists of obtaining a complete history, including a focused obstetric history, performing a targeted physical examination, and monitoring the fetus. Initial fetal assessment following trauma includes an accurate determination of gestational age when possible in conjunction with immediate auscultation of fetal heart tones.

If fetal heart tones are absent, resuscitation of the fetus should not be attempted prior to stabilization of the mother. There were no fetal survivors in a series of 441 pregnant trauma patients with initially absent fetal heart tones (Morris et al., 1996). When fetal heart tones are auscultated by Doppler, gestational age can be estimated by fundal height, history, Leopold's maneuvers, or ultrasound.

Ultrasound remains the most accurate method for determining gestational age and placental location. However, its clinical utility is limited by both availability and clinical expertise. Determining fetal viability is the most important step following documentation of fetal heart tones, noting that this definition is subject to institutional variation. An estimated gestational age of 24 weeks and less commonly an estimated fetal weight (EFW) of at least 500 g are thresholds for fetal viability. All decisions regarding fetal viability are made on the basis of the best gestational age available. Figure 15.2 provides a general algorithm for the management of catastrophic trauma.

Laboratory and Imaging Studies

Laboratory analysis following more significant injuries include a complete blood count (CBC), basic metabolic profile with chemistries and glucose, blood typing, coagulation studies, and urinalysis. Anemia of pregnancy is not unexpected, but profound anemia is abnormal and a source of blood loss should be sought. Abnormal coagulation factors may suggest disseminated intravascular coagulation (DIC) from placental abruption. In addition, there is evidence that low bicarbonate and elevated lactate levels correlate with poor fetal outcome (Aghababian, 2006) so attention to these laboratory values is prudent.

Pregnant trauma patients require the same diagnostic studies and interventions as nonpregnant patients. This includes all indicated radiographic studies such as plain film x-ray, computed tomography (CT), angiography, and magnetic resonance imaging (MRI). The risk of fetal injury is virtually unchanged if the total fetal dosage is less than 10 rad (10,000 millirads). An additional imaging tool is ultrasound, which when combined with the evaluation of the pericardium is often referred to as a Focused Assessment with Sonography for Trauma (FAST scan). This has proven to be an effective

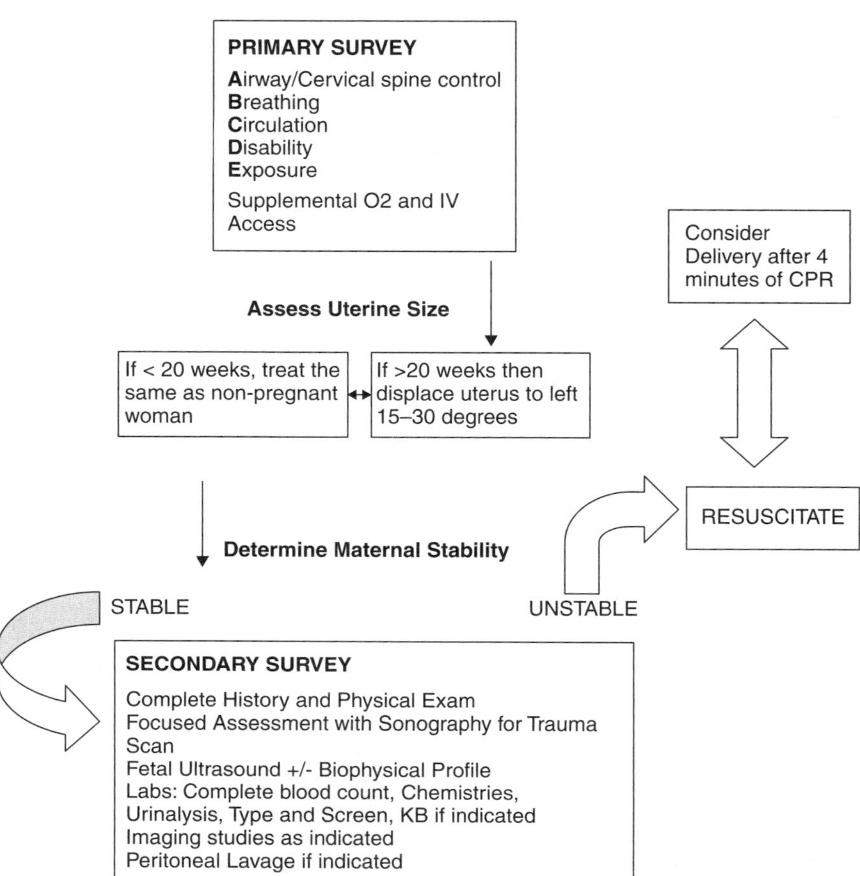

FIGURE 15.2 Algorithm for the management of catastrophic trauma.
Source: Adapted from Muench and Canterino (2007).

screening method that can potentially minimize the need for more costly and potentially hazardous diagnostic modalities.

Clinical Management and Follow-Up

The primary goals in the initial assessment and management of an injured pregnant woman are essentially identical to those in the nonpregnant population. These include stabilization and transfer to a facility with the appropriate level(s) of care. Prevention of supine hypotensive syndrome via left lateral uterine displacement is also essential to optimize maternal and fetal hemodynamics. Aortocaval compression can result in decreased venous return from the lower extremities with a subsequent drop in maternal systolic blood pressure of up to 30 mmHg and a 30% decrease in stroke volume (Grossman, 2004).

Pregnant women presenting in cardiac arrest are managed according to advanced cardiac life support (ACLS) guidelines. Although chest compressions are more difficult than in the nonpregnant individual due to reduced chest wall compliance and the presence of the gravid uterus, there are no guidelines for cardiopulmonary resuscitation (CPR) specific to pregnancy. Thus, closed-chest CPR is routinely performed on pregnant women in the supine position. A thoracotomy and or cesarean delivery are indicated if there is no initial response to therapy after 4 minutes.

In addition to the standard secondary survey, assessment of the injured pregnant patient should include performing pelvic and rectal examinations. Vaginal bleeding, ruptured membranes, and signs or symptoms of labor need to be ruled out. Women also need to be evaluated for the presence of contractions and any abnormal fetal heart rate pattern. Administration of appropriate medications including narcotics and tetanus immunoglobulin and toxoid are safe and appropriate in pregnancy, when indicated.

Urgent cesarean delivery may be appropriate in the setting of imminent maternal death, CPR that has not been effective within 4 minutes, or a stable mother with a nonreassuring fetal heart rate tracing (Morris & Stacey, 2003). Presently, there are no clear guidelines regarding perimortem cesarean delivery. However, fetal survival is not likely if greater than 15 to 20 minutes have transpired since the loss of maternal vital signs. One review suggests that optimum infant and maternal survival are obtained when cesarean delivery is initiated within 4 minutes of maternal cardiac arrest and the fetus is delivered within 5 minutes (Katz, Balderston, & Defreest, 2005). Notably, ineffective resuscitation efforts may become effective following delivery as a result of decreased fetal-placental mass and improved cardiac return to the heart.

PELVIC FRACTURES

Although uncommon, pelvic fractures in the setting of pregnancy carry a particularly high maternal and fetal morbidity given the propensity for massive intraperitoneal hemorrhage and subsequent hypovolemic shock (Mirza et al., 2010). Not surprisingly, both maternal and fetal outcomes are dependent on the degree and extent of the injury. In general, women who sustain pelvic fractures in the third trimester of pregnancy can safely attempt vaginal birth (ACOG, 1998). However, fractures that are extensive, severely dislocated or unstable may preclude a successful vaginal delivery. Vaginal birth was successful in 75% of women who had suffered pelvic fractures during the latter portion of their pregnancy (Leggon, Wood, & Indeck, 2002).

PENETRATING TRAUMA

Penetrating injury is a rare occurrence during pregnancy and consists primarily of gunshots and to a lesser degree, stab wounds. Maternal mortality occurs in less than 5% of penetrating trauma cases and is directly related to the size of the gravid uterus in relation to other intra-abdominal organs (Rudra et al., 2007). Conversely, direct fetal injury is by far more common in this setting with fetal demise occurring in up to 60% of cases of penetrating trauma (Hill & Lense, 1996). The management following penetrating injury is ultimately determined by the entrance location. Injury to the maternal bowel is likely with upper abdominal penetrating injuries, while lower abdominal wounds are more likely to injure the uterus and/or fetus. Of note, the appearance of the entrance wound is not predictive of the extent of internal injury.

The first step in assessing any penetrating injury in the pregnant female regardless of the type or location is to adequately expose the body. Careful and thorough inspection of the entire body facilitates evaluation and timely management of what may be multiple injuries. Operative management is often utilized for entrance wounds above the fundus, while more conservative options such as ultrasound, diagnostic laparoscopy, serial abdominal exams, and diagnostic peritoneal lavage are reserved for those injuries that occur below the uterine fundus. Moreover, the decision to proceed with surgical intervention is dependent on numerous factors including the type and location of the injury, uterine size, fetal status, and maternal vital signs.

BURNS AND ELECTRICAL INJURY

Burns may occur due to either electrical or thermal causes. Regardless of the cause, pregnancy does not alter maternal outcomes following burn injuries. Fetal outcome, however, is largely dependent on the extent of maternal burn as well as the complications resulting from the burn. Direct inhalation injury can result in significant airway compromise and subsequent maternal and fetal hypoxia.

Electrical injuries vary based on type and voltage of current as well as its path through the body. Significant maternal injuries can result due to direct effects of the heat generated by the current in conjunction with associated trauma. However, the greatest risk following electrical injury is to the fetus that is immersed in amniotic fluid, which serves as an excellent conductor for electrical energy.

Aggressive fluid replacement, respiratory support, and initial wound care are the emergency management goals in pregnant burn victims in conjunction with fetal monitoring to assure well-being. Ideally, pregnant women suffering penetrating trauma, significant burns, or electrical injuries, require transfer to a tertiary care setting with the appropriate trauma and intensive care unit personnel available. In addition, all patients with evidence of smoke inhalation require evaluation for carbon monoxide poisoning.

Ultimately, both maternal and fetal outcomes are drastically improved when a multidisciplinary team approach is utilized and thus early transport to a facility capable of evaluating and treating trauma, obstetrical, and neonatal emergencies is critical.

REFERENCES

American College of Obstetrics and Gynecology (ACOG). (2011). Committee on healthcare for underserved women. Sexual assault. Committee opinion no. 499. *Obstetrics and Gynecology, 118*, 396–399.

American College of Obstetricians and Gynecologists (ACOG). ACOG educational bulletin (1998). Obstetric aspects of trauma management. Number 251, September 1998 (replaces Number 151, January 1991, and Number 161, November 1991). *International Journal of Gynecology and Obstetrics, 64*, 87–94.

Aghababian, R. (2006). *Essentials of emergency medicine.* Sudbury, MA: Jones and Bartlett.

Barraco, R. D., Chiu, W. C., Clancy, T. V., Como, J. J., Hess, L. W., Hoff, W. S.... EAST Practice Management Guidelines Work Group. (2010). Practice management guidelines for diagnosis and management of injury in the pregnant patient: The EAST practice management guidelines work group. *Journal of Trauma, 69(1)*, 211–214.

Brown, H. L. (2009). Trauma in pregnancy. *Obstetrics and Gynecology, 114(1)*, 147–160.

Cahill, A., Bastek, J., Stamilio, D., Odibo, A., Stevens, E., & Macones. G. (2008). Minor trauma in pregnancy—Is the evaluation unwarranted? *American Journal of Obstetrics and Gynecology, 198*, 208e2–208e5.

Dahmus, M. A., & Sibai, B. M. (1993). Blunt abdominal trauma: Are there any predictive factors for abruptio placentae or maternal-fetal distress? *American Journal of Obstetrics and Gynecology, 169*, 1054–1059.

Desjardins, G. (2003). Management of the injured pregnant patient. Retrieved from http:www.Trauma.org/resus/pregnancytrauma.html

El-Kady, D., Gilbert, W., Towner, D., & Smith, L. (2004). Trauma during pregnancy: An analysis of maternal and fetal outcomes in a large population. *American Journal of Obstetrics and Gynecology, 190*, 1661–1669.

Grossman, N. B. (2004). Blunt trauma in pregnancy. *American Family Physician, 70*(7), 1303–1310.

Hill, D. A., & Lense, J. J. (1996). Abdominal trauma in the pregnant patient. *American Family Physician, 53*(4), 1269–1274.

Katz, V., Balderston, K., & Defreest, M. (2005). Perimortem cesarean delivery: Were our assumptions correct? *American Journal of Obstetrics and Gynecology, 192*(6), 1916–1920; discussion 1920–1911.

Leggon, R. E., Wood, G. C., & Indeck, M. C. (2002). Pelvic fractures in pregnancy: Factors influencing maternal and fetal outcomes. *Journal of Trauma*;53: 796–804.

Mirza, F. G., Devine, P. C., & Gaddipati, S. (2010). Trauma in pregnancy: A systematic approach. *American Journal of Perinatology, 27*, 579–586.

Morris, J. A., Rosenbower, T. J., Jurkovich, G. J., Hoyt, D. B., Harviel, J. D., Knudson, M. M.,... Bass, J. G. (1996). Infant survival after cesarean section for trauma. *Annals of Surgery, 223*(5), 481–488; discussion 488–491.

Morris, S., & Stacey, M. (2003). Resuscitation in pregnancy. *British Medical Journal, 327(7426)*, 1277–1279.

Muench, M., Bashat, A., Reddy, U., Mighty, H., Weiner, C., Scalea, T., & Harman, C. (2004). Kleihauer-Betke testing is important in all cases o f maternal trauma. *The Journal of Trauma, Injury and Critical Care, 57*, 1094–1098.

Muench, M., & Canterino, J. C. (2007). Trauma in pregnancy. *Obstetrics and Gynecology Clinics of North America, 34*(3), 555–583.

Pearlman, M. D., Tintinallli, J. E., & Lorenz, R. P. (1990). A prospective controlled study of outcome after trauma during pregnancy. *American Journal of Obstetrics and Gynecology, 162*, 1502–1507; discussion 1507–1510.

Rudloff, U. (2007). Trauma in pregnancy. *Archives of Gynecology and Obstetrics, 276(2)*, 101–117.

Rudra, A., Ray, A., Chatterjee, S. Bhattacharya, C., Kirtania, J., Jumar, P.... Roy, V. (2007). Trauma in Pregnancy. *Indian Journal of Anaesthesia, 51*(2), 100–105.

Yost, N., Bloom, S., McIntire, G., & Leveno, K. (2005). A prospective observational study of domestic violence during pregnancy. *Obstetrics and Gynecology, 106*, 61–65.

Severe Preeclampsia or Eclampsia and Hypertensive Issues

16

Agatha S. Critchfield and Asha J. Heard

Acute hypertension in pregnancy is a severe obstetric complication that requires immediate evaluation and treatment. It can occur in the context of a variety of disorders of pregnancy and is associated with significant maternal and fetal morbidity and potential mortality. Hypertension in pregnancy can occur along a spectrum as noted in Table 16.1.

The spectrum of pregnancy-related hypertensive disorders frequently presenting with acute changes in blood pressure control will be presented. The common presenting symptomatology, the initial steps in maternal/fetal evaluation (history, physical examination, and laboratory evaluation) and management in the obstetric triage setting will be covered. In addition, other possible etiologies of acute hypertension, severe preeclampsia, and possible imitators of HELLP (**h**emolysis, **e**levated **l**iver enzymes and **l**ow **p**latelets) syndrome will be discussed.

DEFINITIONS

Hypertension in pregnancy, otherwise known as gestational hypertension (GHTN), is defined as a systolic blood pressure level of 140 mmHg or greater and a diastolic blood pressure level of 90 mmHg or greater (National High Blood Pressure Education Program Working Group, 2000). *Severe* hypertension is defined as persistent systolic blood pressure of 160 mmHg or greater or diastolic blood pressure of 110 mmHg or greater. Severe hypertension is associated with a significantly higher rate of potentially catastrophic maternal and fetal events, including maternal stroke or other central nervous complications and placental abruption with subsequent fetal compromise (Magee and von Dadelszen, 2009). Of note, elevated systolic blood pressure has been more strongly associated with maternal cerebral vascular accident than diastolic blood pressure (Martin et al., 2005).

As many as 25% of women with GHTN will go on to develop *preeclampsia* (Saudan, Brown, Buddle, & Jones, 1998), which is defined as persistent hypertension diagnosed after 20 weeks' gestation with the addition of proteinuria. Preeclampsia occurs in 3% to 10% of all pregnancies (Haddad & Sibai, 2009) and is a disorder of largely unknown etiology that is likely associated with abnormal placentation and subsequent

TABLE 16.1 Pregnancy-Induced Hypertension Spectrum

DISORDER	DEFINITION
GHTN	Persistent hypertension without proteinuria noted in previously normotensive patient after 20 weeks' gestation
Preeclampsia	Persistent hypertension after 20 weeks' gestation with proteinuria. See Exhibit 16.1 for mild versus severe preeclampsia
Chronic hypertension	Hypertension predating the pregnancy/noted prior to 20 weeks' gestation
Eclampsia	Occurrence of seizures not attributable to other causes in patient with preeclampsia

Source: Adapted from ACOG (2002).

wide-reaching vascular and endothelial dysfunction (American College of Obstetricians and Gynecologists [ACOG], 2002). Preeclampsia can be further subdivided into mild and severe forms with *severe preeclampsia* including a variety of signs and symptoms of evolving endothelial dysfunction as noted in Exhibit 16.1. Potential fetal effects of hypertensive disorders in pregnancy include placental dysfunction manifested as poor fetal growth, oligohydramnios, nonreactive fetal heart rate testing, abruption, and intrauterine fetal demise.

Further on the spectrum of hypertensive disorders of pregnancy is *eclampsia* (occurrence of seizures not attributable to other causes in a patient with preeclampsia). In addition, preeclampsia can be accompanied by significant end-organ damage and coagulopathy—as evidenced by the frequent presentation of preeclampsia with *HELLP syndrome*—an acronym which stands for *hemolysis, elevated liver enzymes, and low platelets.* While HELLP syndrome can present without evidence of hypertension and proteinuria (Roberts, 2004), it will be considered in this chapter due to the shared pathophysiologic changes and frequent presentation in the context of severe preeclampsia.

Chronic hypertension is defined as hypertension predating the pregnancy or noted prior to 20 weeks' gestation. Another clinical entity to be considered is *preeclampsia* (either mild or severe) *superimposed on preexisting chronic hypertension* (sometimes referred to simply as "*superimposed preeclampsia*"). Unfortunately, superimposed preeclampsia poses a significant diagnostic conundrum as women affected by chronic hypertension often have some element of baseline renal dysfunction and resultant proteinuria, in addition to elevated blood pressures. However, it is known that maternal and fetal prognosis in the setting of superimposed disease is worse than with other disease processes alone (Roberts, 2004). Therefore, clinicians must be vigilant of any increase in blood pressure or worsening of baseline proteinuria in pregnant women with previously diagnosed chronic hypertension and have a high index of suspicion for superimposed preeclampsia. Maternal risk factors for the development of preeclampsia are noted in Exhibit 16.2.

While the spectrum of hypertensive disorders in pregnancy is often referred to collectively as "pregnancy-induced hypertension," this is not an endorsed term and only disorder-specific terms should be used.

EXHIBIT 16.1

Diagnosis of Severe Preeclampsia

Preeclampsia is considered severe if one or more of the following is present:

1. SBP ≥ 160 or DBP ≥ 110 on two occasions at least 6 hr apart when patient is on bed rest
2. Proteinuria ≥ 5 g in 24-hr urine specimen or ≥ 3+ on two random urine samples collected 4 hr apart
3. Oliguria (≤ 500 mL in 24 hr)
4. Cerebral or visual disturbances
5. Pulmonary edema or cyanosis
6. Epigastric or right upper quadrant pain
7. Impaired liver function
8. Thrombocytopenia
9. Fetal intrauterine growth restriction

Source: Adapted from ACOG (2002).

EXHIBIT 16.2

Maternal Risk Factors for Preeclampsia

1. Nulliparity
2. Teen pregnancy
3. Advanced maternal age
4. History of prior preeclampsia
5. Obesity
6. Pregestational diabetes
7. Thrombophilias
8. Chronic hypertension
9. Renal disease
10. Multiple gestations

Source: Adapted from Roberts (2004); Sibai (2005).

PRESENTING SYMPTOMATOLOGY

Considering the pervasive endothelial dysfunction present in preeclampsia/eclampsia, it is not surprising that the presenting symptomatology often relates to a multitude of organ systems suffering from poor vascular perfusion. Cerebral symptoms most commonly include a persistent headache but can also include dizziness, tinnitus, fever, drowsiness, changes in respiratory rate, and tachycardia. Visual symptoms often present as diplopia, scotoma, blurred vision, and vision loss. Gastrointestinal symptoms are common and usually present with nausea, vomiting, and possible epigastric pain but can also include hematemesis. Renal symptoms may include oliguria, anuria, or hematuria. In addition, many pregnant women will note an increase in edema (extremities, facial). Some women with severe disease suffering from cardiopulmonary compromise and resultant pulmonary edema will report significant shortness of breath. While many of these symptoms are possible, certain symptoms are considered more ominous and indicative of *severe preeclampsia*. These include those signs of hepatic capsular distension (which can present as epigastric pain), dyspnea that is secondary to pulmonary edema, headache indicative of poor cerebral perfusion (and possible impending eclampsia), and retinal artery edema and spasm causing visual changes (Roberts, 2004).

HISTORY AND DATA COLLECTION

The gravid woman presenting to an obstetric triage setting with hypertension warrants immediate evaluation. While initial history and data collection are obtained simultaneously, steps must be taken by the care team to begin treatment of severe range blood pressures and, if present, eclamptic seizure activity. In addition, fetal status must be evaluated as soon as possible with either a modified biophysical profile (mBPP) or biophysical profile (BPP).

Maternal history includes a pertinent history of present illness focusing on classic preeclampsia symptomatology. Maternal past obstetric history (including prior preeclampsia/eclampsia), as well as history of preexisting hypertension or other medical/surgical conditions must be obtained.

Maternal blood pressure needs to be evaluated with an appropriately sized cuff (length 1.5 times the circumference of the upper arm) to minimize inaccurate readings. Ideally, the blood pressure is obtained after a rest period of 10 minutes, without exposure to caffeine or tobacco for 30 minutes (ACOG, 2002). The blood pressure is obtained with a woman sitting upright; however, it can also be evaluated with the patient lying in the left lateral position with the brachial artery at heart level (Magee et al., 2008). While some electronic devices are acceptable, in general mercury sphygmomanometry (manual blood pressure cuff) is preferred due to increased accuracy (ACOG, 2002; Magee & von Dadelson, 2009).

PHYSICAL EXAMINATION

While initial steps toward the treatment of the hypertensive emergency begin and laboratory evaluations are obtained, a thorough physical examination should be performed. Classic physical examination findings of preeclampsia, while not diagnostic, include edema, hyperreflexia, and clonus. Retinal artery changes (due to localized retinal vascular narrowing and segmental spasm) occur in 50% of patients with preeclampsia (Roberts, 2004). Other less common and significantly more ominous findings on physical examination include ascites and hydrothorax (associated with marked edema, increased neck vein distension, and rales on pulmonary examination) consistent with pulmonary edema/congestive heart failure, hepatic enlargement and tenderness indicative of hepatic capsular distension, and petechiae, bruising, or bleeding associated with disseminated intravascular coagulation (DIC).

A complete physical examination is performed, including cardiovascular, pulmonary, abdominal, ophthalmologic, neurologic, skin, and extremity evaluation. A cervical examination is also performed to evaluate the Bishop's score for cervical readiness and possible delivery planning. The fetal status is evaluated as soon as possible using external fetal monitoring and, as outlined below, by ultrasound evaluation.

LABORATORY AND IMAGING STUDIES

Laboratory studies include complete blood count (CBC), creatinine, liver function tests, uric acid, lactate dehydrogenase (LDH), coagulation profile, urinalysis, and urine protein:creatinine ratio. Consideration can be given to sending a urine toxicology screen as sympathomimetic drugs such as amphetamines can elevate blood pressure. Major laboratory changes are usually found in the context of severe preeclampsia or eclampsia, and it is common for women with mild preeclampsia to have proteinuria as the only laboratory abnormality.

The diagnosis of preeclampsia requires the presence of proteinuria—defined as 1+ or greater protein on a urine dip or >300 mg protein/24-hour period noted on a 24-hour urine collection specimen. Proper collection of a 24-hour urine specimen involves discarding the first void of the day followed by complete collection for 24 subsequent hours with an adequate volume of urine obtained. Adequacy is determined by 24-hour urine creatinine excretion equal to 15 to 20 mg/kg prepregnancy body weight. Recently, obstetric providers have adopted the use of the urine spot protein:creatinine ratio, which is a favored method of proteinuria evaluation in the nonpregnant population (Eknoyan et al, 2003) and has gained support in the medical literature as a valid way to evaluate proteinuria in the pregnant population (Côté et al., 2008; Neithardt, Dooley, & Borensztajn, 2002; Papanna, Mann, Kouides & Glantz, 2008). Most providers recommend collection of a 24-hour urine specimen when a urine protein:creatinine ratio is greater than or equal to 0.2 (Côté et al., 2008; Neithardt et al., 2002; Papanna et al., 2008).

Common abnormalities noted on laboratory analysis include evidence of hemoconcentration (elevated hematocrit), hemolysis (thrombocytopenia, elevated LDH), renal compromise (elevated creatinine), hepatic damage (elevated liver function tests), coagulopathy [elevated prothrombin time (PT), elevated international normalized ratio (INR), elevated partial thromboplastin time (PTT), low fibrinogen], and elevated uric acid. Approximately 20% of patients with severe preeclampsia will have HELLP syndrome with laboratory findings as noted in Table 16.2 (Sibai et al., 1993). Frequent laboratory reevaluation in the situation of markedly abnormal maternal labs, changing clinical status, or expectant management of severe preeclampsia needs to be considered.

There are no specific imaging studies required in the context of maternal hypertensive emergencies. While the exact incidence of cerebral hemorrhage in nonfatal eclampsia is unknown, it has been reported that 50% of reversible, pregnancy-related ischemic strokes do occur in the context of preeclampsia

TABLE 16.2 Criteria for the Diagnosis of HELLP Syndrome and Corresponding Laboratory Findings

Hemolytic anemia	Schistocytes on peripheral smear LDH ≥ 600 IU/L Bilirubin ≥ 1.2 mg/dL Haptoglobin ≤ 25mg/dL
Elevated liver enzymes	AST ≥ 70 IU/L
Low platelets	Platelet count < 100,000 cells/microL

Source: Adapted from Sibai et al. (1993).

(Zeeman, 2009). If persistent neurologic changes suspicious for maternal intracranial pathology after resolution of seizure activity are noted, computed tomography (CT) imaging of the head is also indicated. If pulmonary edema is suspected, an urgent chest radiograph is warranted. If congestive heart failure is suspected, arrangements can be made for maternal echocardiogram once the maternal and fetal status is stabilized.

Considering the high risk for fetal morbidity including abruption, growth restriction, and placental insufficiency, fetal evaluation is necessary. Initial fetal testing with nonstress test (NST) and/or BPP is initiated as soon as the clinical situation allows. In addition, ultrasound evaluation of fetal growth, amniotic fluid volume, and umbilical artery systolic-to-diastolic ratios are recommended in the setting of preeclampsia (Maulik, Mundy, Heitmann, & Maulik, 2010).

DIFFERENTIAL DIAGNOSIS

The differential diagnosis of hypertensive emergencies in the obstetric population is broad and must consider both obstetric and nonobstetric etiologies. As discussed above, pregnancy-specific disorders such as GHTN, preeclampsia (mild and severe), and HELLP syndrome must be at the top of all obstetric triage providers' differential list. In addition, consideration must be given to an exacerbation of chronic hypertension with or without superimposed preeclampsia. When a woman presents with findings consistent with severe preeclampsia/HELLP syndrome, it is wise to keep in mind the variety of other disorders that can present in a similar manner. There include, but are not limited to, acute fatty liver of pregnancy (AFLP) and the thrombotic microangiopathies (including thrombotic thrombocytopenic purpura and hemolytic uremic syndrome) or a systemic lupus erythematosus flare (Sibai, 2009).

Other less common but still possible nonobstetric etiologies for hypertensive emergencies in the obstetric triage setting include withdrawal from antihypertensive medication (most pertinent to those women with chronic hypertension), renal artery stenosis, increased adrenergic activity secondary to pheochromocytoma, autonomic dysfunction (e.g., spinal cord injury, Guillian-Barré), or the use of sympathomimetic drugs such as cocaine or amphetamines.

CLINICAL MANAGEMENT

It is essential to initiate prompt treatment of persistent severe range blood pressures to decrease the risk of adverse vascular events—particularly maternal stroke or other central nervous system complications (Magee et al., 2008). The goal of blood pressure management is to expeditiously lower mean arterial blood pressure by no more than 25% initially, with the ultimate goal of lowering and maintaining the blood pressure at less than 160/105 mmHg (Magee & von Dadelszen, 2009). Common parenteral medications used in the obstetric setting include labetalol and hydralazine as noted in Table 16.3.

Labetalol is a beta blocker that also has some alpha-blocking activity. It is avoided in those women with asthma, cardiac disease, or active abuse of sympathomimetic drugs (cocaine, amphetamines). A reasonable initial dose of labetolol is 20 mg given once intravenously (IV). If the desired effect is not obtained within 10 minutes, repeated doses may be given to a maximum of 220

TABLE 16.3 Treatment of Acute Hypertension in Pregnancy

MEDICATION	MECHANISM OF ACTION	DOSE (MG)	ROUTE	FREQUENCY (MIN)	24-HOUR MAXIMUM DOSE (MG)	CAUTION/ CONTRAIN-DICATIONS
Labetalol	Beta blocker (has some alpha-blocking activity)	20→ 40→ 80→ 80	IV	10	220	Asthma, sympatho-mimetic drugs (cocaine), and cardiac disease
Hydralazine	Vasodilator	5–10	IV	20–30	20	Must give by slow IV push. Otherwise possible maternal hypotension
Nifedipine*	Ca^{2+} channel blocker	10	PO	30	120	Cardiac disease. Concurrent use of magnesium sulfate

* *Note*: Not FDA approved use

Source: Adapted from Roberts (2004) and ACOG (2002).

mg total. Labetalol can also be used as a continuous IV drip. Hydralazine is a vasodilator that can be given in 5 to 10 mg IV increments every 20–30 minutes by *slow push* as needed to a total maximum dose of 20 mg. Of note, hydralazine can cause maternal hypotension if not given slowly. The most common oral agent used in the acute setting is nifedipine, which is a calcium channel blocker that comes in short, intermediate, and long-acting forms. The short-acting form of nifedipine can be given in the acute setting when, for example, IV access has yet to be obtained. Of note, the use of short-acting nifedipine in the treatment of acute hypertension is an off-label (non-FDA approved) use. It is used with caution in women with a history of cardiac disease and in those concurrently on magnesium sulfate due to risk of pulmonary edema. Treatment may be initiated with 10 mg by mouth. This can be repeated every 30 minutes to a maximum total dose of 120 mg/day. For severe refractory hypertension, sodium nitroprusside has been recommended in small doses and for a brief duration (in an intensive care setting only). There is a concern for fetal cyanide toxicity if used for prolonged periods (Sass, Itamoto, Silva, Torloni & Atallah, 2007).

Another priority in the treatment of severe preeclampsia is the prevention of eclampsia. Though there is no consensus regarding the use of magnesium sulfate for the prevention of seizures in those women with mild preeclampsia, there is a significant body of evidence to support the use of magnesium sulfate for the prevention of seizures in patients with severe preeclampsia (Altman et al., 2002; Coetzee, Dommisse, & Anthony, 1998). One common protocol is a 4-g loading dose (in 100 mL fluid) given over 20 minutes, followed by 1–2 g per hour as a continuous IV infusion (ACOG, 2002).

For treatment of active seizures, magnesium sulfate is a more effective treatment in the eclamptic population than either phenytoin or diazepam (Eclampsia Trial Collaborative Group, 1995). If treatment with magnesium sulfate has not yet begun, it can be administered with the above regimen. Deep intramuscular (IM) administration in the buttock is acceptable if IV access is yet to be obtained (5 g IM in each buttock). Of note, magnesium sulfate is contraindicated in women with heart block or myocardial damage and must be used with extreme caution in patients with myasthenia gravis or significant renal disease. For women experiencing seizures despite magnesium sulfate treatment, a repeat 2 g magnesium bolus (IV) can be considered. In addition, diazepam (5–10 mg IV every 5–10 min, maximum 20 mg) or lorazepam (4 mg slow IV push, may repeat times 1 after 10 min) can also be administered. Of note, lorazepam has a longer duration of action though it can take up to 2 minutes to take effect. Protection of the airway to prevent aspiration and prevention of maternal injury during seizure activity is also important to consider. Fetal bradycardia will often occur during maternal seizure activity and most often resolves with maternal stabilization.

Providers must also be aware of the potential for magnesium sulfate toxicity. Signs and symptoms include electrocardiogram (ECG) changes, loss of deep tendon reflexes, respiratory suppression, and the possibility for cardiovascular collapse. Treatment of magnesium sulfate toxicity is calcium gluconate 1 g IV and cardiopulmonary support. Most providers recommend frequent evaluation of patient status while on magnesium sulfate to evaluate for toxicity. This includes evaluation of the cardiopulmonary status (cardiac and pulmonary exam, reviewing fluid intake/output, oxygen saturation) and deep tendon reflexes. Provider evaluation every 3 to 4 hours in a stable woman may be appropriate. Many providers would consider evaluation of serum magnesium levels and subsequent titration of magnesium doses in those women who are at high risk for magnesium sulfate toxicity (i.e., those with poor renal function).

Overall, when considering the decision to deliver a woman with preeclampsia, the provider must balance maternal and fetal risks. In general, continued close observation of a woman with mild preeclampsia is appropriate in the context of stable maternal and fetal status, though most providers would recommend delivery at 37 weeks' gestation in this situation. In general, inpatient management of all women with preeclampsia with twice weekly laboratory evaluation and daily fetal testing is recommended. However, consideration can be given to outpatient management of women with mild preeclampsia who are asymptomatic, have reassuring laboratory evaluation and fetal testing, and who are compliant with care. If the woman is deemed a candidate for outpatient management, weekly prenatal visits with twice weekly fetal testing is warranted.

The decision to expectantly manage those women with severe preeclampsia and/or HELLP syndrome remote from term (less than 32 weeks' gestation) to achieve steroid administration has received recent support but should only be attempted under the care of an obstetrician comfortable with this high-risk scenario, in a tertiary care setting (Sibai & Barton, 2007). Indications for *immediate* delivery regardless of gestational age include uncontrolled severe hypertension despite maximum doses of two antihypertensive agents, eclampsia, pulmonary edema, abruption, oliguria (<0.5 mL/kg/hr), persistent headache, vision changes, epigastric/right upper quadrant pain, rapid deterioration of HELLP syndrome, platelets <100,0000/μL, creatinine >1.4 mg/dL, or nonreactive fetal testing (Sibai, 2009). If no indication for immediate delivery exists, women can be admitted to labor and delivery for further fetal and maternal monitoring, magnesium sulfate administration, repeat laboratory evaluation, and steroid administration for fetal lung maturity (dexamethasone 6 mg IM every 12 hr times four doses or betamethasone 12 mg IM every 24 hr for two doses). Those who are very stable may be candidates for expectant management beyond 48 hours, though the general recommendation is for delivery by 34 weeks' gestation in the setting of severe preeclampsia (Sibai & Barton, 2007). Of note, even in those women with an indication for expedited delivery, induction of labor can be attempted if no other contraindications exist. The presence of preeclampsia/eclampsia is not necessarily an indication for delivery by cesarean section.

REFERENCES

Altman, D., Carroli, G., Duley, L., Farrell, B., Moodley, J., Neilson, J., Smith, D., & The Magpie Trial Collaboration Group. (2002). Do women with preeclampsia, and their babies, benefit from magnesium sulfate? The Magpie Trial: A randomized placebo controlled trial. *Lancet, 359 (9321)*, 1877–1890.

American College of Obstetricians and Gynecologists (ACOG). (2002). Diagnosis and management of preeclampsia and eclampsia. ACOG Practice Bulletin, 33. *Obstetrics and Gynecology, 99(1)*, 159–167.

Coetzee, E. J., Dommisse, J., & Anthony, J. (1998). A randomized controlled trial of intravenous magnesium sulfate versus placebo in the management of women with severe preeclampsia. *British Journal of Obstetrics and Gynecology, 105(3)*, 300–303.

Côté, A. M., Brown, M. A., Lan, E., von Dadelszen, P., Firoz, T., Liston, R. M., & Magee, L. A. (2008). Diagnostic accuracy of urinary spot protein:creatinine ratio for proteinuria in hypertensive pregnant women: A systematic review. *British Medical Journal, 336(7651)*, 1003–1006.

Eclampsia Trial Collaborative Group. (1995). Which anticonvulsant for women with eclampsia? Evidence from the collaborative eclampsia trial. *Lancet, 345(8963)*, 1455–1463.

Eknoyan, G., Hostetter, T., Bakris, G.L., Hebert, L., Levey, A. S., Parving, H. H.,... Toto, R. (2003). Proteinuria and other markers of chronic kidney disease: A position statement of the National Kidney Foundation (NKF) and the National Institute of Diabetes and Digestive and Kidney Diseases (NIDDK). *American Journal of Kidney Disease, 42(4)*, 617.

Haddad, B., & Sibai, B. (2009). Expectant management in pregnancies with severe preeclampsia. *Seminars in Perinatology, 33*, 143–151.

Magee L. A., Helewa, M., Moutquin, J. M., & von Dadelszen, P. Hypertension Guideline Committee; Strategic Training Initiative in Research in the Reproductive Health Sciences (STIRRHS) Scholars. (2008). Diagnosis, evaluation, and management of the hypertensive disorders of pregnancy. *Journal of Obstetrics and Gynaecology Canada, 30*(3), S1–S48.

Magee, L. A., & von Dadelszen, P. (2009). The management of severe hypertension. *Seminars in Perinatology, 33*, 138–142.

Martin, J. N., Jr, Thigpen, B. D., Moore, R. C., Rose, C. H., Cushman, J., & May, W. (2005). Stroke and severe preeclampsia and eclampsia: A paradigm shift focusing on systolic blood pressure. *Obstetrics and Gynecology, 105*, 246–254.

Maulik, D., Mundy, D., Heitmann, E., & Maulik, D. (2010). Evidence-based approach to umbilical artery Doppler fetal surveillance in high-risk pregnancies: an update. *Clinical Obstetrics and Gynecology, 33(4)*, 869–878.

National High Blood Pressure Education Program Working Group. (2000). Report of the National High Blood Pressure Education Program Working Group on High Blood Pressure in Pregnancy. *American Journal of Obstetrics and Gynecology, 183*, S1–S22.

Neithardt, A. B., Dooley, S. L. & Borensztajn, J. (2002). Prediction of 24-hour protein excretion in pregnancy with a single voided urine protein-to-creatinine ratio. *American Journal of Obstetrics and Gynecology, 186(5)*, 883.

Papanna, R., Mann, L. K., Kouides, R. W., & Glantz, J. C. (2008). Protein/creatinine ratio in preeclampsia: A systematic review. *Obstetrics and Gynecology, 112*(1), 135.

Roberts, J. M. (2004). Pregnancy related hypertension. In R. K. Creasy, R. Resnick, & J. D. Iams, (Eds.). *Maternal fetal medicine principles and practice* (pp. 859–899). Philadelphia, PA: Saunders.

Sass, N., Itamoto, C. H., Silva, M. P., Torloni, M. R., & Atallah, A. N. (2007). Does sodium nitroprusside kill babies? A systematic review. *Sao Paolo Medical Journal, 125*, 108–111.

Saudan, P., Brown, M. A., Buddle M. L., & Jones, M. (1998). Does gestational hypertension become preeclampsia? *British Journal of Obstetrics and Gynaecology, 105*, 1177–1184.

Sibai, B. M. (2005). Preeclampsia: 3 preemptive tactics. *OBG Management, 17*(2), 20–32.

Sibai, B. M., & Barton, J. R. (2007). Expectant management of severe preeclampsia remote from term: Patient selection, treatment, and delivery indications. *American Journal of Obstetrics and Gynecology, 196*(6), 514.e1–e9.

Sibai, B. M. (2009). Imitators of severe preeclampsia. *Seminars in Perinatology, 33*, 196–205.

Sibai, B. M., Ramadan, M. K., Usa, I., Salama, M., Mercer, B. M., Friedman, S. A. (1993). Maternal morbidity and mortality in 442 pregnancies with hemolysis, elevated liver enzymes, and low platelets (HELLP syndrome). *American Journal of Obstetrics and Gynecology, 169*(4), 1000–1006.

Zeeman, G. G. (2009). Neurologic complications of preeclampsia. *Seminars in Perinatology, 33*, 166–172.

17 Labor Evaluation

Elisabeth D. Howard

The process of childbirth at term is normally initiated by regular uterine contractions, by spontaneous rupture of membranes, or by both (Cunningham, Levino, Bloom, Hauth, & Rouse, 2010). Safe, thorough evaluation of the pregnant woman at term who presents to an obstetric triage setting requires knowledge of the necessary components of maternal and fetal assessment, including history, physical examination, and clinical management. A review of clinical management of the main presenting concerns of women at term including premature rupture of membranes (PROM), latent labor, active labor, and imminent delivery will be presented.

PROM AT TERM

PROM at term occurs in 8% to 10% of all pregnancies (ACOG, 2007) and refers to spontaneous rupture of membranes at term occurring prior to the onset of labor (Cunningham et al., 2010; Hannah et al., 1996). The management of PROM at term remains somewhat controversial. Managed expectantly, 95% of women with PROM will labor and deliver within 72 hours (Hannah et al., 1996). Current data from the American College of Obstetricians and Gynecologists (ACOG, 2007) recommend induction of labor for women with term or near term PROM upon presentation, while the position of the American College of Nurse Midwives (ACNM, 2008) suggests that with appropriate counseling and informed consent, under specific conditions and absence of risk factors, selected patients may be offered expectant management as a safe alternative to induction of labor. This is predicated on the preference of the woman and provider evaluation.

PRESENTING SYMPTOMATOLOGY

A history of a sudden gush of fluid or continued trickling of fluid is suggestive but not confirmatory evidence of ruptured membranes. Time of leakage, color of fluid (i.e., blood tinged, meconium stained), and odor are important to ascertain. Associated cramping, contractions, and presence of fetal movement need to be noted.

HISTORY AND PHYSICAL EXAMINATION

Ruptured membranes are confirmed by visualization of a pool of amniotic fluid in the vaginal vault or leakage of fluid from the cervical os, nitrazine positive fluid in the vagina on speculum examination, and presence of ferning on a dry microscope slide. It is critical to obtain fluid from the vaginal vault rather than the cervical os where mucus may be present and confound findings. Vaginal secretions are normally slightly acidic, whereas amniotic fluid is basic, thus turning nitrazine paper dark blue. Dried amniotic fluid forms crystals (ferning) on a microscope slide, whereas vaginal secretions do not. Cervical dilation and effacement are estimated visually only during the sterile speculum examination (Cunningham et al., 2010).

Maternal vital signs including blood pressure, temperature, and pulse are assessed. In addition, abdominal examination is performed to determine fetal presentation, lie, estimated fetal weight, and presence or absence of contractions. The fetal heart rate (FHR) may be evaluated with a fetoscope, Doppler, or an external fetal monitor for baseline FHR, variability, and presence or absence of decelerations and accelerations. It is critical that confirmation of fetal presentation be obtained. Group B *Streptococcus* (GBS) status will need to be determined.

DIFFERENTIAL DIAGNOSIS

If spontaneous rupture of membranes is not confirmed by examination, other possibilities need to be considered. These include normal leukorrhea of pregnancy, loss of mucous plug, involuntary loss of urine, and vaginal infections.

CLINICAL MANAGEMENT

When PROM is confirmed by physical examination, the risks and benefits of both induction of labor and expectant management may be reviewed with the pregnant woman. The maternal risks of ruptured membranes at term are low (Cunningham et al., 2010; Zlatnik, 1992). The risks to the fetus include ascending infection and umbilical cord compression (ACOG, 2007). In general, these risks may be mitigated with delay of baseline vaginal examination and minimal vaginal examinations (ACNM, 2008).

The largest prospective study to date that has investigated management of PROM is the TermPROM study. This was a multicenter, randomized trial that consisted of over 5,000 women at term with PROM (Hannah et al., 1996). In the expectant management arm of this trial, there was a higher incidence of chorioamnionitis and endometritis (Seaward et al., 1997). The incidence of neonatal infection was not statistically significant in any of the groups. It is recommended that women receive counseling and informed consent about the risks and benefits of induction of labor versus expectant management. According to ACNM (2008), women who select expectant management as a safe alternative to induction of labor must meet the following conditions: a term, uncomplicated, single vertex pregnancy with clear amniotic fluid, absence of identified infection, absence of fever, a Category 1 FHR tracing, and minimization of digital vaginal examinations (including avoiding a baseline vaginal examination).

Visualization and estimation of cervical dilation and length are appropriate for planning for cervical ripening versus pitocin induction, although no studies have proven the superiority of prostaglandin induction over pitocin in the setting of PROM. Confirmation of fetal presentation via abdominal examination and ultrasound are crucial in the absence of a digital examination. Overall recommendation, based on the current evidence with term PROM is that labor should be preferentially induced at the time of presentation (ACOG, 2007). Observation of the woman for the onset of spontaneous labor includes documentation of the rationale of care, informed consent/patient counseling, and clinical circumstances (ACNM, 2008).

There are times when the woman's stated history of spontaneous rupture is inconsistent with the physical examination findings, yet the history is compelling. If examination results are equivocal, it may be appropriate to repeat the sterile speculum examination in 20 to 30 minutes or longer after the woman has been reclining, to assess for reaccumulation of pooling, ferning, and repeat nitrazine testing.

LATENT LABOR

The latent phase of labor is complex and not well understood or well studied. There is a wide range of variation in the duration of the latent phase. This is partially due to the subjective nature of patient's perception as to the onset of contractions. In addition, this is the time when the clinician makes the determination between early and false labor (Braxton Hicks contractions).

Clinically, it is important to recognize when a woman is still in the latent phase of labor and not yet active (Greulich & Tarrant, 2007). Incorrectly identifying the latent phase as active may result in unnecessary interventions, such as administration of oxytocics or operative birth for abnormal labor progress (Greulich & Tarrant, 2007).

PRESENTING SYMPTOMATOLOGY

Women may present with regular contractions that are still infrequent in timing. The contractions may be irregular and the intervals between them long. Discomfort may be chiefly in the lower abdomen and is likely to be relieved by sedation. In early labor, the contractions, though infrequent, are becoming coordinated and increasing in intensity.

PHYSICAL EXAMINATION

A review of the medical record reviewing the past medical and obstetric histories is obtained. Additional data collection include the following: the frequency, duration and intensity of contractions, time established when they first became uncomfortable, the degree of discomfort, any mitigating factors, status of membranes, vaginal bleeding, and leakage of fluid. Maternal coping resources are reviewed and these include the amount of recent sleep, support persons available, level of hydration, and alimentation. Vital signs including blood pressure, temperature, and pulse are noted, as well as an abdominal examination to determine fetal presentation and position. The FHR is evaluated and a cervical examination is performed.

CLINICAL MANAGEMENT

Pregnant women in the latent phase of labor need support, encouragement, and advice if and when they are discharged from an obstetric triage unit (Greulich & Tarrant, 2007). Ideally, the discussion of latent labor takes place prenatally, and healthy pregnant women are encouraged to spend the latent phase at home (Greulich & Tarrant, 2007). Anticipatory guidance on the length of latent phase, comfort measures, and guidelines regarding when to call the provider are helpful for the pregnant woman to have. It is important to review the risks of early admission including pitocin augmentation, need for epidural anesthesia, and the potentially higher cesarean section rate. Suggested comfort measures for women in latent labor include tub baths, hydration, alimentation, ambulation, and support of family. In addition to support, women may benefit from the following medications for outpatient support as noted in Table 17.1.

PROLONGED LATENT PHASE

Approximately 5% of women may experience a prolonged latent phase (Cunningham et al., 2010). There are no current diagnostic guidelines, therefore, most clinicians refer to Friedman's (1967) definition of prolonged latent phase as greater than 20 hours in nulliparas and greater than 14 hours in multiparas. However, one recent study on the natural course of normal labor suggests that active labor begins later than first presumed (Zhang, Landy et al., 2010). In addition, when the position of the fetus is occiput posterior, the duration of the latent phase is often prolonged (Simkin, 2010; Simkin & Ancheta, 2011). These are often the patients seen multiple times for latent phase labor evaluation in obstetric triage.

There are times when women may benefit from inpatient support services, particularly when they are fatigued and have exhausted existing coping resources (Austin & Calderon, 1999). The clinical management options include therapeutic rest, uterotonic drugs or amniotomy, and induction/augmentation

TABLE 17.1 Outpatient Therapeutic Rest: Pharmacologic Regimens

MEDICATION	BRAND NAME	DOSE (mg)	COMMENTS
Promethazine	Phenergan	12.5–25	Antiemetic, sedating properties without significant maternal or newborn side effects
Hydroxyzine	Vistaril	50–100 (PO or IM)	Has antianxiety and sedative properties. Maternal sedation is achieved without significant maternal or newborn side effects
Diphenhydramine	Benadryl	50 (PO)	Hypnotic and may help with rest
Zolpidem	Ambien	5–10 (PO)	Hypnotic and may help with rest

Source: Adapted from Greulich & Tarrant (2007).

of labor (Austin & Calderon, 1999). In general, a woman with an unfavorable cervix may benefit from relief measures and therapeutic rest in an inpatient setting. Morphine may be administered subcutaneously (15–20 mg) or intramuscularly (10 mg; Anderson, 2011). Approximately 85% of women provided therapeutic rest will progress to the active phase of labor, 10% will have diminished contractions, and 5% with a persistent dysfunctional pattern (Greulich & Tarrant, 2007). Women with prolonged latent phase who are greater than 41 weeks' gestation have a favorable cervix and desire labor stimulation, or have contraindications to expectant management, should be offered pitocin. The favorability of the cervix is determined by the Bishop's score, which includes a digital examination ascertaining cervical dilation, effacement, position, and consistency of the cervix and station. Each component is assigned a numeric value. In general, a Bishop's score of 6 or greater is considered favorable in a multiparous woman and 8 or greater is favorable in a nulliparous woman (Cunningham et al., 2010). For determining the Bishop's score, refer to Table 17.2.

ACTIVE LABOR

Labor is a normal physiologic process characterized by sequential and rhythmic changes that result in birth of the newborn. While it is a continuous process that takes place over time, it is divided into first, second, and third stage of labor. This section will address the diagnosis of the active first stage of labor.

Whereas latent labor is characterized by slow changes in cervical effacement, dilation, and station, the active phase is associated with a faster rate of dilation, generally beginning at 4 cm (Cunningham et al., 2010). The Emergency Medical Treatment and Active Labor Act (EMTALA) comes into play in an obstetric triage or emergency setting when transfer becomes necessary. For example, in an actively laboring woman, the decision to transfer is based on the clinical assessment that there is adequate time to effect a safe transfer to another hospital before delivery.

Recent evidence on the natural progress of labor suggests that for primigravidas, this active phase actually begins at 5 cm and in multiparous women, 6 cm (Zhang, Troendle, Mikolajczykk et al., 2010). The average duration of active labor in healthy women is 7.7 hours for nulliparas and 5.6 hours in multiparas (Albers, 1999).

PRESENTING SYMPTOMATOLOGY

Women presenting in active labor will give a history of contractions occurring at regular time intervals that are gradually shortening. The discomfort may

TABLE 17.2 Assessment of Cervical Ripeness (The Bishop's Score)

PARAMETER/SCORE	0	1	2	3
Position	Posterior	Intermediate	Anterior	–
Consistency	Firm	Intermediate	Soft	–
Effacement	0%–30%	31%–50%	51%–80%	>80%
Dilation	0 cm	1–2 cm	3–4 cm	>5 cm
Fetal station	–3	–2	–1, 0	+1, +2

Source: Adapted from Bishop (1964).

be located in the back or abdomen. The intensity has increased over time, and the discomfort has not been stopped by sedation. Most notably, the cervix will efface and dilate over time. It is crucial to inquire about presence of fetal movement, any leakage of fluid, or vaginal bleeding experienced. Ultimately, labor is a clinical diagnosis, determined by history, cervical change by examination, and uncomfortable uterine contractions.

CLINICAL MANAGEMENT AND FOLLOW-UP

The goals of the initial physical examination are to establish maternal coping/pain control, baseline cervical status, review prenatal record, assess for presence of GBS colonization, and evaluate vital signs. A woman with regular uterine contractions who has demonstrated cervical change or is at least 4 cm is considered in active labor (Cunningham et al., 2010). Contemporary review of labor patterns suggest that active labor starts at 6 cm (Zhang, Troendle, Mikolajczykk et al., 2010). Attempts to define the norms and limits of labor duration have yielded variable results, as labor is difficult to systematically measure (Neal et al., 2010). Clinical decision making takes into account maternal coping, contraction pattern, fetal well-being, and cervical dilation. It is important to keep in mind EMTALA rules, particularly if the emergency setting requires transfer to a hospital with an obstetric unit.

LABORATORY TESTS

A complete blood count (CBC) and blood typing are ordered on actively laboring women. Women who do not have a documented human immunodeficiency virus (HIV) need a rapid HIV drawn, and documentation of hepatitis B screening performed if not available in the medical record. Women with a history of herpes simplex virus are assessed for evidence of prodromal symptoms in addition to an evaluation via sterile speculum examination to visualize for any lesions. Additional laboratory tests will be dependent on maternal history (e.g., diabetes, hypertension) and changes in maternal/fetal status. The GBS status is noted and if appropriate, GBS prophylaxis is initiated as noted in Figure 17.1.

IMMINENT DELIVERY

MANAGING A DELIVERY IN THE OBSTETRIC TRIAGE/EMERGENCY SETTING

Most normal births occur with excellent outcomes, even when the birth occurs outside of a fully equipped labor and delivery unit. Imminent delivery of the newborn requires an understanding of the second stage of labor and the mechanisms of delivery. The second stage of labor begins when the cervix has reached full dilation and is completed with expulsion of the infant.

PRESENTING SYMPTOMATOLOGY

There are common factors that may cause rapid or precipitous delivery, including multiparity and spontaneous rupture of membranes. Signs of imminent

CDC RECOMMENDED REGIMENS FOR INTRAPARTUM ANTIBIOTIC PROPHYLAXIS FOR PREVENTION OF EARLY-ONSET GROUP B STREPTOCOCCAL (GBS) DISEASE*

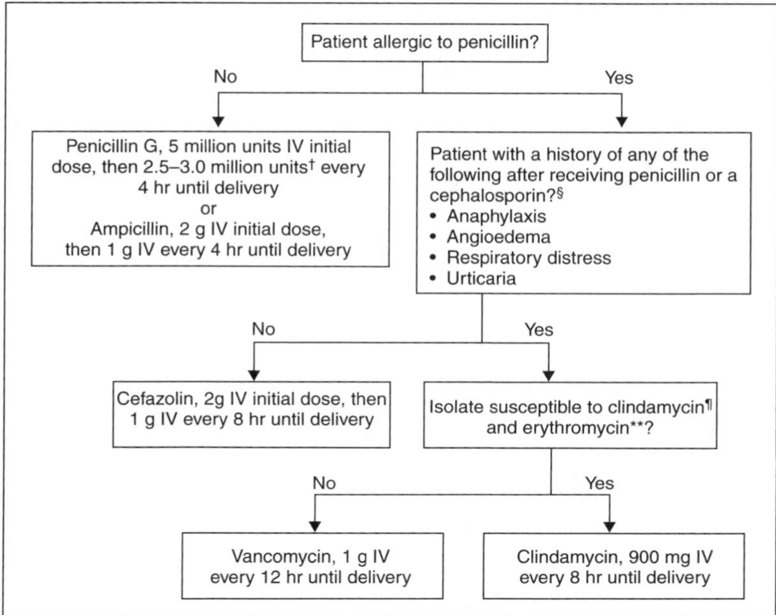

Abbreviation: IV = intravenously.

* Broader spectrum agents, including an agent active against GBS, might be necessary for treatment of chorioamnionitis

† Doses ranging from 2.5 to 3.0 million units are acceptable for the doses administered every 4 hours following the initial dose. The choice of dose within that range should be guided by which formulations of penicillin G are readily available to reduce the need for pharmacies to specially prepare doses.

§ Penicillin-allergic patients with a history of anaphylaxis, angioedema, respiratory distress, or urticaria following administration of penicillin or a cefazolin for GBS intrapartum prophylaxis. For penicillin-allergic patients who do not have a history of those reactions, cefazolin is the preferred agent because pharmacologic data suggest it achieves effective intraamniotic concentrations. Vancomycin and clindamycin should be reserved for pencillin-allergic women at high risk for anaphylaxis.

¶ If laboratory facilities are adequate, clindamycin and erythromycin susceptibility testing (Box 3) should be performed on prenatal GBS isolates from penicillin-allergic women at high risk for anaphylaxis. If no susceptibility testing is performed, or the results are not available at the time of labor, vancomycin is the preferred agent for GBS intrapartum prophylaxis for penicillin-allergic women at high risk for anaphylaxis.

** Resistance to erythromycin is often but not always associated with clindamycin resistance. If an isolate is resistant to erythromycin, it might have inducible resistance to clindamycin, even if it appears susceptible to clindamycin. If a GBS isolate is susceptible to clindamycin, resistant to erythromycin, and testing for inducible clindamycin resistance has been performed and is negative (no inducible resistance), then clindamycin can be used for GBS intrapartum prophylaxis instead of vancomycin.

FIGURE 17.1 Centers for Disease Control and Prevention Guidelines for GBS prophylaxis (CDC, 2010).

delivery include maternal urge to push, involuntary bearing down, separation of labia, bulging perineum, passage of stool, and the maternal declaration that the "baby is coming."

CLINICAL MANAGEMENT

If there is reason to believe that delivery is imminent and there will not be time to transfer the patient, help is requested. The most critical information to ascertain includes the following: when is the due date, what number pregnancy is this, has prenatal care been received, any health problems or pregnancy-related problems. The equipment needed includes gloves, gown, goggles, blankets, bulb syringe, sterile clamps, and sterile scissors. It is important to support the birthing woman by remaining calm, giving gentle, directive, concise communication in addition to reassurance. An additional provider is designated to obtain fetal heart tones. It is critical to keep birth safe by positioning women in either a semi-Fowler's or side-lying position and keeping the room controlled. Universal precautions must be observed at all times. A pediatric provider is called to participate. If membranes are ruptured, any meconium should be noted.

The birth is controlled by providing a calm environment and assisting the mother with gentle breathing. The delivery of the fetal head may be controlled with flexion of the infant's head with nondominant hand, allowing controlled extension of head and supporting the perineum with the opposite hand. As the fetal head extends, a nuchal cord is assessed and if present, gently reduced. As the infant delivers, if the bed makes it difficult to clear the shoulders, then place a bed pan or blanket roll under the woman's buttocks or realign the woman to a lateral position.

Immediate care of the newborn includes keeping the infant warm via skin-to-skin contact with mother, drying, stimulating, and clearing the airway. The umbilical cord may be cut and clamped following delivery and the apgars assigned.

It is critical that the obstetric triage unit have a coordinated drill in place for deliveries that take place prior to transfer to the labor floor. Simulations, practice drills, and team training can ensure that imminent delivery can take place in a calm, safe environment.

REFERENCES

American College of Nurse Midwives (ACNM). (2008). *Position statement. Premature rupture of membranes (PROM) at term*. Retrieved from www.acnm.org

American College of Obstetricians and Gynecologists (ACOG). (2007). Committee on practice bulletin no. 80. Premature rupture of membranes. American College of Obstetricians and Gynecologists. *Obstetrics and Gynecology, 109*, 1007–1019.

Albers, L. L. (1999). The duration of labor in healthy women. *Journal of Perinatology, 19*(2), 114–119.

Anderson, D. (2011). Review of systemic opioids commonly used for labor pain relief. *Journal of Nurse Midwifery and Women's Health, 56*(3), 222–239.

Austin, D. A., & Calderon, L. (1999). Triaging patients in the latent phase of labor. *Journal of Nurse Midwifery, 44*(6), 585–591.

Bishop, E. H. (1964). Pelvic scoring for elective induction. *Obstetrics and Gynecology,* 24*266–268.

Center for Disease Control. (2010). *2010 guidelines for the prevention of perinatal group B streptococcal disease*. Retrieved from www.cdc.gov

Cunningham, F. G., Leveno, K. J., Bloom, S. L., Hauth, J. C., & Rouse, D. J. (2010). Antepartum assessment. In F. G. Cunningham, K. J. Leveno, S. L. Bloom, J. C. Hauth, & D. J. Rouse (Eds.), *Williams obstetrics* (pp. 334–348, 23rd ed.). Columbus, OH: The McGraw-Hill Companies, Inc.

Friedman, E. A. (1967). Labor: Clinical evaluation and management. New York: Appleton-Century-Crofts.

Greulich, B., & Tarrant, B. (2007). The latent phase of labor: Diagnosis and management. *Journal of Midwifery and Women's Health, 52*(3), 190–198.

Hannah, M. E., Ohlsson, A., Farine, D., Hewson, S. A., Hodnett, E. D., Myhr, T. L.,... Willan, A. R. (1996). Induction of labor compared with expectant management for prelabor rupture of membranes at term. TERMPROM Study Group. *New England Journal of Medicine, 334*, 1005.

Neal, J. L., Lowe, N. K., Ahijevych, K. L., Patric, T. E., Cabbage, L., & Corwin, E. J. (2010). "Active Labor" duration and dilation rates among low-risk, nulliparous women with spontaneous labor onset: A systematic review. *Journal of Midwifery and Women's Health, 55*(4), 308–318.

Seaward, P. G., Hannah, M. E., Myhr, T. L., Farine, D., Ohlsson, A., Wang, E. E.,... Hodnett, E. D. (1997). International Multicentre Term Premature Rupture of Membranes Study: Evaluation of predictors of clinical chorioamnionitis and postpartum fever in patients with premature rupture of membranes at term. *American Journal of Obstetrics and Gynecology, 177*(5), 1024–1029.

Simkin, P., & Ancheta, R. (2011). The labor progress handbook (3rd ed.). Hoboken, NJ: Wiley Blackwell.

Simkin, P. (2010). The fetal OP positions. *Birth, 37*(1), 67–71.

Zhang, J., Landy, H. J., Branch, W., Burkman, R., Haberman, S., Gregory, K. D.,... Consortium on Safe Labor. (2010). Contemporary patterns of spontaneous labor with normal neonatal outcomes. *Obstetrics and Gynecology, 116*(6), 1281–1287.

Zhang, J., Troendle, J., Mikolajczykk, R., Sundaram, R., Beaver, J., & Fraser, W. (2010). The natural history of the normal first stage of labor. *Obstetrics and Gynecology, 115*(4), 705–710.

Zlatnik, F. J. (1992). Management of premature rupture of membranes at term. *Obstetrics and Gynecology Clinics of North America, 19*(2), 353–364.

Severe Medical Complications in Pregnancy 18

Lucia Larson and Karen Rosene-Montella

Pregnant women with potentially serious medical illnesses are a challenge to the clinician. Women can develop new medical illnesses coincidental to pregnancy or may have underlying medical disease that worsens with the physiologic changes of pregnancy. Women are increasingly delaying pregnancy until they are older and there are also more medical complications associated with increasing age and the obesity epidemic. An approach to evaluating pregnant women in the obstetric (OB) triage unit is outlined and complications that could represent serious medical illness (and not illness) are noted. Topics that are addressed include headache, shortness of breath (SOB) and pulmonary disease, chest pain and cardiovascular disorders, as well as selected causes of abdominal pain.

HEADACHE

Headache is a common complaint in pregnancy and the majority of women presenting to OB triage have migraine, tension type headaches, or headaches related to preeclampsia. Other serious and potential life-threatening causes of headaches that must be diagnosed and treated promptly are noted in Table 18.1.

Though most headaches caused by preeclampsia do not cause neurologic impairment or death, a subset of women with preeclampsia will have associated subarachnoid hemorrhage, intracerebral bleeding, or posterior reversible encephalopathy syndrome (PRES). The risk for subarachnoid hemorrhage from rupture of cerebral aneurysms and arteriovenous malformations is increased in pregnant women. The gravida is also at risk for cerebral vein thrombosis and benign increased intracranial hypertension (pseudotumor cerebri). Tumor can also present as headache during pregnancy.

Migraine headaches often worsen in the beginning of pregnancy, paralleling the hormonal changes of the early pregnancy and are described as headaches with characteristics similar to prepregnancy headaches. The presence of an aura, unilateral throbbing, and nausea and vomiting are suggestive of a migraine. Triggering factors such as certain foods (nuts, aged cheeses, and caffeine), change in sleep pattern, or stress may be identified. Since many women eliminate caffeine intake with pregnancy, caffeine withdrawal may trigger headaches early in pregnancy, as well. Tension type headaches are

TABLE 18.1 Selected Causes of Headache in Pregnant Women Presenting to Obstetric Triage/Emergency Department

CAUSE OF HEADACHE	DISTINGUISHING FEATURES	COMMENTS	TREATMENT
Most Common			
Tension Type	Bilateral, nonthrobbing steady mild to moderate pain. Not worsened by physical activity	May be associated with muscular tenderness. Medication may have been discontinued	Acetaminophen preferred analgesic
Migraine	Unilateral, throbbing headache, associated with nausea, vomiting, photophobia, phonophobia. May be preceded by aura (typically visual but may have other neurologic manifestation)	Patients may be able to identify specific triggers. Migraine frequency typically decreases as pregnancy progresses but worsens postpartum. Medication may have been discontinued	Acetaminophen (can be combined with beverage containing caffeine), metoclopramide, prochlorperazine, IV magnesium
Most Serious			
Preeclampsia/Eclampsia • Intracerebral bleed • Subarachnoid bleed • Cerebral edema and ischemia • PRES	May have abnormal preeclampsia labs. Headache migrainous in nature and may be associated with focal neurologic signs and symptoms. Seizures may occur	Head CT and/or brain MRI can be useful	Careful blood pressure control Caution with fluids Delivery when appropriate
Subarachnoid Hemorrhage • Cerebral aneurysm • Arteriovenous malformation (AVM) • Preeclampsia/eclampsia	Sudden onset thunderclap headache. With sentinel bleed headache can improve but with continued bleeding, declining mental status develops	Rupture of aneurysm and AVM increased in pregnancy. Noncontrast head CT best to identify blood. MRI to identify specific lesions. Not 100% diagnostic so lumbar puncture (LP) to identify blood in cerebral spinal fluid (CSF) required in patient with sudden onset headache and negative imaging. Associated with high mortality	

Cerebral Vein Thrombosis	Variable presentation: only headache that may be mild to sudden onset severe. May worsen with reclining or Valsalva. Have focal signs and symptoms, seizures or declining mental status	Diagnosis requires MRI with venous imagining (MRV) Increased incidence in pregnancy. May be associated with hypercoagulable states	Treatment usually entails anticoagulation with LMWH
Pseudotumor Cerebri	Headache migraine, tension or have associated visual symptoms, photopsia or diplopia. May have pulsatile tinnitus. Papilledema present and may have visual field cut and/or 6th nerve palsy	MRI should be obtained to rule out lesion. LP reveals elevated opening pressure. Formal visual fields critical to monitor optic nerve involvement as vision loss is a serious complication	Acetazolomide, steroids or serial LPs to decrease opening pressure
Tumor Meningioma, Malignancy	Headaches may be focal, worse in a.m. and improve during the day, progressive and associated with nausea. Focal neurologic signs and symptoms develop	CT scan or MRI	
Meningitis	Global severe headache in ill patient presenting with fever and nuchal rigidity. Altered mental status common in acute bacterial meningitis	Emergent lumbar puncture diagnostic. Head CT prior to LP is only necessary if there is concern for mass lesion as suggested by focal neurologic findings on exam	Antibiotics as soon as possible and should include ampicillin for *Listeria* coverage in pregnant women. Typical regimen vancomycin, a third generation cephalosporin, plus ampicillin

Continued

TABLE 18.1 Selected Causes of Headache in Pregnant Women Presenting to Obstetric Triage/Emergency Department *Continued*

CAUSE OF HEADACHE	DISTINGUISHING FEATURES	COMMENTS	TREATMENT
Pituitary Apoplexy	Sudden onset headache associated with ophthalmoplegia and change in mental status	Caused by sudden hemorrhage or infarct in pituitary gland with pituitary adenoma. Macroadenomas increase in size in pregnancy	
Other Causes Worth Considering			
Rebound Headaches	Occurs in patients with headache who have been taking analgesics more than 2 to 3 days per week. Headaches develop with awakening and occur daily		Stop offending agent. Administer prophylaxis for underlying headache disorder
Obstructive Sleep Apnea (OSA)	Morning headaches associated daytime somnolence, snoring, or other symptoms of OSA	OSA can develop in pregnancy and may be related to weight gain and/or edema of upper airways	

typically tight, squeezing headaches that worsen later in the day and are not associated with aura, visual or other neurologic signs or symptoms, or nausea or vomiting. Alerts that suggest more serious causes of headache include sudden onset (thunder clap), new or different type of headache, worsening upon awakening in the morning or waking up at night, onset with exertion, association with neurologic impairment, or fever. In addition, victims of domestic violence may present with chronic complaints including headaches.

When migraine or severe tension headache is not relieved by acetaminophen alone the addition of caffeine (such as coffee or a cola drink) and/or metoclopramide or prochlorperazine may be helpful. Narcotics are frequently suboptimally effective and are also associated with rebound headaches (Goadsby, Goldberg, & Silberstein, 2008). Despite this, they can be helpful in the acute setting. Intravenous (IV) magnesium (1–2 g) is useful for relief of acute migraines in nonpregnant women and it is reasonable to assume it may be effective and safe during pregnancy. If acute treatment does not provide adequate control of headache, prophylactic medication such as beta blockers and tricyclic antidepressants are an option.

RESPIRATORY ISSUES

Shortness of Breath

Dyspnea is a common complaint in normal pregnancy experienced by up to 50% of women. However, pathologic cardiopulmonary causes are essential to distinguish as noted in Table 18.2.

The pregnant woman with dyspnea of pregnancy has symptoms at rest but not with exertion and may describe the need to "take deep breaths" or frequent "sighs." There may also be SOB while talking on the telephone. These women are thought to be particularly sensitive to the normal increased tidal volume of pregnancy. Deconditioning or SOB associated with progressing pregnancy and weight gain may cause dyspnea on exertion but the history and physical exam are otherwise reassuring. The presence of wheezing, chest tightness, cough, or nocturnal awakening suggests asthma as a cause of dyspnea. A history of pulmonary or cardiac disease predating pregnancy suggests the possibility of worsening disease or an inability to tolerate pregnancy physiologic changes. SOB that presents at the peak of blood volume (28–32 weeks) may be due to underlying cardiac disease exacerbated by increased volume. Associated symptoms which suggest concerning underlying pathology include fever, cough, chest tightness or chest pain, orthopnea (though this can be present in normal pregnant women secondary to the elevated diaphragm), and paroxysmal nocturnal dyspnea (PND). Physical exam findings mandating a more extensive workup for underlying cardiopulmonary disease include increased respiratory rate, decreased pulse oximetry at rest or with exertion, tachycardia, abnormal lung exam, elevated jugular venous pulsation (JVP), loud murmurs or gallops on cardiac exam. An initial workup includes a complete blood count (CBC), shielded anterior-posterior (AP) and lateral chest x-rays (CXR), and an electrocardiogram (ECG). Evaluation for pulmonary embolism (PE) with chest CT pulmonary angiogram (CTPA) and lower extremity Doppler or ventilation perfusion scan (VQ scan), underlying structural heart abnormalities with an echocardiogram, or other lung pathology with pulmonary function tests may be indicated.

TABLE 18.2 Selected Causes of Shortness of Breath (SOB) in Pregnant Women Presenting to Obstetric Triage/Emergency Department

ETIOLOGY	FEATURES	COMMENTS
Dyspnea of Pregnancy	Experience of "air hunger" or the need to take a deep breath. Patients note the need to "catch their breath" while talking on the phone. There are no symptoms or physical exam findings suggestive of underlying cardiac or pulmonary disease	Thought to be caused by awareness of the increased ventilation in pregnancy. Begins early in pregnancy at an average of 18 weeks' gestation. Tends to improve later in pregnancy
Asthma	Complaints of chest tightness, dyspnea and nocturnal awakening. Cough is common. May identify triggers such as cigarette smoke, gastroesophageal reflux, or sinusitis. Exam reveals wheezing	Pulmonary function tests and peak flow measurements useful. CXR is normal, if obtained. Treatment includes beta agonists and steroids as per the National Asthma Guideline Recommendations (National Asthma Education and Prevention Program, 2007)
Pneumonia	Cough, fever, and SOB are typical presenting features. Physical exam reveals evidence of lung consolidation	Chest x-ray reveals pneumonia. Most gravidas with pneumonia require admission to monitor for progression and to ensure oxygen saturations remain above 95%
Pulmonary Embolism (PE)	Variable presentation which may include SOB, dizziness, sudden onset pleuritic chest pain, hemoptysis, and palpitations. Exam may or may not reveal tachycardia, hypotension, hypoxia, pleural rub or evidence of lower extremity DVT	ECG may reveal sinus tachycardia of right heart strain but often normal. Chest x-ray may be normal. CTPA done in combination with lower extremity Dopplers or VQ scanning is diagnostic. D-dimers not validated in pregnancy Treatment is anticoagulation with LMWH or unfractionated heparin. Patients may require IVC filter if near term, unable to tolerate anticoagulants, have failed anticoagulants or have large clot burden
Pulmonary Edema	SOB associated with crackles on lung exam. Look for underlying disorder associated with pulmonary edema such as preeclampsia, sepsis or pyelonephritis, abnormal cardiac exam if associated underlying cardiac disease	May respond readily to diuresis with furosemide and treatment of underlying precipitating disorder. Physiologic changes which predispose to pulmonary edema include increased blood volume and lower oncotic pressure. With preeclampsia there is associated endothelial damage and further lowering of oncotic pressure. If there is infection, there may be increased effects of endotoxin

Continued

TABLE 18.2 Selected Causes of Shortness of Breath (SOB) in Pregnant Women Presenting to Obstetric Triage/Emergency Department *Continued*

ETIOLOGY	FEATURES	COMMENTS
Pulmonary Hypertension	Progressive SOB which may or may not be associated with chest pain and syncope. Cardiac exam may reveal persistent S2 splitting and there may be evidence of right sided heart failure on exam in severe cases	ECG may reveal right heart strain. Echo elevated pulmonary artery pressures but cardiac catheterization is necessary for accurate measurement. Search for secondary causes including PE is crucial. Pulmonary hypertension has a very high mortality in pregnancy
Valvular Heart Disease	Progressive SOB with cough, orthopnea, PND, and exertional symptoms suggest cardiac disease. May have elevated JVP, cardiac murmur and gallop, crackles on lung exam, and lower extremity edema.	Cardiac echo is diagnostic. The physiologic demands of pregnancy may unmask previously well compensated valvular heart disease.
Peripartum Cardiomyopathy	In addition to progressive dyspnea, cough, orthopnea, and PND, patients may present with palpitations or syncope secondary to an arrhythmia. Exam reveals elevated JVP, displaced point of maximal impulse, gallop, crackles on lung exam, and edema	Cardiac echo reveals ventricular dysfunction. Presents later in pregnancy and no other causes of cardiomyopathy is identified. Preeclampsia must be differentiated. Causes of death include arrhythmia, thromboembolic disease, and progressive heart failure
Myocardial Ischemia/Infarct (MI)	Classic presentation includes substernal chest tightness that radiates to left shoulder/arm and jaw and is associated with SOB, nausea, vomiting, and diaphoresis. Atypical presentations are common in women so high index of suspicion is necessary	ECG and cardiac enzymes used for diagnosis. Women may not have traditional risk factors such as diabetes, hypertension, hyperlipidemia, and smoking. Mechanism may be coronary artery dissection, thrombosis in a normal coronary artery, or vasospasm, in addition to coronary artery disease. Cocaine should be considered

Pulmonary Embolism (PE)

PE in pregnancy is a leading cause of maternal death in developed nations (Zeitlin & Mohangoo, 2008). Factors contributing to the increased risk of thrombosis in pregnancy include venodilation secondary to hormonal and mechanical factors, increase in prothrombotic and decrease in fibrinolytic factors, and venous trauma at labor and delivery. Risk factors for thrombosis in pregnancy include history of thrombophilia, smoking, elevated body mass index particularly in the setting of antepartum immobilization, age, parity, cesarean delivery, preeclampsia, and assisted reproductive techniques (Jacobson, Skejeldestad, & Sandset, 2008; James, Jamison, & Brancazio, 2006; van Walraven et al., 2003).

There is no one clinical sign or symptom that is consistently seen in gravidas with PE and a high index of suspicion is needed to prevent missing this potentially fatal diagnosis. Women may or may not present with chest pain, SOB, tachypnea, tachycardia, hypoxia, abnormal CXR, or ECG. In one study, over half of pregnant women with documented PE had normal pO_2 on arterial blood gas and normal A-a gradients (Powrie et al., 1998). In the nonpregnant population, the Wells' criteria (Wells et al., 2000) and Geneva criteria (Le Gal et al., 2006) are useful clinical decision tools for determining the probability of PE but elements of these tools, such as heart rate, are altered by pregnancy physiology. Further, the use of D-dimers is hampered by increasing levels as gestation progresses and cannot be considered reliable to rule out PE in the gravida without further studies.

Since these tools have not been validated in pregnancy, diagnostic imaging is the cornerstone for the diagnosis of PE in pregnant women. The initial evaluation includes a CXR that may reveal an alternate diagnosis with minimal radiation exposure. PE can then be definitively diagnosed with either a ventilation perfusion scan (VQ scan) or CTPA. An advantage of the CTPA is the potential to identify an alternate diagnosis with lower fetal radiation exposure. However, the risk for maternal breast cancer may be increased because CTPA exposes the maternal breasts to as much as 2 to 5 rads of radiation (Miller et al., 2011). Some centers use breast shields to mitigate this risk. In addition, CTPA is more likely to be technically limited in pregnancy because the increased blood volume and cardiac output affect the arrival of contrast to the pulmonary artery. The VQ scan has a strong negative predictive value for PE and fetal radiation exposure is still well within an acceptable range. Some clinicians prefer it to CPTA particularly for women who have had previous CT scans or who are otherwise at increased risk for breast cancer. Local expertise in interpreting the results of VQ or CTPA is also a driving force in determining the best test to order. In the pregnant woman with symptoms of PE and findings suggest a lower extremity deep vein thrombosis (DVT), a lower extremity Doppler ultrasound is a reasonable first test. If a DVT is identified, PE can be presumed and therapeutic anticoagulation is indicated regardless.

The mortality of untreated PE is 30% and death can occur from a recurrent PE within several hours of the initial event. Since anticoagulation decreases mortality to 2% to 8%, it is crucial to begin treatment quickly (Kearon et al., 2008). In women with a high suspicion for PE and low risk for bleeding, anticoagulation is begun immediately so as not to delay for the results of testing. Stable women with a potential alternative diagnosis in whom testing is performed quickly can be treated after the results of investigations are known. The preferred initial treatment for PE is low molecular weight heparin (LMWH) because of its proven mortality benefits, associated decreased recurrence of thrombosis, better bioavailability, ease of administration, and decreased risk of heparin induced thrombocytopenia. IV unfractionated heparin still has an important role for use in women at high risk for bleeding, near delivery, with significant hypotension, obesity, or renal insufficiency, and in whom thrombolytics may be considered.

Though the use of thrombolytics has been reported in pregnancy with a risk of bleeding similar to that of nonpregnant women, thrombolytics are most likely to be beneficial in the hemodynamically unstable gravida with refractory hypoxemia (Leonhardt et al., 2006). Inferior vena cava (IVC) filters may be considered for use in pregnant women with PE who have contraindications to anticoagulation or in whom a large clot burden has been identified in the lower extremities or pelvis, which could potentially cause a fatal recurrent PE.

Asthma

Asthma is a common medical condition in pregnancy affecting approximately 3.7% to 8.4% of pregnancies in the United States (Kwon, Belanger & Bracken, 2003). Though asthma does not necessarily worsen in pregnancy, approximately one-third of women will develop asthma exacerbations during gestation. Exacerbations are more likely to occur in women who have more severe asthma prior to pregnancy (Schatz et al., 2003). Factors specific to pregnancy that may contribute to exacerbations include hormonal changes, noncompliance with medications, increased gastroesophageal reflux, and possible triggering by rhinitis of pregnancy.

Gravidas with an asthma exacerbation present with SOB, wheezing, cough, and/or chest tightness. Physical exam may reveal increased respiratory and heart rate, hypoxia, wheezing, and decreased air flow. Use of accessory muscles of respiration and paradoxical breathing portend respiratory failure. Peak flows are helpful to determine severity of attack if performed with proper technique. Though pulse oximetry determines oxygenation, an arterial blood gas is necessary in women suspected of having more serious exacerbations to assess maternal $PaCO_2$. In pregnancy, the normal maternal PaO_2 is 100 to 105 mmHg and average $PaCO_2$ is 30 mmHg. For fetal well-being, it is necessary to maintain the pregnant woman's oxygenation saturation greater than 95% or the maternal pO_2 at at least 70 mmHg of oxygen. The pregnant asthmatic with a $PaCO_2$ of 35 mmHg is already retaining CO_2 and signifies impending respiratory failure. Because of the increased rates of aspiration and failed intubation in pregnancy, it is critical to anticipate the possible need for intubation in advance so that equipment and experienced personnel are as prepared as possible.

Supplemental oxygen, short acting beta agonists (SABA), and steroids are used for treatment of acute asthma exacerbations in pregnant women as in the nonpregnant population (National Asthma Education and Prevention Program, 2007). Albuterol can be administered by nebulizer or metered dose inhaler and is initially given every 20 minutes for three doses followed by hourly doses as needed. Women who do not respond quickly to SABA or who are already taking steroids require the addition of methylprednisolone or prednisone. Ipratropium is added for severe exacerbations. CXR is indicated if there is concern about an underlying pulmonary process such as pneumonia. Women can be discharged with close outpatient follow up if the peak expiratory flow rate is greater than or equal to 70% of predicted, there is a sustained response 60 minutes after the last treatment, no supplemental oxygen is required to keep oxygen saturation greater than 95% at rest or with exertion, there is no distress and physical exam is normal. A low threshold for admission in pregnancy is prudent if there is any concern since pregnant women have less respiratory reserve and higher oxygen saturation requirements than nonpregnant women.

CARDIAC AND VASCULAR ISSUES

Chest Pain

The causes of chest pain in pregnancy range from benign and self-limiting to potentially life-threatening. An initial history and physical exam help to narrow the differential. Often, the clinician is able to tell patients what the pain "isn't" with more certainty than what the pain "is." It can be reassuring that once the life-threatening causes are eliminated, it is unlikely that the cause of the chest pain will be harmful to either the pregnant woman or fetus and will likely resolve quickly. Many causes of chest pain also cause SOB and the evaluation for these disorders overlap. The most serious causes of chest pain that must not be missed include PE, myocardial ischemia, and aortic dissection. Table 18.3 provides an overview of key points for chest pain in pregnancy.

Myocardial Ischemia and Infarction

The risk for myocardial infarct (MI) is increased by 3- to 4-fold in pregnancy as compared with the nonpregnant state (James, Jamison, & Biswass, 2006). Pregnant women with myocardial ischemia may present with classic substernal chest tightness associated with dyspnea, nausea and diaphoresis but they can also present atypically so a high index of suspicion is needed. Risk factors for MI in pregnancy include maternal age over 35, hypertension, diabetes mellitus, obesity, eclampsia, and severe preeclampsia (Ladner, Danielsen, & Gilbert, 2005). In one study of the coronary arteries of 103 women with MI in pregnancy, only 40%were found to have atherosclerotic disease while 27% had coronary artery dissection, 8% had thrombus in a normal coronary artery, 2% had spasm, 2% had emboli, and 13% were found to be normal (Roth & Elkayam, 2008). Treatment includes oxygen, aspirin, beta blockers, heparin, and nitrates. Cardiac catheterization is preferred over thrombolysis because of the increased incidence of coronary artery dissection.

Vascular Issues

Pregnant women have an increased risk for arterial dissections and this is thought to be related to the hormonal and hemodynamic changes of pregnancy. Examples include the increased incidence of cerebral aneurysm rupture and coronary artery dissection. In addition, women with Marfan's syndrome and dilated aortic roots greater than 4.0 to 4.5 cm are at very high risk of aortic dissection. Beta blockers are used in these women to decrease shear forces on the vasculature. The pain associated with aortic dissection is typically described as a severe tearing pain radiating to the back. Ehlers Danlos Type IV has a high maternal mortality not only secondary to arterial rupture but there is also a significant risk for bowel and uterine rupture in pregnancy. Splenic artery aneurysms are more likely to occur in women and are not necessarily associated with portal hypertension. Rupture is more likely to happen in the third trimester and is associated with high maternal and fetal mortality. Early diagnosis with ultrasound or CT scan with prompt intervention may be lifesaving. The diagnosis needs consideration in any pregnant woman presenting with severe upper abdominal pain especially if hemodynamicaly unstable (Sadat, Dar, Walsh, & Varty, 2008).

Palpitations

Palpitations are commonly reported by pregnant women and while the majority of them do not have serious medical causes, recognizing those who have serious arrhythmias is crucial. A previous history of cardiac disease, such as congenital heart disease, increases the likelihood of finding an

TABLE 18.3 Selected Causes of Chest Pain in the Pregnant Women Presenting to Obstetric Triage/Emergency Department

ETIOLOGY	FEATURES	COMMENTS
Musculoskeletal	Tenderness found on palpation. Pain associated with movements. May have bruising or swelling noted associated with trauma	Careful questioning about domestic violence which increases during pregnancy is indicated as women may be reluctant to disclose. PE may have chest wall tenderness
Gastroesophageal Reflux (GERD)	Retrosternal burning pain often associated with food intake. Squeezing may represent esophageal spasm	Common in pregnancy secondary to decreased lower esophageal tone and delayed gastric emptying. Antireflux measures, antacids, metoclopramide, and ranitidine helpful. Omeprazole may be considered if these measures inadequate
Pericarditis	Pain typically improves with sitting up and leaning forward. Often sharp and pleuritic in nature	ECG evolves and can show PR depression, widespread ST elevation, T wave inversions. Cardiac echo may show pericardial effusion. Elevated troponin and CPK signals associated myocarditis
Myocardial Ischemia/Infarct (MI) [See Table 18.2]	SOB, nausea, vomiting, and diaphoresis classic associated symptoms of MI. Women often present with atypical symptoms so high index of suspicion is necessary	ECG, cardiac enzymes are initial workup. Cardiac echo may be useful. Pregnant women with myocardial ischemia may have traditional risk factors for coronary artery disease but risk factors may be absent in those with coronary artery dissection, thrombosis within a normal coronary artery and vasospasm, all of which occur as a cause of MI in pregnancy. Cocaine should also be considered
Aortic Dissection	Acute onset of severe tearing or ripping pain in chest that may radiate to back. Associated signs and symptoms may be seen from involvement of branches of the aorta. These include stroke, myocardial infarction, paraplegia, and loss of pulses. New aortic insufficiency may be heard on cardiac exam and discrepancy of 20 mg Hg between arms may be noted	Life threatening emergency. CXR may show widened mediastinum or aorta. ECG may be normal or show ischemia. CT scan, MRI, or transesophageal echo diagnostic. Increased incidence in pregnancy. Associated with Marfan's, Turner's syndromes, and coarctation of the aorta. Also bicuspid aortic valve, Ehlers- Danlos syndrome, vasculitis, trauma, and crack cocaine

Continued

TABLE 18.3 Selected Causes of Chest Pain in the Pregnant Women Presenting to Obstetric Triage/Emergency Department *Continued*

ETIOLOGY	FEATURES	COMMENTS
Pulmonary Embolus (PE) [See Table 18.2]	Sudden onset of chest pain that is classically pleuritic but may be constant. May be associated with SOB, hemoptysis, or palpitation but presentation is variable and requires high index of suspicion. Exam may or may not reveal tachycardia, hypotension, hypoxia, pleural rub or evidence of lower extremity DVT	ECG most likely to reveal sinus tachycardia. It may also show right heart strain but more often it is normal. Chest x-ray may be normal. CTPA done in combination with lower extremity Dopplers or VQ scanning is diagnostic. D-dimers are not validated for the diagnosis of venous thromboembolism in pregnancy (Miller et al., 2011)
Pneumonia	Cough, fever, and SOB typical presenting features. May have history of antecedent viral illness. Physical exam reveals evidence of lung consolidation	Chest x-ray reveals pneumonia. Most gravidas with pneumonia require admission to monitor for progression and to ensure oxygen saturations remain above 95%
Pneumothorax	Abrupt onset of pleuritic chest pain and SOB. Decreased breath sounds may be noted on affected side. Patient may have a previous history of pneumothorax. Smoking is a risk factor	Upright chest x-ray diagnostic. Tension pneumothorax is associated with hypoxia, tachycardia and hypotension and requires immediate aspiration
Herpes Zoster	Pain may be described as burning, stabbing, or throbbing and can precede the vesicular rash. Hypoesthesia in the dermatomal distribution is sometimes present	Rash may develop as long as 30 days after pain
Preeclampsia/ Eclampsia/HELLP/ Acute Fatty Liver of Pregnancy	Not typically associated with chest pain but it can occur	Rarely preeclampsia/eclampsia is associated with MI. Pain originating in the liver can occasionally be felt as chest or epigastric pain

arrhythmia requiring intervention. Supraventricular arrhythmias are more common but ventricular arrhythmias also occur with increased frequency in pregnancy. The history of a sudden onset rapid rhythm with sudden termination is suggestive of supraventricular tachycardia whereas a slow resolution is more suggestive of sinus tachycardia. A rapid irregular rhythm suggests atrial fibrillation. A dangerous ventricular arrhythmia may present with presyncope or sudden syncope and it is particularly concerning if there is a family history of premature or sudden death. Physical exam may reveal an abnormal rate and heart sounds which are clues to underlying cardiac disease. The cardiac monitor and 12 lead ECG may reveal the rhythm abnormality but may be normal if the symptoms have resolved. Abnormalities on the ECG may be suggestive of underlying cardiac disease, a bypass tract, or

TABLE 18.4 Causes of Palpitations in Pregnant Women Presenting to Obsteric Triage

ARRHYTHMIA	FEATURES	COMMENTS
Sinus Tachycardia	Often asymptomatic but in the symptomatic patient gradually improves with treatment of underlying disorder	Look for underlying causes including anemia, pulmonary embolism, thyroid disease, infection/sepsis, hypotension, fever, hypoxia, dehydration, myocardial ischemia, heart failure, drugs, pain, pheochromocytoma, anxiety
Supraventricular Tachycardia, Including Wolfe-Parkinson-White (WPW) Syndrome	Sudden onset of rapid regular rhythm that may or may not be associated with presyncope/syncope, chest pain, and SOB	Vagal maneuvers should be tried first; IV adenosine, beta-blockers, calcium channel blockers can be used. Direct current (DC) cardioversion can be used if indicated
Atrial Fibrillation or Flutter	Rapid irregularly irregular rhythm that may or may not be associated with presyncope/syncope, chest pain, and SOB	Beta blockers, calcium channel blockers, digoxin, procainamide can be used safely. Amiodarone should be avoided if possible because of concern for the fetal thyroid. Anticoagulation with LMWH may be appropriate in some cases to prevent thromboembolic disease. Consider underlying precipitating causes such as PE, thyroid disease, and infection
Ventricular Tachycardia	Rapid rhythm associated with syncope/presyncope, chest pain, and/or SOB	DC cardioversion if indicated. Lidocaine preferred over amiodarone secondary to concern for fetal thyroid function

reveal a prolonged QT interval that is associated with ventricular arrhythmia. Women at risk for serious arrhythmia require admission to a telemetry unit even if symptoms have resolved and the ECG is normal. Those at low risk may be further evaluated with an outpatient holter monitor or event monitor. An echocardiogram is necessary to assess for structural heart abnormalities in women with true arrhythmia. Most of the medications used to treat nonpregnant women can be used safely in pregnancy. Direct current (DC) cardioversion can and should be used when indicated (Adamson & Nelson-Piercy, 2007). Table 18.4 summarizes the causes of palpitations in pregnant women.

SELECTED CAUSES OF ABDOMINAL PAIN

Cholelithiasis, appendicitis, and bowel obstruction in pregnancy are covered elsewhere in this book. However, selected causes of abdominal pain that are less common but important or unusual will be discussed here. Epigastric pain that radiates to the back, improves with leaning forward, and is associated with nausea and vomiting is typical of pancreatitis. Specific pregnancy associated causes of pancreatitis include cholelithiasis and hypertriglyceridemia. Supportive laboratories are elevated amylase and lipase and ultrasound may be helpful to identify gallstones, inflammation or psuedocyst. Thrombosis of mesenteric, pelvic, and hepatic vessels also occurs in pregnancy. Typically this pain is difficult to localize but helpful diagnostic tests include abdominal/pelvic CT scan or magnetic resonance imaging (MRI) taken with images to evaluate the arteries and veins. An elevated lactic acid is ominous signaling bowel ischemia. Women who note the sudden onset of pain associated with trauma, cough, or sudden movement may have a rectus sheath hematoma. Physical exam reveals tenderness on palpation and ultrasound is helpful for diagnosis. The mechanical changes of pregnancy are likely responsible for the predisposition to rectus sheath hematoma but hypertension and anticoagulation are also risk factors. The sudden onset of abdominal pain in association with hypovolemic shock may be caused by aneurysm rupture but spontaneous hemoperitoneum has also been reported from bleeding of superficial veins of the uterus or parametrium (Brosens, Fusi, & Brosens, 2009). A history of endometriosis and nulliparity appear to be risk factors. Though not necessarily a primary abdominal disorder, diabetic ketoacidosis (DKA) can present with abdominal pain that may be associated with nausea, vomiting, polyuria, polydipsia, and altered mental status. Glucose is typically elevated but a significant number of pregnant women with DKA present with glucose less than 200. Chemistries reveal an elevated anion gap, creatinine may be elevated, and serum ketones are positive. Immediate hydration, IV insulin, correction of electrolyte abnormalities, and a search for the underlying cause of DKA are imperative to decrease maternal and fetal morbidity and mortality.

The clinician caring for the pregnant woman presenting to the OB triage unit or emergency room with medical illness must consider a broad differential of disorders including those that occur coincidental to pregnancy, those that may be affected by the pregnant state, and those unique to pregnancy itself. The management of pregnant women with severe medical illness often requires an interdisciplinary team which includes the obstetrician/maternal fetal medicine physician, OB internist, surgeon, and other subspecialists.

REFERENCES

Adamson, D. L., & Nelson-Piercy, C. (2007). Managing palpitations and arrhythmias during pregnancy. *Heart, 93*, 1630–1636.

Brosens, I. A., Fusi, L. & Brosens, J. J. (2009). Endometriosis is a risk factor for spontaneous hemoperitoneum during pregnancy. *Fertility and Sterility, 92*, 1243–1245.

Goadsby, P. J., Goldberg, J., & Silberstein, S. D. (2008). Migraine in pregnancy. *BMJ, 336*(7659), 1502–1504.

Jacobson, A. F., Skejeldestad, F. E., & Sandset, P. M. (2008). Ante- and postnatal risk factors of thrombosis: A hospital-based case control study. *Journal of Thrombosis and Haemostasis, 6*, 905–912.

James, A. H., Jamison, M. G., Bisswas, M. S., et al. (2006) Acute myocardial infarction in pregnancy: A United States population based study. *Circulation, 113*(12), 1564–1571.

James, A. H., Jamison, M. G., Brancazio, L. R., et al. (2006). Venous thromboembolism during pregnancy and the postpartum period: Incidence, risk factors, and mortality. *American Journal of Obstetrics & Gynecology, 194*, 1311–1315.

Kearon, C., Kahn, S. R., & Agnelli, G, et al. (2008) Antithrombotic therapy for venous thromboembolic disease: American College of Chest Physician Evidence-Based Clinical Practice Guidelines (8th edition). *Chest*, *133*(Suppl. 6):454S–545S. Erratum in Chest 2008;*134*(4), 892.

Kwon, H. L., Belanger, K., & Bracken, M. B. (2003). Asthma prevalence among pregnant and child-bearing age women in the United States: Estimates from national health surveys. *Annals of Epidemiology, 13,* 317–324.

Ladner, H. D., Danielsen, B., & Gilbert, W. M. (2005). Acute myocardial infarction in pregnancy and the puerperium: A population based study. *Obstetrics & Gynecology, 105*(3), 480–484.

Le Gal, G., Righini, M., Roy, P. M., et al. (2006). Prediction of pulmonary embolism in the emergency department: The revised Geneva score. *Annals of Intern Medicine, 144,* 165–171.

Leonhardt, G., Gaul, C., Nietsch, H. H., et al. (2006). Thrombolytic therapy in pregnancy. *Journal of Thrombosis & Thrombolyis, 21,* 271–276.

Miller, M. A., Chalhoub, M., & Bourjeily, G. (2011). Peripartum pulmonary embolism. *Clinincs in Chest Medicine, 32,* 147–164.

National Asthma Education and Prevention Program Expert Panel Report 3. (2007). Guidelines for the Diagnosis and Management of Asthma. NIH Publication Number 08–5846. October. Retrieved on November 5, 2011, from www.nhlbi.nih.gov/guidelines/asthma/asthsumm.html

Powrie, R. O., Larson, L., Rosene-Montella, K., Abarca M., Barbour, L., & Trujillo, N. (1998). Alveolar-arterial oxygen gradient in acute pulmonary embolism in pregnancy. (Erratum appears in *Am J Obstet Gynecol, 181*(2), 510.) *American Journal of Obstetrics and Gynecology, 178*(2), 394–396.

Roth, A., & Elkayam, U. (2008). Acute myocardial infarction associated with pregnancy. *Journal of the American College of Cardiology, 52*(3), 171–180.

Sadat, U., Dar, O., Walsh, S., & Varty, K. (2008). Splenic artery aneurysms in pregnancy: A systematic review. *The Indian Journal of Surgery, 6*(3), 261–265.

Schatz, M., Dombrowski, M. P., Wise, R., et al. (2003). Asthma morbidity during pregnancy can be predicted by severity classification. *The Journal of Allergy and Clinical Immunology, 112*(3), 283–288.

van Walraven, C., Mamdani, M., Cohn, A., et al. (2003). Risk of subsequent thromboembolism for patients with pre-eclampsia. *BMJ, 326,* 791–792.

Wells, P. S., Anderson, D. R., Rodger, M., et al. (2000). Derivation of a simple clinical model to categorize patients probability of pulmonary embolism: increasing the models utility with the SimpliRED D-dimer. *Thrombosis and Haemostasis, 83,* 416–420.

Zeitlin, J., & Mohangoo, A. (2008). European perinatal health report by the European Peristat project: (better statistics for better health for pregnant women and their babies): data from 2004. Retrieved December 14, 2011, from www.europeristat.com/index.shtml

Vaginal Bleeding in Pregnancy

19

Robyn A. Gray

Throughout pregnancy vaginal bleeding can cause adverse maternal, fetal, and neonatal outcomes. Although vaginal bleeding is more common in early pregnancy, during the latter half, it complicates approximately 5% of pregnancies (Clark, 2004). The major causes of antepartum bleeding include "bloody show" associated with labor or cervical insufficiency, abruptio placenta (30%), placenta previa (20%), uterine rupture, and vasa previa (which is very rare) (Clark, 2004).

Vaginal bleeding is a common presenting complaint to emergency departments, and especially to an obstetric triage unit. Expeditious and thorough evaluation of vaginal bleeding during pregnancy in the acute setting is crucial to overall maternal and fetal well-being. This review will focus on the major causes of vaginal bleeding in the second and third trimester, specifically beyond viability (gestational age of at least 24 weeks 0 days), as well as the approach to diagnosis and management.

ABRUPTIO PLACENTA

PRESENTING SYMTOMATOLOGY

Classically, pregnant women with abruptio placenta will present with vaginal bleeding and abdominal pain, but occasionally the pain will be mild. The vaginal bleeding can be acute and heavy, or it can be chronic with intermittent acute episodes of bleeding noted. Often, pregnant women will have vague complaints of spotting, mild abdominal pain/cramping, and/or back pain. Less than 5% of abruptions will present with leaking of fluid in addition to vaginal bleeding (Ananth et al., 2005).

Occasionally, pregnant women present without specific complaints, but rather for evaluation due to concerns surrounding an injury for example, fall, motor vehicle accident, or physical assault. Symptoms of abruption may evolve during the period of monitoring for these injuries.

HISTORY AND DATA COLLECTION

A medical history is obtained in the pregnant women with a specific focus on the current pregnancy, and any risk factors for abruption, which may exist.

Exhibit 19.1 lists factors that increase the risk for a placental abruption. When available, the prenatal record is reviewed for blood type and Rh status (for Rh immune globulin, as needed), hemoglobin and hematacrit, and all ultrasound reports, especially assessing for placental location.

The amount of blood loss prior to presentation can be estimated by a pad count, as well as the amount and size of clots. Symptoms of excessive blood loss such as dizziness, loss of consciousness, mental status changes, or shortness of breath need to be documented. Any prior episodes of bleeding and any prior hospitalizations, which may have required tocolysis and/or corticosteroids for fetal lung maturity, need to be elicited and noted. Evaluation of pain includes a description of quality, onset, location, severity and radiation. The relationship between onset of pain and bleeding is important to document.

PHYSICAL EXAMINATION

Pallor, hypotension, mental status changes and/or tachycardia may be indicative of orthostatic changes and a severe hemorrhage, and must prompt an expeditious, focused physical examination. If ultrasound records are easily located, confirmation that there is no known placenta previa must be noted, before performing a digital examination. Immediate bedside ultrasound is performed in these cases by qualified individuals if needed to assess for placenta previa. The pelvic exam includes visualization of external genitalia, noting lesions, lacerations, masses, or hematoma. On speculum exam, the amount of blood in the vaginal vault is observed, and the cervical os is visualized to determine dilatation or any active bleeding, as well as polyps or cervicitis. It is important to note that the amount of vaginal bleeding has not been shown to correlate well with the degree of placental separation (Clark, 2004). Therefore, it is not recommended to base potential maternal and fetal outcome on bleeding alone. If bleeding is light, continuation of the exam will include a

EXHIBIT 19.1

Risk Factors for Abruptio Placenta

- Trauma
- Preterm premature rupture of membranes/spontaneous rupture of membranes
- Multifetal gestation
- Hydramnios
- Abnormal placentation (placenta previa, uterine anomaly, leiomyomata)
- Chorioamnionitis
- Chronic hypertension
- Preeclampsia
- History of abruption
- Inherited thrombophilia
- Cocaine
- Cigarrette smoking

Source: Adapted from Ananth et al. (2004); Pariente et al. (2011).

wet mount to rule out bacterial vaginosis, trichomoniasis, and candidiasis as possible causes of vaginal bleeding.

Continuous external fetal monitoring is necessary in the setting of vaginal bleeding with any pregnancy beyond viability. Contractions in the setting of an abruption are classically high frequency and low in amplitude. Tachysystole, defined as more than five contractions in 10 minutes averaged over a 30 minute window, or an elevated resting uterine tone may be seen if an abruption is in progress. An abnormal uterine contraction pattern can point to a diagnosis of a concealed abruption in the women with severe abdominal pain and absent to mild vaginal bleeding. Concealed abruptions comprise approximately 10% to 20% of all placental abruptions (Oyelese & Ananth, 2006).

LABORATORY AND IMAGING STUDIES

In the setting of vaginal bleeding, immediate assessment of blood type and screen are noted and a complete blood count (CBC) and hold tubes are obtained. A urine drug screen may be indicated, with cocaine being the greatest risk factor. When there is concern for hemorrhage or disseminated intravascular coagulopathy (DIC), coagulation studies can be obtained, including prothrombin time (PT), partial thrombin time (PTT), International Normalized Ratio (INR), and fibrinogen. Kleihauer-Betke (KB) can be ordered for pregnant women who are Rh (D) immune globulin negative. The utility of obtaining a KB in the diagnosis and management of abruption is questionable (Oyelese & Ananth, 2006). However, a KB can be useful in determining the correct dose of Rh immune globulin.

If vaginal bleeding is thought to result secondary to preeclampsia with a resultant abruption, then a CBC, creatinine and liver function test including serum glutamic-oxalocetic transaminase (AST/SGOT) and serum glutamic-pyruvic transaminase (ALT/SGPT), and urine protein-creatinine ratio (preferably obtained by a straight catheterization) can be added to the laboratory studies.

If a pregnant woman is unstable, a bedside ultrasound can be utilized, whereas a more complete or formal ultrasound can be pursued if required. Although ultrasound for abruption has a low sensitivity, when noted, it is highly predictive of abruption (Oyelese et al., 2004). Ultrasound has shown to have a 100% positive predictive value when a retroplacental hematoma was noted; however, only 25% of cases have these findings (Glantz & Purnell, 2002). Figure 19.1 shows the irregular, heterogeneous area behind the placenta consistent with a placental abruptio (retroplacental hematoma).

Ultrasounds can provide additional valuable information, including placental location, fetal presentation, fetal biometry, and assessment of amniotic fluid. This information may be integral in adding data to the management plan.

DIFFERENTIAL DIAGNOSIS

The differential diagnosis of vaginal bleeding after viability can be divided into obstetric and nonobstetric causes. Exhibit 19.2 notes nonobstetric causes only. However, the leading causes of vaginal bleeding in pregnancy include placenta previa, abruptio placenta, preterm labor, cervical insufficiency, placenta accreta, vasa previa, and uterine rupture.

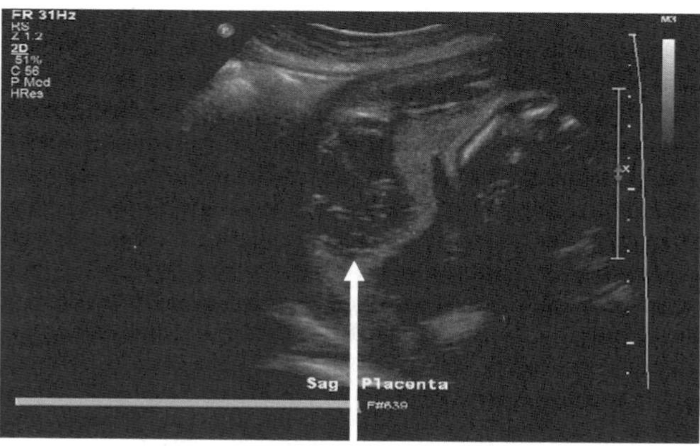

FIGURE 19.1 Ultrasound of abruption with retroplacenatal hematoma.
Source: Courtesy of Department of Radiology, Women & Infants Hospital, Providence, RI.

Urinary and rectal sources of bleeding must be considered in women presenting to an emergency setting with the complaint of vaginal bleeding. The differential diagnosis includes urinary tract infections, nephrolithiasis, hemorrhoids, and rectal fissures

CLINICAL MANAGEMENT AND FOLLOW-UP

Placental abruptio can place the mother and fetus at significant risk for poor outcomes, as shown in Exhibit 19.3. Placental abruption complicates 1% of pregnancies (Oyelese & Ananth, 2006) and is defined as decidual hemorrhage leading to the premature separation of the placenta from the uterine wall, most often due to rupture of maternal vessels prior to delivery of the fetus. The hematoma that results can be small, self-limited, or can be complete, all of which limit the exchange of gases and nutrients to the fetus. Therefore, risks to the fetus are both related to severity of abruption and gestational age at delivery. Oyelese and Ananth (2006) have examined complications associated with placental abruptio, as shown in Exhibit 19.3.

Acute Obstetric Hemorrhage

All pregnant women presenting with vaginal bleeding regardless of etiology must be assessed as to whether they are clinically stable. If hemodynamically unstable, they must undergo immediate therapy to stabilize vital signs with intravascular fluid rescusitation with one to two large bore intravenous lines, replacement of blood products, coagulation factors (fresh frozen plasma, cryoprecipitate, platelets) and delivery by surgical intervention when gestational age is greater than 34 weeks (Reed et al., 2008). Even when gestational age is less than 34 weeks, maternal and/or fetal instability warrants immediate delivery, often by cesarean section, prior to completion of antenatal corticosteroids.

EXHIBIT 19.2

Nonobstetric Causes of Vaginal Bleeding

Gynecologic
- Vaginal laceration
- Cervical trauma
- Infectious
  - Vaginitis
  - Cervicitis (trichomoniasis, bacterial vaginosis)
  - Sexually transmitted (chlamydia, gonorrhea)
- Postcoital
- Cervical polyps
- Malignancy

Urinary
- Urinary tract infection
- Nephrolithiasis
- Rectal
- Hemorrhoids
- Rectal fissures
- Crohns', ulcerative colitis
- Infectious colitis
- Malignancy

Medical
- Thrombophilia
- Anti-coagulation

Source: Adapted from Hoffman (2008).

Management of Stable Abruptio Placenta

The approach to placental abruption will vary depending on the type of bleeding at the time of presentation. An area of debate exists over tocolysis in the setting of abruption. Tocolysis is usually contraindicated in setting of an abruption. The only indication for administration of tocolysis is to prolong pregnancy to allow for fetal lung maturation. If tocolytics are being administered then care should be taken to avoid beta-mimetics, due to adverse cardiovascular effects, i.e., tachycardia.

Occasionally women will present with contractions and pain only, with a presumed diagnosis of preterm labor. There must be a high index of suspicion for abruption with even minor bleeding in a stable patient in the setting of uterine contractions and abdominal pain. Concealed abruption is an example of how the amount of vaginal bleeding may not equal the extent of placental separation (Clark, 2004). Only 10% to 20% of abruptions are concealed (Clark, 2004; Oyelese & Ananth, 2006). Close maternal and fetal monitoring are indicated in these scenarios.

When gestational age is at least 34 weeks the plan should be for delivery. It is reasonable to attempt vaginal delivery if mother and fetus are stable.

EXHIBIT 19.3

Complications Associated With Placental Abruption

Fetal

- Growth restriction (chronic abruption)
- Preterm delivery, and associated morbidity
- Perinatal mortality
- Fetal hypoxemia or asphyxia

Maternal

- Hypovolemia secondary to blood loss
- Blood transfusion
- Disseminated intravascular coagulopathy (DIC)
- Cesarean hysterectomy, and associated morbidity
- Renal failure
- Acute respiratory distress syndrome (ARDS)
- Multisystem organ failure (MOF)
- Death

Source: Adapted from Oyelese & Ananth (2006)

When women are not in labor but are clinically stable, then induction can be considered. However, delivery by cesarean section at any time during induction for maternal or fetal compromise should be expeditious. In the presence of coagulopathy, cesarean section carries high maternal morbidity. Most providers will begin correction of any coagulopathy with aggressive transfusion of red blood cells, fresh frozen plasma, cryoprecipitate and platelets, while moving toward cesarean section.

If the gestational age is between 24 and 34 weeks, and there is no longer active bleeding (in setting of acute or chronic abruptio) with reassuring fetal testing, expectant management is acceptable. Corticosteroids are administered for lung maturity secondary to increased risk of preterm delivery with chronic abruption. Routine fetal surveillance with serial growth scans and biophysical profiles (BPP) or nonstress tests (NST) are performed as either inpatient or outpatient management. Delivery occurs in these cases between 37 and 38 weeks' gestation, due to increased risk for stillbirth (Oyelese et al., 2004).

With chronic abruptio, women often present with intermittent episodes of vaginal bleeding, noted as "acute abruption or chronic abruption." It is reasonable to consider giving a "rescue course" of antenatal corticosteroids if gestational age is less than 32 weeks 6 days, previous steroid course is greater than 2 weeks prior and delivery is anticipated within 7 days (ACOG 2011; Garite et al., 2009). A multicenter randomized placebo-controlled trial showed improved neonatal outcome with rescue steroids without apparent increased risk (Garite et al., 2009).

When fetal demise has occurred due to placental abruption, vaginal delivery is the optimal route of delivery with close monitoring of maternal vital signs, blood loss and laboratory values. Cesarean delivery in these cases should only result when there is maternal compromise or if vaginal delivery is contraindicated for reasons such as previous classical cesarean section.

PLACENTA PREVIA

PRESENTING SYMPTOMATOLOGY

The classic presentation of placenta previa is sudden, painless vaginal bleeding in approximately 80% of pregnant women. An additional 10% to 20% of women will present with bleeding in the setting of uterine contractions (Silver et al., 2006). Symptomatic vaginal bleeding occurs before 30 weeks in roughly one-third of pregnancies, another third between 30 and 36 weeks and 10% will reach term/delivery without any episodes of bleeding (Silver et al., 2006).

HISTORY AND DATA COLLECTION

In all settings of acute vaginal bleeding, the same information, as noted for abruption, is necessary, therefore the history process will be identical to that of a suspected abruption. Questions to consider include how much bleeding has occurred, is there a prior ultrasound or diagnosis to account for bleeding, and is the woman experiencing symptoms of significant blood loss such as light headedness. If available, the prenatal record is obtained and reviewed. Exhibit 19.4 lists the most common risk factors for placenta previa.

PHYSICAL EXAMINATION

The physical examination will initially focus on any signs of significant blood loss such as pallor, hypotension, mental status changes, and/or tachycardia.

EXHIBIT 19.4

Risk Factors for Placenta Previa

- Endometrial scarring
  - Prior cesarean section (associated risk of accreta)
    - Unscarred uterus, 1% to 5%
    - One previous cesarean section, 11% to 25%
    - Two previous cesarean section, 35% to 47%
    - Three previous cesarean section, 40%
    - Four plus previous cesarean section, 50% to 70%
  - Uterine surgery (e.g., myomectomy, uterine septum resection)
  - Increasing number of prior curettages
- Increasing parity
- Maternal smoking
- Multiple gestation
- Infertility treatments
- Advanced maternal age

Source: Adapted from Faiz & Ananth, (2003); Rosenberg et al., (2011); Silver et al., (2006).

If placental location is unknown or immediate documentation is unavailable, bimanual exam is delayed. Immediate bedside ultrasound can be performed in these cases. Digital examinations may exacerbate bleeding in the case of placenta previa, and cause an emergent, life threatening hemorrhage, and are thus not performed on women with placenta previa. Continuous external fetal monitoring is appropriate in the setting of vaginal bleeding beyond viability.

LABORATORY AND IMAGING STUDIES

The initial blood work includes type and screen, CBC, and a hold tube. When bleeding is clinically significant, a cross match for packed red blood cells is added. When concern for hemorrhage or DIC is high, coagulation studies are obtained.

Ultrasound imaging is essential for the evaluation of placental location during pregnancy. Transabdominal ultrasound for initial assessment of placental location in the obstetric triage setting for initial presentation of vaginal bleeding can be performed. It is important to note that transabdominal ultrasound has several limitations. A posterior, placenta previa at term can be difficult to visualize, especially when the fetal head is low in the maternal pelvis. Similarly, a complete noncentral previa displaced laterally may be difficult to visualize. When the findings are uncertain and vaginal bleeding is minimal, transperineal or transvaginal ultrasound is performed to define placental position. Figure 19.2 shows the placenta completely covering the internal os, consistent with a complete placenta previa. Figure 19.3 shows that the placental edge extends to the level of the internal os, consistent with the diagnosis of marginal previa.

Magnetic resonance imaging (MRI) has limited utility in diagnosis of placenta previa due to high cost, limited availability, and established accuracy of transvaginal ultrasound. There is some potential benefit to MRI in setting of a questionable posterior placenta or to assist in the diagnosis of a placenta accreta, in the setting of a placenta previa, especially when anterior.

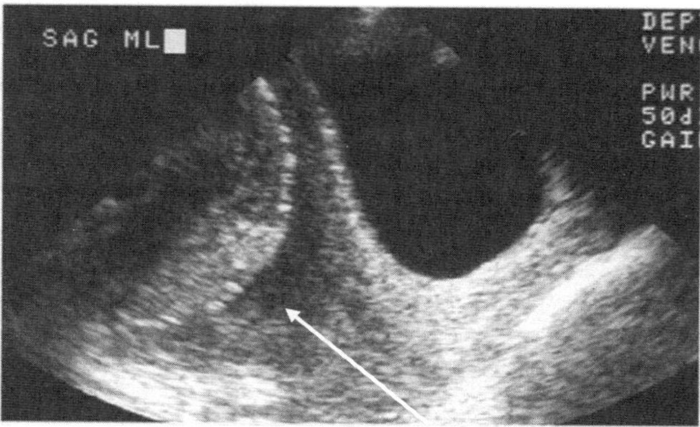

FIGURE 19.2 Ultrasound of placenta previa, complete. Arrow showing placenta covering entire cervix.

Source: Courtesy of Department of Radiology, Women & Infants Hospital, Providence, RI.

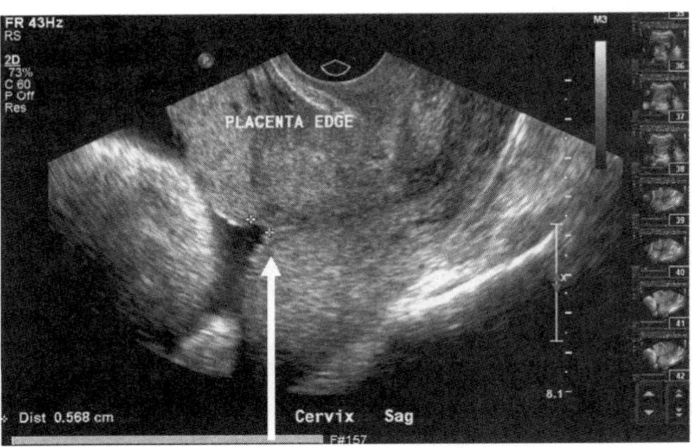

FIGURE 19.3 Ultrasound of placenta previa, marginal. Arrow showing placenta edge from internal os of cervical canal.

Source: Courtesy of Department of Radiology, Women & Infants Hospital.

CLINICAL MANAGEMENT AND FOLLOW-UP

When pregnant women with a bleed from a placenta previa are hemodynamically stable and have reassuring fetal testing, immediate delivery may not be necessary. Reed et al. (2008) determined that 50% can be managed with supportive care and the pregnancy may be prolonged for up to 4 weeks. A randomized controlled trial by Wing et al. (1996) looked at expectant management comparing safety and costs for inpatient versus outpatient management. No significant differences were determined when comparing outcomes in this study.

If delivery is anticipated in the first 12 hours from presentation, and gestational age is less than 31 weeks and 6 days, it is recommended to begin magnesium sulfate for fetal neuroprotection against cerebral palsy (Rouse et al., 2008). Recent systematic reviews and meta-analysis of antenatal administration of magnesium sulfate for prevention of cerebral palsy have supported the use of magnesium with few exclusions: intrauterine fetal demise, maternal severe preeclampsia, fetus with lethal anomalies, and maternal contraindications, e.g., myasthenia gravis, renal failure (Conde-Agudelo & Romero 2009; Reeves et al., 2011).

The current recommendations for management of asymptomatic and/or stable symptomatic placenta previa (whether inpatient or outpatient) involves pelvic rest and serial ultrasounds for growth and placental location every 4 weeks. There are also recent data to suggest that placenta previa does not increase the risk for intrauterine growth restriction (IUGR), regardless of type of previa (Harper et al., 2010). There are no data to support antepartum testing in asymptomatic patients, but it may be indicated with other coexisting conditions of pregnancy such as intrauterine growth restriction, preterm premature rupture of membranes, preterm labor, and medical co-morbidities, i.e., hypertensive disorders, diabetes, gestational diabetes.

VASA PREVIA

Vasa previa is rare and seen with a prevalence of 1 in 2500 deliveries (Francois et al., 2003). Pregnant women with increased risk factors for vasa previa

TABLE 19.1 Vasa Previa Management Considerations

CONSIDERATION	MANAGEMENT	LEVEL OF EVIDENCE
Low lying placenta	Evaluation cord insertion	II-2B
Velamentous insertion Bilobate/succenturiate placenta Vaginal bleeding	Transvaginal ultrasound	II-2B
Vasa previa suspected	Transvaginal ultrasound with Doppler flow	II-2B
Antenatal diagnosis	Elective cesarean section	II-1A
Preterm delivery	Antenatal corticosteroids between 28 and 32 weeks	II-2B
Preterm delivery	Inpatient management between 30 and 32 weeks until delivery	II-2B
Bleeding or PROM	Urgent cesarean section	III-B
Antenatal diagnosis	Transfer to tertiary care facility	II-3B

Source: Adapted from Gagnon et al. (2009).

include those with a history of a resolved placenta previa or the rare patient in whom an accessory placenta can be identified on ultrasound. Vasa previa is difficult to diagnose in an asymptomatic, pregnant woman. A comparison of women diagnosed antenatally and those without vasa previa showed neonatal survical rates of 97% and 44%, respectively (Gagnon et al., 2009). Given that most cases will present with acute hemorrhage and fetal tracing abnormalities (classically sinusoidal pattern), emergent cesarean delivery is indicated to prevent the fetus from potentially exsanguinating. Any woman presenting with brisk vaginal bleeding in the setting of ruptured membranes must have an ultrasound evaluation to confirm placenta previa from vasa previa, when

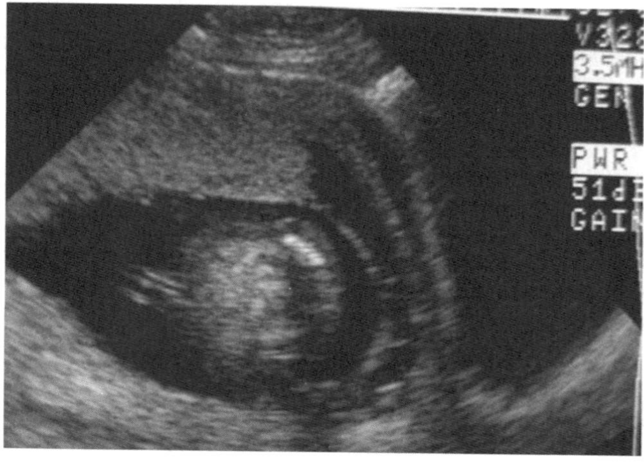

FIGURE 19.4A Ultrasound of vasa previa.

Source: Courtesy of Department of Radiology, Women & Infants Hospital, Providence, RI.

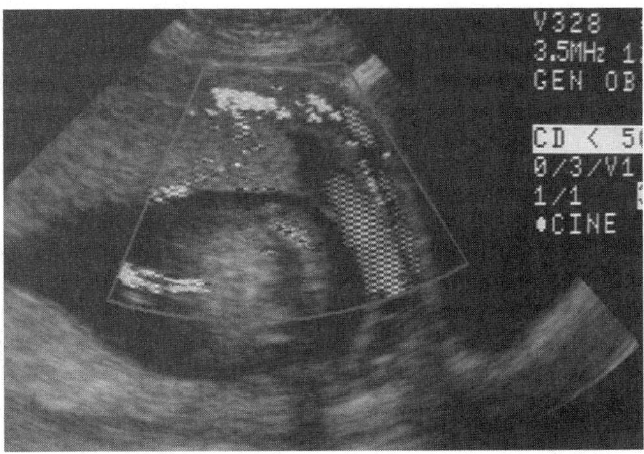

FIGURE 19.4B Ultrasound of vasa previa, Doppler flow.

Source: Courtesy of Department of Radiology, Women & Infants Hospital, Providence, RI.

clinically stable. Table 19.1 shows recommendations for clinical management of pregnant women with vasa previa.

Figure 19.4a illustrates how difficult it may be to diagnose a vasa previa. When color Doppler is applied, as in Figure 19.4b, the diagnosis becomes more obvious.

REFERENCES

ACOG Committee Opinion No 475. (2011). Antenatal corticosteroid therapy for fetal maturation. *Obstetrics & Gynecology, 117*, 422–424.

Ananth, C. V., Oyelese, Y., Yeo, L., Pradhan, A., & Vintzileos, A. M. (2005). Placental abruption in the United States, 1979 through 2001: Temporal trends and potential determinanats. *American Journal of Obstetrics & Gynecology, 192*(1), 191–198.

Ananth, C. V., Oyelese, Y., Srinivas, N., Yeo, L., & Vintzileos, A. M. (2004). Preterm premature rupture of membranes, intrauterine infection, and oligohydramnios:risk factors of placental abruption. *Obstetrics & Gynecology, 104*(1), 71–77.

Clark, S. L. (2004). Placenta previa and abruption placentae. In R. K. Creasy, & Resnik, R., (Eds.). *Maternal fetal medicine* (5th ed., p. 715). Philadelphia, PA: WB Saunders.

Conde-Agudelo, A., & Romero, R. (2009). Antenatal magnesium sulfate for the prevention of cerebral palsy in preterm infants less than 34 weeks' gestation: A systematic review and meta-analysis. *American Journal of Obstetrics & Gynecology, 200*(6), 595–609.

Faiz, A. S., & Ananth, C. V. (2003). Etiology and risk factors for placenta previa: An overview and emeta-analysis of observational studies. *The Journal of Maternal-Fetal & Neonatal Medicine, 13,* 175–190.

Francois, K., Mayer, S., et al. (2003). Association of vasa previa at delivery with a history of second-trimester placenta previa. *The Journal of Reproductive Medicine, 48*(10), 771–774.

Gagnon, R. et al. (2009). Guidelines for the management of vasa previa. *Journal of Obstetrics and Gynaecology Canada, 31*(8), 748–760.

Garite, T. J., Kurtzman, J., Maurel, K., & Clark, R. (2009). Impact of a 'rescue course' of antenatal corticosteroids: A multicenter randomized placebo-controlled trial. *American Journal of Obstetrics and Gynecology, 200,* 248 e1–e9.

Glantz, C., & Purnell, L. (2002). Clinical utility of sonography in the diagnosis and treatment of placental abruption. *Journal of Ultrasound in Medicine, 21,* 837–840.

Harper, L. M., Odibo, A. O., Macones, G. A., Crane, J. P., & Cahill, A. G. (2010). Effect of placenta previa on fetal growth. *American Journal of Obstetrics and Gynecology, 203,* 330.e1–e5.

Hoffman, B. L. (2008). Abnormal uterine bleeding. In Schorge, J. O., Schaffer, J. I., Halvorson, L. M., Hoffman, B. L., Bradshaw, K. D., & Cunningham, F. G. (Eds.), *Williams gynecology* (pp. 174–196). New York, NY: McGraw-Hill.

Oyelese, Y., Catanzarite, V., Prefumo, F., Lashley, S., Schachter, M., Tovbin, Y., Goldstein, V., & Smulian, J. C. (2004). Vasa previa: The impact of prenatal diagnosis on outcomes. *Obstetrics & Gynecology, 103,* 937–942.

Oyelese, Y., & Ananth, C. V. (2006). Placental abruption. *Obstetrics & Gynecology, 108*(4), 1005–1016.

Pariente, G., Wiznitzer, A., Sergienko, R., Mazor, M., Holcberg, G., & Sheiner, E. (2011). Placental abruption: Critical analysis of risks factors and perinatal outcomes. *Journal of Maternal Fetal Neonatal Medicine, 24*(5), 698–702.

Reed, B., Cypher, R., & Shields, A. (2008). Diagnosis and management of placenta previa. *Postgraduate Obstetrics & Gynecology, 28*(20), 1–5.

Reeves, S. A., Gibbs, R. S., & Clark, S. L. (2011). Magnesium for fetal neuroprotection. *American Journal of Obstetrics & Gynecology, 204,* 202.e1–e4.

Rosenberg, T., Pariente, G., Sergienko, R., Wiznitzer, A., & Sheiner, E. (2011). Critical analysis of risks factor and outcomes of placenta previa. *Archives of Gynecologic Obstetrics, 284*(1), 47–51.

Rouse, D. J., Hirtz, D. G., Thom, E., Varner, M. W., Spong, C. Y., Mercer, B. M., . . . Eunice Kennedy Shriver NICHD Maternal-Fetal Medicine Units Network. (2008). A randomized, controlled trial of magnesium sulfate for the prevention of cerebral palsy. *New England Journal of Medicine, 359*(9), 895–905.

Silver, R. M., Landon, M. B., Rouse, D. J., Leveno, K. J., Spong, C. Y., Thom, E. A., . . . National Institute of Child Health and Human Development Maternal-Fetal Medicine Units Network. (2006). Maternal morbidity associated with multiple repeat cesarean deliveries. *Obstetrics & Gynecology, 107,* 1226–1232.

Wing, D. A., Paul, R. H., & Millar, L. K. (1996). Management of the symptomatic placenta previa: A randomized, controlled trial of inpatient versus outpatient expectant management. *American Journal of Obstetrics & Gynecology, 174,* 806–811.

Common General Surgical Emergencies in Pregnancy

Chelsy Caren and David A. Edmonson

Abdominal discomfort is a common presenting complaint in pregnancy, and often it has a benign, physiologic etiology. However, severe pain, or pain associated with peritoneal signs on physical examination, is not considered to be normal in pregnancy. The differential diagnosis of such pain in a pregnant woman is extensive, as shown in Table 20.1 by abdominal quadrant. Table 20.2 describes differential diagnoses for acute pain in pregnancy by abdominal location. Both tables include obstetric and nonobstetric conditions. Emergent general abdominal surgery is performed approximately in 0.2% of pregnant women, most commonly for acute appendicitis, acute cholecystitis, and bowel obstructions (Gilo, Amini, & Landy, 2009). Each of these conditions will be discussed in detail.

GENERAL SURGICAL CONSIDERATIONS DURING PREGNANCY

Several considerations need to be taken into account during the evaluation, diagnosis, and treatment of a pregnant woman for any disorder that may require emergent surgical intervention. Foremost are the anatomic and physiologic changes that take place as a result of being pregnant. These changes may alter the presentation of a given disease or make a certain diagnosis more or less likely. Obstetric complications, when present, may have an effect on these factors, as well.

Evaluation of Fetal Well-Being

The status of the fetus must be addressed throughout the evaluation of a pregnant woman presenting with acute abdominal pain, as well as during any general surgery that is deemed necessary. This can be challenging, especially in light of the fact that a delay in diagnosis or treatment can jeopardize the health or life of the mother and/or fetus. Hemodynamic stability of the pregnant woman does not necessarily imply adequate placental perfusion or fetal oxygenation. Therefore, the American College of Obstetricians and Gynecologists (ACOG) recommends that a fetal heart rate be documented before and after any surgical procedure for a woman pregnant with a previable fetus.

TABLE 20.1 Differential Diagnoses for Acute Pain in Pregnancy by Abdominal Quadrant

RUQ:

Severe preeclampsia
HELLP syndrome ± hepatic distension/rupture
Acute fatty liver of pregnancy (AFLP)
Acute hepatitis (viral or toxic)
Perihepatitis (Fitz-Hugh-Curtis syndrome)
Biliary colic
Acute cholecystitis
Ascending cholangitis
Gallstone pancreatitis
Budd-Chiari syndrome
Hepatic congestion, tumor or abscess
Pneumonia (RLL)
Pleuritis
Empyema
Pulmonary infarction
Perforated peptic ulcer
Appendicitis
Pyelonephritis
Perinephritis
Costochondritis
Rib fracture
Herpes zoster
Leiomyoma degeneration

LUQ:

Splenomegaly
Splenic infarction, abscess or rupture
Ruptured splenic artery aneurysm
Gastritis
Perforated gastric ulcer
Pancreatitis
Pyelonephritis
Perinephritis
Pneumonia (LLL)
Pleuritis
Empyema
Pulmonary infarction
Chostochondritis
Rib fracture
Herpes zoster
Diverticulitis of the jejunum or splenic flexure
Leiomyoma degeneration

RLQ:

Spontaneous/septic abortion
Ectopic pregnancy
Round ligament pain
Placental abruption
Uterine rupture
Ruptured uterine artery
Leiomyoma degeneration
Pelvic inflammatory disease
Ruptured ovarian cyst
Ovarian torsion
Acute appendicitis
Torsion of appendix epiploica
Pyelonephritis
Nephrolithiasis
Intestinal obstruction
Inguinal hernia
Right-sided, cecal or Meckel's diverticulitis
Crohn's disease
Acute enterocolitis
Mesenteric adenitis
Gallstone disease
Psoas abscess
Herpes zoster

LLQ:

Spontaneous/septic abortion
Ectopic pregnancy
Round ligament pain
Placental abruption
Uterine rupture
Ruptured uterine artery
Leiomyoma degeneration
Pelvic inflammatory disease
Ruptured ovarian cyst
Ovarian torsion
Pyelonephritis
Nephrolithiasis
Intestinal obstruction
Inguinal hernia
Diverticulitis
Crohn's disease
Acute enterocolitis
Ischemic/ulcerative colitis
Mesenteris adenitis
Psoas abscess
Herpes zoster

Source: Adapted from Vandeven et al. (2010) and Matthews & Hodin (2006).

TABLE 20.2 Differential Diagnoses for Acute Pain in Pregnancy by Abdominal Location

Epigastric:

Labor (late term)
Chorioamnionitis
Placental abruption
Uterine rupture
Peptic ulcer
Pancreatitis
Biliary colic
Acute cholecystitis
Ascending cholangitis
Gallstone pancreatitis
Gastroenteritis
Gastritis/gastroesophageal reflux disease
Early appendicitis
Severe preeclampsia
HELLP syndrome ± hepatic distension/rupture
Acute hepatitis (viral ot toxic)
Acute fatty liver of pregnancy (AFLP)
Perihepatitis (Fitz-Hugh-Curtis syndrome)
Leiomyoma degeneration
Ruptured abdominal aortic aneurysm

Periumbilical:

Labor (late term)
Chorioamnionitis
Placental abruption
Uterine rupture
Early appendicitis
Pancreatitis
Gastroenteritis
Mesenteric ischemia
Bowel obstruction
Leiomyoma degeneration
Ruptured abdominal aortic aneurysm

Midline lower abdominal:

Cystitis
Urinary retention
Spontaneous/septic abortion
Labor
Ectopic pregnancy
Placental abruption
Uterine rupture
Bowel obstruction
Ruptured ovarian cyst
Ovarian torsion
Pelvic inflammatory disease
Leiomyoma degeneration
Crohn's disease
Acute enterocolitis
Diverticulitis

Diffuse or poorly localized:

Spontaneous/septic abortion
Ruptured ectopic pregnancy
Labor
Chorioamnionitis
Placental abruption
Uterine rupture
Spontaneous rupture of a uterine artery
Ruptured abdominal aortic aneurysm
Early or perforated appendicitis
Bowel obstruction
Perforated peptic ulcer
Perforated diverticulitis
Gastroenteritis
Irritable bowel syndrome
Mesenteric adenitis/ischemia
Crohn's disease
Pancreatitis
Sickle cell crisis
Pelvic/hepatic/mesenteric/ovarian vein thrombosis
Diabetic coma
Acute porphyria
Tuberculosis peritonitis
Malaria/familial Mediterranean fever
Food poisoning
Heavy metal poisoning
Acute leukemia
Primary peritonitis

Source: Adapted from Vandeven et al. (2010) and Matthews & Hodin (2006).

Continuous fetal monitoring is advised when the fetus is viable, as long as the surgery is amenable to safe interruption or modification to allow for an urgent delivery. ACOG also recommends that indicated surgery be performed at an institution where appropriate obstetric, neonatal, and pediatric services are available, in the event that an emergent cesarean section becomes necessary. If these services are not available, then electronic fetal heart rate and contraction monitoring are advised immediately before and after the procedure, to allow for documentation of fetal well-being as well as the presence or absence of contractions (ACOG, 2011).

Diagnostic Imaging

When diagnostic imaging is indicated in a pregnant woman, the safety of fetal radiation exposure must be weighed against the risk to the pregnant woman and/or fetus of a delayed diagnosis. In most instances, the latter is greater. Most commonly used diagnostic imaging studies expose the fetus to significantly less than 5 rads of ionizing radiation, below which there is no evidence for an increased risk of pregnancy loss, fetal anomalies, fetal growth restriction, or developmental delay (CDC, 2011). For instance, a routine chest radiograph exposes the fetus to less than 1 mrad, while an abdominal flat plate exposes the fetus to 140 mrad. Both are considered acceptable in pregnancy.

Graded compression ultrasonography (US) is the initial imaging modality of choice for acute abdominal or pelvic pain in pregnant women. This is because it involves no discernable radiation exposure, employs no contrast agents, and there has been no documentation of any biological effects to mother or fetus over a long history of use (Gilo et al., 2009; Long, Long, Lai, & Macura, 2011). In addition, US is generally readily available and results are rapid. When US is not sufficient to make an accurate diagnosis, noncontrast magnetic resonance imaging (MRI) is the next recommended study. MRI utilizes the magnetic properties of tissues to create images, and therefore, like US, involves no fetal exposure to ionizing radiation. However, MRI is not yet available in all institutions and/or at all hours. Computed tomography (CT) is recommended when US is nondiagnostic and MRI is unavailable. CT scans are readily available and have proven diagnostic capabilities in the abdomen and pelvis. Although the fetus is exposed to ionizing radiation and iodinated contrast (approximately 20 mrad for a chest CT with abdomen shielded, 150–200 mrad for an abdominal CT with uterus shielded, and 2 rad for a pelvic CT), protocols that decrease fetal radiation exposure without affecting performance are available and advocated for pregnant women (Long et al., 2011; Vandeven, Adzick, & Krupnick, 2011).

Timing of Surgical Intervention

Urgently indicated surgery is acceptable in a pregnant woman regardless of trimester. Alternatively, elective surgery is best deferred until the postpartum period. Nonurgent but indicated surgery is best deferred to the early to mid-second trimester, as indicated in the recent ACOG Committee Opinion (ACOG, 2011). Surgery is performed in the second trimester when adverse pregnancy outcomes are at the lowest rate. In addition, by following these guidelines, the fetus would not be exposed to potentially harmful anesthetic agents during the period of organogenesis, though no currently used anesthetic agents have been shown to have any teratogenic effects when standard concentrations are used at gestational age. Finally, the gravid uterus may obliterate the operative field in the third trimester and make surgery more technically difficult at later gestational ages.

Route of Surgery and Complication Rates

Laparoscopic surgery is considered safe in pregnancy and is therefore a viable alternative to laparotomy for most general surgical emergencies (Vandeven et al., 2011). In addition, despite the fact that complications are occasionally seen with negative diagnostic surgeries, the overall rates of complications for common nonobstetric surgeries in pregnant women are not increased above those for nonpregnant women (McGory et al., 2007; Silvestri et al., 2011; Vandeven et al., 2011).

Anesthesia

A full discussion of the issues encountered by the anesthesiologist in managing pregnant women is outside the scope of this chapter. Briefly, the risks and benefits of the type of anesthesia and individual medications chosen are carefully weighed in conjunction with current obstetric and pediatric knowledge in preparing for the indicated surgery. Aspiration prophylaxis is administered preoperatively, and regional anesthesia is preferred when possible.

Additional Considerations

In preparation for general surgery at or near viability, tocolytics are not recommended prophylactically, but only for the treatment of preterm labor when present. Prophylactic glucocorticoids may be considered for surgeries that occur between 24 and 34 weeks' gestation if the underlying process or procedure is thought to put the pregnant woman at increased risk of preterm labor, and if systemic infection is absent. Antibiotics are administered according to the guidelines specific to the procedure, with avoidance of medications with associated fetal toxicities or teratogenic effects when alternatives are available. Finally, deep venous thrombosis (DVT) prophylaxis with sequential compression devices is implemented during surgery of any type or duration, as pregnancy is a well-known hypercoagulable condition.

ACUTE APPENDICITIS

Acute appendicitis is the most common general surgical emergency among pregnant women, and it accounts for 25% of nonobstetric surgery performed during pregnancy (Gilo et al., 2009). An incidence as high as 1 in 1,400 deliveries has been reported, which is similar to the incidence in nonpregnant women (Gilo et al., 2009). Appendiceal rupture is more likely when surgery is delayed more than 20 to 24 hours from symptom onset (Bickell, Aufses, Rojas, & Bodian, 2006; Yilmaz, Akgun, Bac, & Celik, 2007). Elevated rates of maternal sepsis and preterm labor are seen under these circumstances (Corneille et al., 2010); therefore, a timely diagnosis is crucial.

PRESENTING SYMPTOMATOLOGY

The classic presentation of acute appendicitis includes a report of vague periumbilical pain thought to be due to luminal obstruction of the appendix by a fecalith or by lymphoid hyperplasia. This is a referred pain relayed by visceral mechanisms as a result of the increased pressure in the appendix. It is followed by anorexia, nausea, and vomiting, also mediated by visceral mechanisms. As the inflammatory process progresses beyond the appendix itself and affects the overlying peritoneum of the right lower quadrant or pelvis, the pain shifts to that region. This is reported to be the most common presenting symptom of appendicitis in pregnancy (Mourad, Elliot, Erickson, & Lisboa, 2000; Yilmaz et al., 2007). Fever often follows, generally low-grade unless the appendix is perforated. Diffuse abdominal pain is also more common with perforation. Additional symptoms that may be present include urinary complaints, diarrhea, or constipation, allowing to the proximity of the bladder and bowel to the inflamed appendix. Though microscopic hematuria, pyuria, or bacteriuria are present in one-third to more than one-half of patients with acute appendicitis (Yilmaz et al., 2007), a complaint of frank hematuria is rare.

In the pregnant woman, especially with advancing gestational age, the presentation may be less classic, though perhaps not as much as originally thought. Though the growing uterus shifts, the location of the appendix a few centimeters superiorly during the pregnancy, the right lower quadrant pain has been found to be in close proximity to McBurney's point regardless of the gestational age of the pregnancy (Hodjati & Kazerooni, 2003; Mourad et al., 2000). This is in contrast to the classic teaching that the pain is displaced superiorly as well. However, since the uterus lifts the anterior abdominal wall away from the appendix as it grows, thereby preventing direct contact between the area of inflammation and the anterior parietal peritoneum, the presentation of the pain may be significantly less pronounced. Gastrointestinal (GI) symptoms may also be more subtle, since the uterus intervenes between the appendix and the bladder and bowel in many cases. Although 58% to 77% of pregnant women with appendicitis report some degree of nausea and vomiting, complaints may consist only of simple indigestion, mild bowel irregularity, or generalized malaise (Vandeven et al., 2011).

HISTORY AND DATA COLLECTION

A complete review of systems is recommended including special attention to pain assessment and upper GI symptoms. In particular, certain urinary or bowel symptoms may make an alternate diagnosis more likely, since pregnancy-induced physiologic changes render these organs highly susceptible to compromise. Inquiry regarding pregnancy and fetal status is also crucial. A history of vaginal bleeding or abdominal trauma coincident with the onset of pain would clearly increase concern for an obstetric etiology for the presenting symptoms. In pregnancies that have reached fetal viability, fetal heart rate abnormalities may also add to the concern for pregnancy-related causes of abdominal pain, though they can occur with nonobstetric etiologies as well.

PHYSICAL EXAMINATION

Pregnant women with acute appendicitis appear variably uncomfortable, depending how early in the process they present for care. A documented low-grade fever and elevated heart rate, in addition to the common presenting complaints, would support a diagnosis of early acute appendicitis. A fever above 39.4°C (103°F) is especially concerning for a perforated appendix.

On abdominal examination, while the point of maximal tenderness in the right lower quadrant is consistently close to McBurney's point (1.5–2 in. from the anterior superior iliac spine in the direction of the umbilicus), rebound and guarding are inconsistently found (Vandeven et al., 2011). Additional peritoneal signs that are less sensitive, and variably influenced by the intervening uterus, are listed in Table 20.3.

Cervical motion tenderness may be present on pelvic examination, as may pelvic tenderness upon rectal examination, especially in the case of a retrocecal or pelvic appendix.

LABORATORY AND IMAGING STUDIES

While the diagnosis of appendicitis is based primarily upon clinical findings, a complete blood count (CBC) is usually obtained to screen for leukocytosis. However, a normal white cell count in a pregnant woman ranges from 6,000 to 13,0000 cells/mm^3 in the first and second trimesters, up to 16,000 cells/mm^3 by term, and may reach the 20,000 to 30,000 cells/mm^3 range during labor (Vandeven et al., 2011). This is in contrast to a normal nonpregnant white cell count, which ranges from 4,000 to 11,000 cells/mm^3.

A retrospective review of the pregnancies of over 66,000 consecutive deliveries at a single hospital was performed in the late 1990s. The mean leukocyte count among expectant mothers with confirmed appendicitis in this study was found to be 16,400 cells/mm^3 compared with 14,000 cells/mm^3 for those found to have a normal appendix (Mourad et al., 2000). A left shift or bandemia in the differential, thought previously to favor appendicitis or another infectious process, was found to be nondiagnostic in the same study. These findings complicate the interpretation of an elevated white cell count in pregnancy and suggest the need for increased reliance upon other elements in the evaluation of a pregnant woman presenting with acute abdominal pain. However, it should be noted that appendicitis is unlikely when the overall white count is normal, while a white count above 20,000 cells/mm^3 in the absence of labor raises concern for an appendiceal perforation (Vandeven et al., 2011).

TABLE 20.3 Peritoneal Signs on Physical Examination Suggestive of Acute Appendicitis

Dunphy's sign	Increased pain with coughing or movement
Rovsing's sign	Pain in the right lower quadrant with palpation of the left lower quadrant, indicative of right-sided peritoneal irritation
Psoas sign	Right lower quadrant pain with passive hip extension, indicative of retrocecal inflammation (likely related to a retrocecal appendicitis)
Obturator sign	Right lower quadrant pain with passive flexion of the right hip and knee followed by internal rotation of the right hip, indicative of internal obturator inflammation (likely related to a pelvic appendicitis)

Source: Adapted from Matthews & Hodin (2006).

As previously mentioned, urinalysis in a woman with appendicitis may show microscopic hematuria or pyuria, and this should not discount the diagnosis. In addition, in the absence of biliary disease, mild elevations in serum bilirubin (>1.0 mg/dL) have been associated with a perforated appendix (Sand et al., 2009).

Though an experienced examiner may be able to diagnose appendicitis based on history, physical examination, and laboratory findings alone, imaging is recommended when the diagnosis is not certain. The diagnosis of appendicitis is made by US with 86% sensitivity and 81% specificity (Teresawa, Blackmore, Bent, & Kohlwes, 2004) if a thick-walled, noncompressible, blind-ended tubular structure, with a diameter greater than 6 mm, is present in the right lower quadrant, as shown in Figure 20.1.

If a normal appendix is not clearly visualized by US, additional imaging with MRI is advised, where available (Long et al., 2011). In the largest study to date, the sensitivity and specificity of MRI in the detection of appendicitis were 100% and 93%, respectively. A negative predictive value of 100% was also noted (Pedrosa, Lafornara, Pandharipande, Goldsmith, & Rofsky, 2009). The diagnostic finding of an enlarged (>6 mm), fluid-filled appendix on MRI is shown in Figure 20.2.

When clinical evaluation and US results are inconclusive, or MRI is not readily available, computed tomography (CT) is recommended (Long et al., 2011). CT is available in most institutions and has well-established diagnostic value for appendicitis in the general population, with a sensitivity of 94% and a specificity of 95% (Teresawa, Blackmore, Bent, & Kohlwes, 2004). A meta-analysis of three retrospective studies in pregnant women reported sensitivity of 85.7% and a specificity of 97.4% (Basaran & Basaran, 2009). The main findings suggestive of appendicitis on CT are an enlarged (>6 mm) nonfilling or occluded tubular structure, inflammation as manifested by appendiceal wall thickening or enhancement, and/or periappendiceal fat stranding in the right lower quadrant, as seen in Figure 20.3.

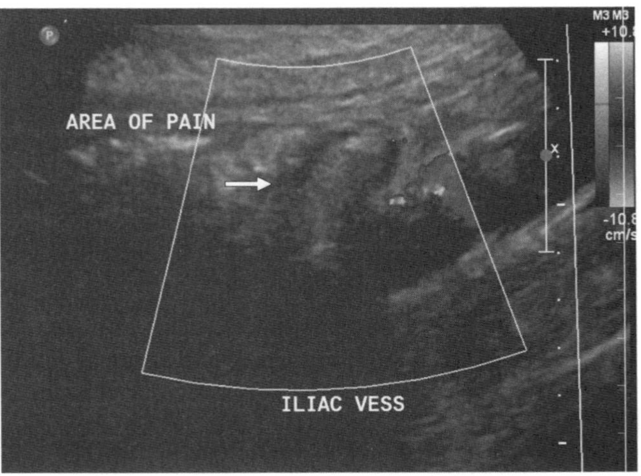

FIGURE 20.1 Ultrasound appearance of acute appendicitis.

Source: Courtesy of Department of Radiology, Women & Infants Hospital, Providence, RI.

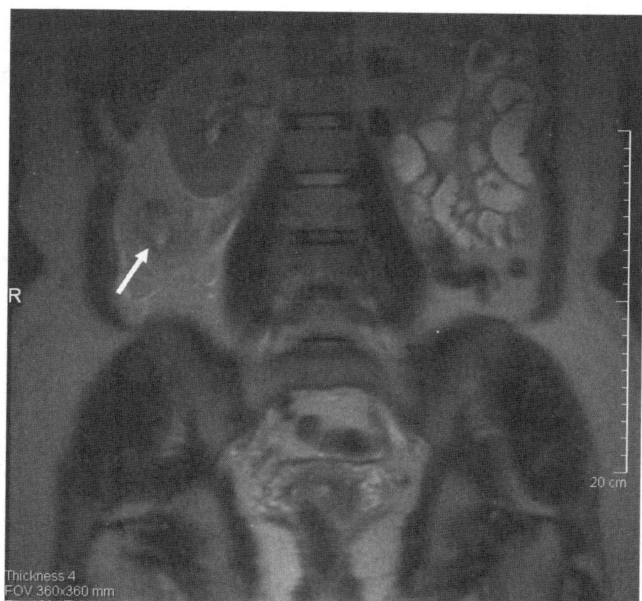

FIGURE 20.2 MRI appearance of acute appendicitis.

Source: Courtesy of Department of Radiology, Women & Infants Hospital, Providence, RI.

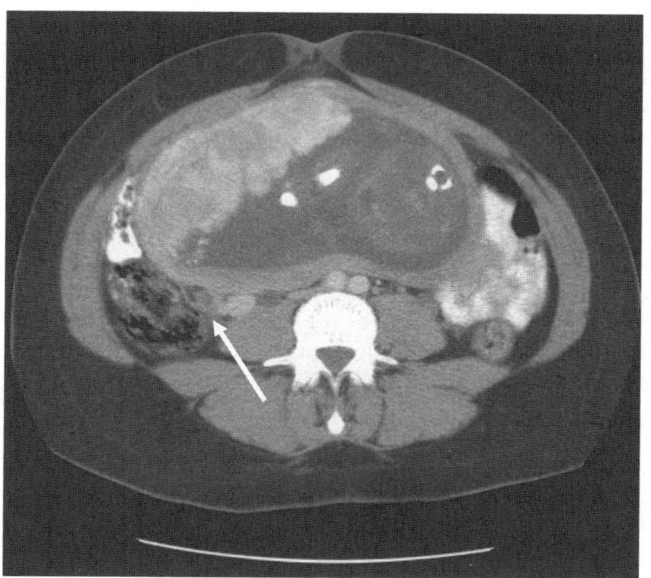

FIGURE 20.3 CT appearance of acute appendicitis.

Source: Courtesy of Department of Radiology, Women & Infants Hospital, Providence, RI.

In addition, in 25% of cases, an appendicolith is visualized (Whitley, Sookur, McLean, & Power, 2009). An appendiceal lumen with air or contrast present on CT essentially rules out the diagnosis, though a nonvisualized appendix does not.

DIFFERENTIAL DIAGNOSIS

The differential diagnosis of appendicitis in pregnancy is extensive. Cecal and Meckel's diverticulitis deserve special mention, however, as they may present identically to appendicitis. Diagnosis of these conditions is usually the result of imaging studies and/or exploratory surgery to evaluate for appendicitis.

CLINICAL MANAGEMENT AND FOLLOW-UP

When acute appendicitis is strongly suspected or diagnosed by ultrasound, MRI, or CT, a general surgeon must be consulted immediately. Due to the high risk of appendiceal perforation with a delay over 20 to 24 hours, an indicated appendectomy should be performed expeditiously regardless of the gestational age (Bickell et al., 2006; Yilmaz et al., 2007). In equivocal cases, a short period of observation may be recommended. In cases where perforation is known to have occurred already, and the woman is stable, medical management may be considered by the consulting surgeon (Young, Hamar, Levine, & Roque, 2009). In practice, general surgeons have been seen to tolerate a higher negative surgical intervention rate in pregnant women, 4% to 50% as opposed to 10% to 15% in the general population (Gilo et al., 2009; Yilmaz et al., 2007). This is due to the high rates of maternal sepsis, preterm labor and delivery, and fetal loss when perforation occurs. Though complication rates are low with these surgeries, preterm labor and fetal loss do occur (McGory et al., 2007; Vandeven et al., 2011; Yilmaz et al., 2007). Of note, the long-term prognosis for women who undergo surgery for acute appendicitis during pregnancy is good, and there does not appear to be an increased risk for infertility or other complications (Viktrup & Hee, 1998).

ACUTE CHOLECYSTITIS

Acute cholecystitis is the second most common indication for general abdominal surgery during pregnancy, and it is more common in pregnant than in nonpregnant women. It is usually a result of gallstone disease, occurring when a stone completely obstructs the cystic duct and leads to inflammation of the gallbladder. Additional serious complications of gallstone disease occur when stones enter the common bile duct (choledocholithiasis) and duodenum and result in the life-threatening emergencies known as ascending cholangitis and gallstone pancreatitis. Although these most serious sequelae of gallstone disease develop in fewer than 10% of symptomatic women, they are associated with a high rate of additional complications such as gangrene (20%) and perforation (2%) of the gallbladder, along with a 15% risk of maternal mortality and a 60% risk of fetal mortality if they are not treated appropriately and in a timely fashion (Vandeven et al., 2011).

Gallstone disease in general is more common in pregnancy due to the elevated circulating estrogen levels, which increase the saturation of bile (Everson, 1992). Gallstones are found in approximately 4% of gravid women early in pregnancy and in as many as 12.2% immediately following delivery. However, the incidence of acute cholecystitis in pregnancy is only 0.01% to 0.08% (Ko, Beresford, Schulte, Matsumoto, & Lee, 2005). This relative discrepancy is likely due to the fact that progesterone, also elevated during pregnancy,

TABLE 20.4 Most Common Differential Diagnoses for Acute Appendicitis, Acute Cholecystitis, and Bowel Obstruction in Pregnancy

Acute Appendicitis	Cecal and Meckel's diverticulitis Acute gastroenteritis/mesenteric lymphadenitis, bacterial or viral etiology Inflammatory bowel disease: Crohn's disease/acute terminal ileitis/ulcerative colitis Pyelonephritis Nephrolithiasis Acute cholecystitis/choledocholithisis/ascending cholangitis/gallstone pancreatitis Bowel obstruction Colonic pseudo-obstruction Ruptured ovarian cysts Ovarian torsion *Obstetrical causes most common first trimester:* Ruptured ectopic pregnancy (first trimester) Spontaneous or septic abortion Hyperemesis gravidarum (most common in first trimester) Pelvic inflammatory disease (most common in first trimester) *Obstetrical causes most common second and third trimester:* Round ligament pain Preterm labor/labor Chorioamnionitis Placental abruption Uterine rupture
Acute Cholecystitis	Choledocholithiasis Ascending cholangitis Gallstone pancreatitis Acute viral hepatitis Peptic ulcer disease Nonbiliary pancreatitis Acute appendicitis Bowel obstruction Paralytic ileus Pyelonephritis Right-sided pneumonia Acute myocardial infarction *Obstetrical causes most common first trimester:* Hyperemesis gravidarum Fitz-Hugh-Curtis syndrome (gonorrhea-induced perihepatitis) *Obstetrical causes most common second and third trimester:* Acute fatty liver of pregnancy Severe preecalmpsia/HELLP syndrome Preterm labor/labor Placental abruption Uterine rupture Chorioamnionitis

Continued

TABLE 20.4 Most Common Differential Diagnoses for Acute Appendicitis, Acute Cholecystitis, and Bowel Obstruction in Pregnancy *Continued*

Bowel Obstruction	Paralytic ileus Colonic pseudo-obstruction Acute appendicitis and corresponding differential diagnoses Acute cholecystitis and corresponding differential diagnoses *Obstetrical causes most common first trimester:* Ruptured ectopic pregnancy Spontaneous or septic abortion Hyperemesis gravidarum Pelvic inflammatory disease/Fitz-Hugh-Curtis syndrome *Obstetrical causes most common second and third trimester:* Round ligament pain Preterm labor/labor Placental abruption Uterine rupture Chorioamnionitis Acute fatty liver of pregnancy Severe preecalmpsia/HELLP syndrome

Source: Adapted from Vandeven et al. (2010) and Matthews & Hodin (2006).

inhibits gallbladder motility, so that while stones and sludge may form, the contractions of the gallbladder are too weak to cause cystic duct obstruction. After delivery, when progesterone levels drop, obstruction is more likely and, in fact, an increased prevalence of acute cholecystitis is seen during the first year postpartum as well (Ko et al., 2005).

PRESENTING SYMPTOMATOLOGY

The symptoms of acute cholecystitis are related to the inflammation of the gallbladder and are similar in pregnant and nonpregnant women. Abdominal pain is usually reported in the right upper quadrant or epigastric region, and may radiate to the back or shoulder. It is often described as severe, crampy or sharp, intermittent or spasmodic, and it generally lasts longer than 4 to 6 hours. Movement usually worsens the pain. Nausea, vomiting, or anorexia may be present. Subjective or documented fever may be reported.

HISTORY AND DATA COLLECTION

When a pregnant woman presents with the above symptoms, it is crucial to inquire further about the setting in which the abdominal pain began. The pain of both gallstones and acute cholecystitis tends to begin an hour or more following ingestion of fatty foods. Pain that begins sooner than 1 hour after eating does not suggest biliary disease. It is also important to ask about a history of similar episodes in the past that have resolved spontaneously or a documented history of gallstones. Associated symptoms such as fevers or chills are essential to elicit as well.

PHYSICAL EXAMAMINATION

Pregnant women with acute cholecystitis tend to appear ill. They are often noted to lie quite still on the examining table, as the inflammation of the gallbladder extends to the overlying peritoneum and makes movement more painful. Fever and tachycardia are commonly documented. Jaundice is not typically seen with uncomplicated acute cholecystitis, but it is consistent with common bile duct obstruction.

In addition to both voluntary and involuntary guarding, the abdominal examination in acute cholecystitis is usually significant for distinct right upper quadrant tenderness, as a result of the local inflammation there. "Murphy's sign," increased discomfort and/or inspiratory arrest with deep palpation in the region of the gallbladder fossa, is the physical examination finding pathognomonic for the condition (Vandeven et al., 2011). The inflamed gallbladder is occasionally palpable as a mass, though guarding often masks this finding even in a nonpregnant woman, as can the size of the uterus in the second or third trimester in a pregnant woman. Detection of Murphy's sign, as well as the other common peritoneal signs, varies with maternal habitus and gestational age.

LABORATORY AND IMAGING STUDIES

Laboratory evaluation of a pregnant woman suspected of having acute cholecystitis includes a CBC with differential and liver and pancreatic function testing. As with acute appendicitis, the typically elevated white blood cell count found with acute cholecystitis may be difficult to interpret in light of the normal leukocytosis of pregnancy. An elevated alkaline phosphatase is normally found in pregnancy as well but significant elevations of the transaminases or bilirubin levels are consistent with common bile duct obstruction. Slight elevations in serum transaminases and amylase may be seen with uncomplicated cholecystitis, due to the passage of small stones or sludge, while significant elevations of amylase and lipase increase suspicion for gallstone pancreatitis.

Women presenting with the symptoms and clinical findings suggestive of acute cholecystitis in pregnancy often require imaging to confirm the diagnosis. Echogenic shadowing, indicative of the presence of gallstones, is consistent with but not diagnostic of acute cholecystitis. Gallbladder wall thickening, greater than 4 to 5 mm, edema, and pericholecystic fluid are pathognomonic. These findings are shown, along with gallstones, in Figure 20.4. A "sonographic Murphy's sign," pain with visualized compression of the gallbladder by the ultrasound transducer, confirms the presence of inflammation. US is over 97% accurate in making the diagnosis, though it may not detect small stones or sludge (Vandeven et al., 2011).

Magnetic resonance cholangiography (MRCP) is an imaging modality currently being studied in clinical trials for use in the diagnosis of acute cholecystitis. There are no clear guidelines for its use in pregnancy; however, it is generally considered to be safe and can be particularly useful in complicated cases, such as when symptomatic choledocholithiasis or gallstone pancreatitis are suspected (Date, Kaushal, & Ramesh, 2008). Endoscopic retrograde cholangiopancreatography (ERCP) is a minimally invasive procedure that has also been proposed for the evaluation of symptomatic choledocholithiasis or gallstone pancreatitis and can be performed with no direct exposure of the

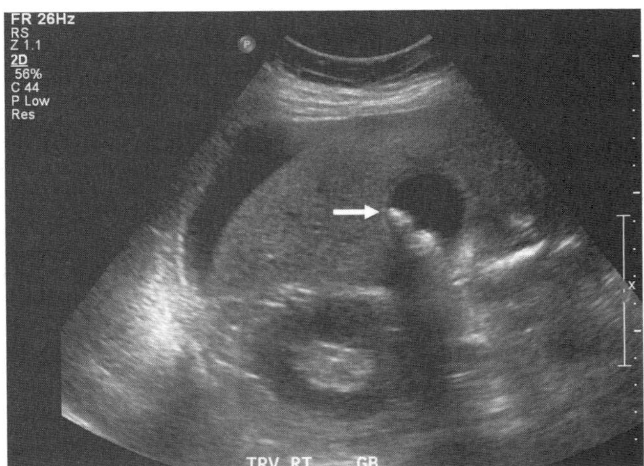

FIGURE 20.4 Ultrasound appearance of acute cholecystitis.

Source: Courtesy of Department of Radiology, Women & Infants Hospital, Providence, RI.

fetus to radiation. The additional benefit of ERCP relative to MRCP is its therapeutic capability. It is possible, during the course of the procedure, to retrieve gallstones from their respective points of obstruction in the common bile duct and thereby alleviate the symptoms of the various gallstone-related disorders (Date et al., 2008; Tham et al., 2003).

DIFFERENTIAL DIAGNOSIS

Cholelithiasis or bilary colic are the most common conditions to consider in the differential diagnosis of acute cholecystitis in pregnancy. Contractions of the gallbladder following a fatty meal push any stones present up against the entrance to the cystic duct and cause visceral pain due to the increase in pressure that results inside the gallbladder. As the gallbladder relaxes, the stones commonly fall back, and the pain completely resolves within a few hours. As mentioned above, the pain of acute cholecystitis does not typically follow this crescendo-decrescendo pattern, but tends to be more constant and severe, lasting longer than 4 to 6 hours. In addition, constitutional symptoms such as fever and malaise are present much more frequently with acute cholecystitis than with biliary colic alone, as is leukocytosis (Gilo et al., 2009).

CLINICAL MANAGEMENT AND FOLLOW-UP

When acute cholecystitis is diagnosed, a general surgical evaluation is obtained to determine whether medical or surgical management is indicated. In the past, medical management was the definitive treatment for acute cholecystitis in pregnancy. However, while initial relief of symptoms is common with medical management (85%), recurrence prior to delivery in pregnant women is common, with hospitalization required for management of the relapses 90% of the time (Vandeven et al., 2011). In addition, progression of disease including choledocholithiasis and gallstone pancreatitis may occur with future attacks and are associated with high rates of maternal and fetal morbidity and mortality (Date et al., 2008; Vandeven et al., 2011). Therefore, while conservative management is often enacted initially, the definitive treatment for acute cholecystitis in both pregnant and nonpregnant populations is surgery.

The Society of Gastrointestinal and Endoscopic Surgeons (SAGES) published treatment guidelines in 2007 that state, "laparoscopic cholecystectomy is the treatment of choice in the pregnant patient with gallbladder disease, regardless of trimester." They assert that, "compared to the open approach, the laparoscopic approach has equivalent outcomes and the well established benefits of laparoscopy" (Kuy, Roman, Desai, & Sosa, 2009). Neither type of surgery has been shown to increase maternal or fetal mortality rates in pregnancy and both can prevent progression of disease (Cohen-Kerem, Railtom, Oren, Lishner, & Koren, 2005; Silvestri et al., 2011). Cholecystectomy is therefore currently recommended during a pregnant woman's initial hospitalization for acute cholecystitis, generally within 72 hours of presentation and within 24 to 48 hours after antibiotics, hydration, and supportive care have been initiated. Immediate surgery is indicated if the woman appears septic or there is concern for gangrene or perforation of the gallbladder.

If surgery is not possible or desirable, percutaneous cholecystostomy has been proposed as a temporizing measure during pregnancy, to provide biliary decompression until a postpartum cholecystectomy can be performed (Allmendinger, Hallisey, Ohki, & Straub, 2005). In addition, as mentioned above, evaluation and treatment of symptomatic choledocholithiasis or gallstone pancreatitis in pregnancy is possible via ERCP.

BOWEL OBSTRUCTION

The incidence of intestinal obstruction during pregnancy is most recently reported to be 1 in 2,500 to 3,500 deliveries. It was reported to be as low as 1 in 68,000 deliveries in the 1930s (Vandeven et al., 2011). This dramatic rise is related to the increased number of women who have undergone laparotomies for various medical conditions prior to becoming pregnant. Intra-abdominal adhesions formed as a result are the most common cause of intestinal obstruction in the gravid woman. Obstruction due to intestinal volvulus is less common, though it is more common in pregnancy than in the general population. Intussusception, hernia incarceration, and intestinal carcinoma are even less frequent causes.

There are three stages of pregnancy during which intestinal obstruction is most likely to present. The first is during the fourth to fifth months, when the growing uterus enters the "true" abdominal cavity and begins to stretch any adhesions that exist there. The second is during the eighth to ninth month, when the infant "drops," with a resultant slight decrease in size of the uterus, and the third is after delivery, when the uterine size decreases dramatically. At each of these times, the relationship of the abdominal viscera to the intra-abdominal adhesions is altered by a change in size of the uterus, and obstruction may occur. In cases of volvulus, an already redundant sigmoid colon (most frequently) or mobile cecum is raised out of the pelvis by the growing uterus and twists around its point of fixation. Of note, incarcerated inguinal hernias, the second most common cause of small bowel obstruction (SBO) in the general population, are rare in pregnancy due to the small bowel being similarly elevated out of the pelvis *and, therefore, away from the inguinal region.*

PRESENTING SYMPTOMATOLOGY

The symptoms of intestinal obstruction in the pregnant woman include abdominal pain and vomiting. Reports of abdominal distension, however, are less consistent owing to the presence of the gravid uterus. Poorly localized, crampy, upper abdominal pain with frequent emesis is more typical of proximal SBO, while lower abdominal pain with less frequent, and possibly feculent, emesis is consistent with colonic obstruction. Obstipation is more common with distal bowel obstruction as well (Vandeven et al., 2011).

In addition to the above GI complaints, individuals with bowel obstruction often present with symptoms that are consistent with progressive hypovolemia, the "hallmark" of the condition. Especially with SBO, dilation, and bacterial overgrowth occur in the proximal bowel. The resulting edema and loss of absorptive function of the bowel wall then cause fluid sequestration in the bowel lumen and, ultimately, loss of this fluid into the peritoneal cavity. In addition to the fluid losses from vomiting, this results in severe dehydration. Pregnant women may report dizziness, lightheadedness, fatigue, and/or shortness of breath above baseline. They may also note significantly decreased urine output. As the intraluminal pressure increases, perfusion to the bowel may be compromised and necrosis may occur. In this case, diffuse, constant abdominal pain and fever may be reported as well.

HISTORY AND DATA COLLECTION

A history of prior abdominal surgery is essential to obtain in any individual who presents with symptoms concerning for bowel obstruction. In particular, a history of gynecologic pelvic surgery, appendectomy, gastric bypass surgery, or bowel resection, especially when the latter is due to prior obstruction or intra-abdominal malignancy, should raise concern for a current obstruction (Kakarla, Dailey, Marino, Shikora, Chelmow, 2005; Vandeven et al., 2011). A history of Crohn's or other inflammatory bowel disease in a pregnant woman also increases the risk due to the increased prevalence of adhesions with these disorders.

PHYSICAL EXAMINATION

Upon presentation, a pregnant woman with a bowel obstruction may be found to be hypotensive and/or tachycardic owing to dehydration. Oliguria is likely. A fever raises the suspicion for bowel necrosis and/or strangulation.

Abdominal examination includes notation of any surgical scars present, as well as the presence of distension that is not consistent with the woman's gestational age, both of which raise suspicion for bowel obstruction. Auscultation and percussion of the abdomen for the high-pitched, hypoactive or absent bowel sounds characteristic of obstruction are increasingly difficult as the pregnancy progresses, and findings may not be reliable. Surgical scars are palpated, as are the umbilical, inguinal, and femoral regions, to check for hernias. Peritoneal signs including localized or rebound tenderness and guarding are variable in pregnancy, as discussed above, and are worrisome when present. Finally, a rectal examination is necessary to search for masses as well as gross or occult blood, which may be consistent with ischemia, intussusception, or neoplasm.

No laboratory studies are diagnostic of bowel obstruction, though they can be helpful in evaluating the degree of dehydration present. Blood urea nitrogen (BUN), creatinine, and hematocrit elevations reflect poor hydration status. Since creatinine usually decreases during pregnancy, even a normal nonpregnant creatinine level may be considered elevated. Leukocytosis with a left shift may be a sign of bowel ischemia or perforation, as may an elevated serum lactate (sensitivity 90%–100%, specificity 42%–87%; Markogiannakis et al., 2007).

Upright and flat abdominal radiographs are the imaging studies of choice when bowel obstruction is suspected, both in the pregnant and nonpregnant population. Distended loops of bowel with multiple air-fluid levels are generally seen with SBO, as shown in Figure 20.5, but may also be seen with colonic obstruction. A grossly dilated loop may be seen with volvulus. Though these films may be nonspecific or equivocal 30% to 50% of the time with early obstruction (Markogiannaki et al., 2007; Vandeven et al., 2011), serial films that show progressive changes confirm the diagnosis, while air in the colon or rectum makes a complete obstruction less likely. An upright chest film is also helpful to evaluate for free air under the diaphragm, suggestive of perforation, if this is not seen clearly on abdominal film.

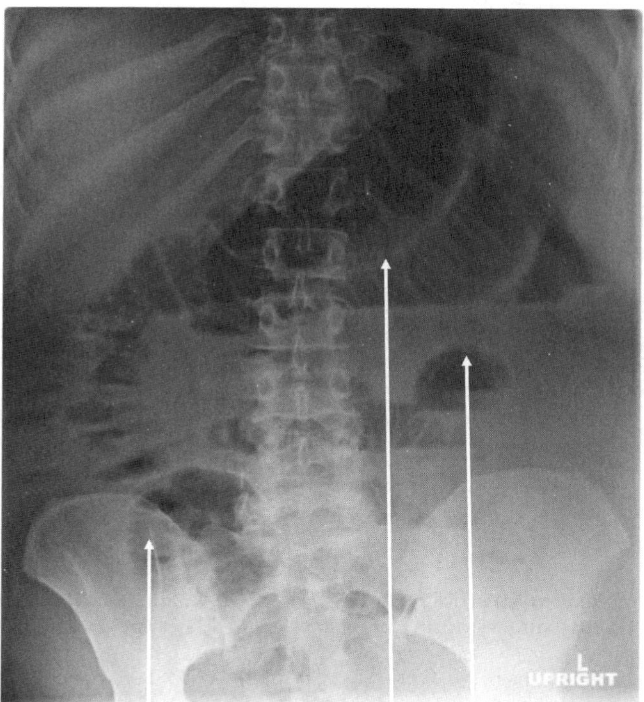

FIGURE 20.5 Abdominal x-ray of SBO.

Source: Courtesy of Department of Radiology, Women & Infants Hospital, Providence, RI.

When plain abdominal films are not diagnostic, a small bowel series with water-soluble contrast or a CT scan with dilute barium- or water-soluble contrast may be performed. The former is the gold standard study for determining partial versus complete obstruction, while the latter is superior at detecting closed-loop obstructions and providing information as to the etiology of the obstruction. Although not as informative as CT, ultrasound is more sensitive and specific than plain films and does not expose the fetus to contrast agents, so may be useful in pregnant women as well (Suri et al., 1999).

DIFFERENTIAL DIAGNOSIS

The clinical symptoms and signs of mechanical bowel obstruction overlap with those of both acute appendicitis and acute cholecystitis but are most similar to those of paralytic ileus and colonic pseudo-obstruction. The latter are functional obstructions due to underlying alterations in the motility of the GI tract. They have many etiologies including electrolyte abnormalities and metabolic conditions. Laboratory testing and imaging studies are critical to help differentiate among these conditions.

CLINICAL MANAGEMENT AND FOLLOW-UP

A general surgery consultation is indicated when any type of bowel obstruction is suspected in a pregnant woman. The initial treatment is likely to include aggressive fluid resuscitation as well as decompression of the distended bowel. The fluid deficit at presentation can range from 1 to 6 L, depending on the stage of the process (Vandeven et al., 2010). In the pregnant woman, this is especially worrisome, since hypovolemia results in decreased blood flow to the uterus and can lead to fetal distress or demise. If the fetus is viable, continuous monitoring should be in progress throughout resuscitation. Decompression is with a nasogastric tube for SBO and with a rectal tube for sigmoid volvulus. Surgery is required for decompression of cecal volvulus.

Initial improvement, and even resolution, is often seen with conservative management for SBO and sigmoid volvulus described above. However, surgical intervention for all types of bowel obstruction is seen sooner and more frequently in pregnant women than in the general population due to the high rates of ischemia, necrosis, and perforation seen with conservative management (Markogiannakis et al., 2007). Furthermore, "aggressive surgical treatment has been credited with reducing maternal and fetal mortality rates from 20% to 50%, respectively, in the 1930s, to 6% and 26% today" (Vandeven et al., 2010).

REFERENCES

ACOG Committee on Obstetric Practice. (2011). ACOG Committee Opinion No. 474: Nonobstetric surgery during pregnancy. *Obstetrics & Gynecology, 117*(2 Pt 1), 420–421.

Allmendinger, N., Hallisey, M., Ohki, S., & Straub, J. (1995). Percutaneous cholecystostomy treatment of acute cholecystitis in pregnancy. *Obstetrics & Gynecology, 86*, 653–654.

Basaran, S. A., & Basaran, M. (2009). Diagnosis of acute appendicitis during pregnancy: A systematic review. *Obstetrics and Gynecological Survey, 64*, 481–488.

Bickell, N., Aufses, A., Jr., Rojas, M., & Bodian, C. (2006). How time affects the risk of rupture in appendicitis. *Journal of American College of Surgeons*, 202, 401–406.

Centers for Disease Control (CDC). 2011. Radiation and pregnancy: A fact sheet for clinicians. Retrieved from www.bt.cdc.gov/radiation/prenatalphysician.asp (accessed December 20, 2011).

Cohen-Kerem, R., Railtom, C., Oren, D., Lishner, M., & Koren, G. (2005). Pregnancy outcome following non-obstetric surgical intervention. *American Journal of Surgery, 190*, 467–473.

Corneille, M., Gallup, T., Bening, T., Wolf, S. E., Brougher, C., Myers, J. G. . . . Stewart, R. M. (2010). The use of laparoscopic surgery in pregnancy: Evaluation of safety and efficacy. *American Journal of Surgery, 200*, 363–367.

Date, R., Kaushal, M., & Ramesh, A. (2008). A review of the management of gallstone disease and its complications in pregnancy. *American Journal of Surgery, 196*, 599–608.

Everson, G. (1992). Gastrointestinal motility in pregnancy. *Gastroenterology Clinical North America, 21*, 751–776.

Gilo, N., Amini, D., & Landy, H. (2009). Appendicitis and cholecystitis in pregnancy. *Clinical Obstetrics and Gynecology, 52*, pp. 586–596.

Hodjati, H., & Kazerooni, T. (2003). Location of the appendix in the gravid patient: a re-evaluation of the established concept. *International Journal of Gynaecology and Obstetrics, 81*, 245–247.

Kakarla, N., Dailey, C., Marino, T., Shikora, S. A., & Chelmow, D. (2005). Pregnancy after gastric bypass surgery and internal hernia formation. *Obstetrics & Gynecology, 105*, 1195–1198.

Ko, C., Beresford, S., Schulte, S., Matsumoto, A. M., & Lee, S. P. (2005). Incidence, natural history and risk factors for biliary sludge and stones during pregnancy. *Hepatology, 41*, 359–365.

Kuy, S., Roman, S., Desai, R., & Sosa, J. (2009). Outcomes following cholecystectomy in pregnant and nonpregnant women. *Surgery, 146*, 358–366.

Long, S., Long, C., Lai, H., & Macura, K. (2011). Imaging strategies for right lower quadrant pain in pregnancy. *American Journal of Roentgenology, 196*, 4–12.

Markogiannakis, H., Messaris, E., Dardamanis, D., Pararas, N., Tzertzemelis, D., Giannopoulos, P., . . . Bramis, I. (2007). Acute mechanical bowel obstruction: Clinical presentation, etiology, management and outcome. *World Journal of Gastroenterology, 13*, 432–437.

Matthews, J., & Hodin, R. (2006). Chapter 74: Acute Abdomen and Appendix. In M. Mulholland, K. Lillimoe, G. Doherty, R. Maier, G. Upchurch (eds.), *Greenfield's Surgery, Scientific Principles and Practice* (pp. 1209–1222). Philadelphia, PA: Lippincott, Williams and Wilkins.

McGory, M., Zingmond, D., Tillou, A., Hiatt, J. R., Ko, C. Y., & Cryer, H. M. (2007). Negative appendectomy in pregnant women is associated with a substantial risk of fetal loss. *Journal of. American College of Surgery, 205*, 534–540.

Mourad, J., Elliot, J., Erickson, L., & Lisboa, L. (2000). Appendicitis in pregnancy: New information that contradicts long-held clinical beliefs. *American Journal of Obstetrics and Gynecology, 182*, 1027–1029.

Pedrosa, I., Lafornara, M., Pandharipande, P., Goldsmith J. D., & Rofsky, N. M. (2009). Pregnant patients suspected of having acute appendicitis: Effect of MR imaging on negative laparotomy rate and appendiceal perforation rate. *Radiology, 250*, 749–757.

Sand, M., Bechara, F., Holland-Letz, T., Sand, D., Mehnert, G., Mann, B. (2009). Diagnostic value of hyperbilirubinemia as a predictive factor for appendiceal perforation in acute appendicitis. *American Journal of Surgery, 198*, 193–198.

Silvestri, M., Pettker, C., Brousseau, C., Dick M. A., Ciarleglio, M. M., & Erekson, E. A. (2011). Morbidity of appendectomy and cholecystectomy in pregnant and nonpregnant women. *Obstetrics and Gynecology, 118*, 1261–1270.

Suri, S., Gupta, S., Sudhakar, P., Venkataramu, N. K., Sood, B., & Wig, J. D. (1999). Comparative evaluation of plain films, ultrasound and CT in the diagnosis of intestinal obstruction. *Acta Radiologica, 40*, 422–428.

Teresawa, T., Blackmore, C., Bent, S., & Kohlwes, R. (2004). Systematic review: Computed tomography and ultrasonography to detect acute appendicitis in adults and adolescents. *Annals of Internal Medicine, 141*, 537.

Tham, T., Vandervoort, J., Wong, R., Montes, H., Roston, A. D., Slivka, A.... D. L. Carr-Locke. (2003). Safety of ERCP during pregnancy. *American Journal of Gastroenterology, 98*, 308–311.

Vandeven, C., Adzick, N., & Krupnick, A. (2010). Chapter 110: The pregnant patient. In M. Mulholland, K. Hemoe, G. Doherty, R. Maier, & G. Upchurch (eds.), *Greenfield's Surgery, Scientific Principles and Practice* (pp. 1983–1998). Philadelphia, PA: Lippincott, Williams and Wilkins.

Viktrup, L., & Hee, P. (1998). Fertility and long-term complications four to nine years after appendectomy during pregnancy. *Acta Obstetricia et Gynecologica Scandinavica, 77*, 746–752.

Whitley, S., Sookur, P., McLean, A., & Power, N. (2009). The appendix on CT. *Clinical Radiology, 64*,190.

Yilmaz, H., Akgun, Y., Bac, B, & Celik, Y. (2007). Acute appendicitis in pregnancy—Risk factors associated with principal outcomes: A case control study. *International Journal of Surgery, 5*, 192–197.

Young, B., Hamar, B., Levine, D., & Roque, H. (2009). Medical management of ruptured appendicitis in pregnancy. *Obstetrics and Gynecology, 114*, 453–456.

21 Management of Biohazardous Exposure in Pregnancy

Dotti C. James, Mary Ann Maher, and Robert J. Blaskiewicz

At any point in time in the United States, 3 million women are pregnant. A biohazard exposure, deliberate or accidental, poses a unique challenge and requires careful assessment and prompt treatment to prevent harm to the woman or infant. Physiologic changes during pregnancy can change the safety and efficacy of medications and vaccines for pregnant women. In addition, the potential effect of many of these measures on the fetus is unknown (Cono, Cragan, Jamieson, & Rasmussen, 2006). Biohazards in pregnancy will be evaluated, specifically smallpox, Lassa fever, ebola, plague, and anthrax, and symptomology and treatment options that may become necessary in the obstetric triage or emergency setting will be discussed.

BIOLOGIC AGENTS

The working group on civilian bio-defense identified a number of biologic agents including smallpox virus and some of the hemorrhagic fever viruses that are more severe during pregnancy (CDC, 2006b). These agents must be considered if exposure is known or suspected.

SMALLPOX

Smallpox, a formerly eradicated disease, has become a bioterrorism threat. One confirmed case of smallpox is a public health emergency. An intense worldwide public health initiative resulted in no documented naturally occurring case of this highly infectious disease occurring since October 26, 1977. The World Health Organization (WHO) officially declared smallpox eradicated in 1980 (Hogan, Harchelroad, & McGovern, 2010). Only two laboratories in the world are known to house smallpox virus: the Centers for Disease Control and Prevention (CDC) in Atlanta, Georgia, and the State Research Center of Virology and Biotechnology in Koltsovo, Russia. If these stores are weaponized, mass vaccination would be needed.

During pregnancy, the woman's susceptibility to infections is altered. Hormonal, cellular, and humoral changes suppress the immune response (White, Henretig, & Dukes, 2002). Circulating white cell count is slightly increased, neutrophil chemotaxis and adherence, cell-mediated immunity and natural killer cell activity decrease.

Clinical experience with smallpox (variola virus) indicates that pregnant women are more susceptible to variola infection and have more severe disease, resulting in an increased smallpox case-fatality rate. They are also more likely to have hemorrhagic smallpox (purpura variolosa) (Jamieson, Theiler, & Rasmussen, 2006).

The CDC, the Department of Defense (DOD), and the Food and Drug Administration (FDA) monitor the outcomes of pregnancy in women exposed to smallpox vaccines in the National Smallpox Vaccine in Pregnancy Registry (CDC, 2003a). In this group, most (77%) were vaccinated near the time of conception, before pregnancy was confirmed. Outcome evaluations have not revealed higher-than-expected rates of pregnancy loss (11.9%), preterm birth (10.7%), or birth defects (2.8%). No cases of fetal vaccinia have been identified (Ryan & Seward, 2008). If terrorism threats become real in the United States, more people, especially the military, will need to be vaccinated.

HISTORY AND PHYSICAL EXAMINATION

Pregnant women are more susceptible to hemorrhagic smallpox or purpura variolosa. Symptoms include fever, backache, diffuse coppery-red rash, and a rapid decline in the health status of mother and infant. Information on the presentation and progression of smallpox is summarized in Exhibit 21.1.

Within 24 hours of the onset of symptoms, a woman will likely develop spontaneous ecchymoses, epistaxis, bleeding gums, an intense erythematous rash, and subconjunctival hemorrhages. Laboratory analysis during this period may demonstrate thrombocytopenia, increased capillary fragility, and depletion of coagulation factors and fibrinogen (Constantin, Martinelli, & Strickland, 2003; Suarez & Hankins, 2002; White, Henretig, & Dukes, 2002). Death would generally result from sepsis.

EXHIBIT 21.1

Smallpox: Presentation and Progression

Clinical Presentation

- Fever, chills
- Body aches, headache
- Backache
- Rash appears 48 to 72 hours after initial symptoms
- Turns into virus-filled sores, later scabs over, process can take 2 weeks

Progression

- Virus enters respiratory tract
- Multiplies, spreads to regional lymph nodes
- Incubation period (12 days)
- Skin eruptions (lesions occur in the mouth, spread to the face, to the forearms and hands, and finally to lower limbs and trunk)

Source: Adapted from CDC NCID (2011); Rao, Prahlad, Swaminathan, & Lakshmi (1963).

Variola virus can cross the placenta and infect the fetus. It is suggested that during pregnancy, there is an increased susceptibility to the variola infection with greater severity of illness. Maternal mortality approaches 50%, compared with 30% for men and nonpregnant women (CDC, 2009, 2007, 2003a, 2003b; White, Henretig, & Dukes, 2002).

If infection occurs during the first trimester, it can result in high rates of fetal loss. During the latter half of pregnancy, infection is associated with increased rates of prematurity. For initial screening, the CDC has developed an interactive algorithm that can be quickly completed by the provider online. This algorithm indicates the risk of the situation being smallpox (CDC, 2007).

FETAL VACCINIA

Smallpox vaccine comes from a live virus related to smallpox called vaccinia, not smallpox virus (variola).The question remains whether to immunize pregnant women if a release of a biological agent is confirmed or suspected (Jamieson, Theiler, & Rasmussen, 2006). There is a rare, serious infection of the fetus, called fetal vaccinia, which can occur following vaccination for smallpox. Congenital variola ranges from 9% to 60% during epidemics of the disease. It is characterized by giant dermal pox and diffuse necrotic lesions of viscera and placenta. Fetal vaccinia typically results in stillbirth or death of the infant. There may be maternal immunity that protects the fetus. Smallpox vaccine is not known to cause congenital malformations but if vaccinated, the woman ought to avoid pregnancy for a month, waiting until the vaccination site has completely healed and the scab has fallen off before trying to become pregnant.

Unvaccinated pregnant women were three times more likely to die (Rao, Prahlad, Swaminathan, & Lakshmi, 1963). Therefore, it is recommended that pregnant women receive the smallpox vaccine only when exposed to a diagnosed case of smallpox because there is a greater risk from the disease than from the vaccine. It is advised that pregnant women not come into contact with anyone who has been recently vaccinated.

If a breastfeeding mother (who has close contact with someone recently vaccinated) develops a rash, it is recommended that the health care provider be contacted to determine if the rash is related to the smallpox vaccine. If a vaccine-related rash occurs, the CDC recommends against breastfeeding until all scabs from the rash have healed. A woman who desires to maintain an adequate milk supply may continue to pump breast milk, but the milk must be discarded until scabs fully separate (CDC, 2009).

Vaccinia immune globulin (VIG) is an alternate treatment for people who have serious reactions to smallpox vaccine. It is an immune globulin from the blood of people who have gotten the smallpox vaccine more than once (usually many times). Antibodies are removed, purified, and stored with the resulting product being VIG. It is administered intravenously and the licensed product is called "VIG-intravenous" (VIG-IV). IV-VIG is available from CDC under Investigational New Drug (IND) protocol that will have guidelines for dosage and administration.

It is recommended that women contact their health care provider regarding use of VIG. Currently, CDC's Advisory Committee on Immunization Practices does not recommend preventive use of VIG for pregnant women. If a woman has another complication from smallpox vaccine that could be treated with VIG, it would be appropriate that it be given while the woman

EXHIBIT 21.2

Lassa Fever: Treatment

- Ribavirin (Virazole)
  - 30 mg/kg IV (maximum, 2 g) loading dose
  - 16 mg/kg IV (maximum, 1 g/dose) q 6 h for 4 days
  - 8 mg/kg IV (maximum, 500 mg/dose) q 8 h for 6 days

Source: Adapted from May (2009).

is pregnant. The few cases of reported fetal vaccinia infection have occurred after an accidental primary vaccination in early pregnancy, or the woman becoming pregnant within 28 days of vaccination. Smallpox vaccine is not known to cause congenital malformations (CDC, 2003b).

LASSA FEVER

Lassa fever is an arenavirus infection that occurs mostly in Africa and can be fatal. It may involve multiple organ systems but spares the central nervous system (CNS). The first reported case of Lassa fever was described in a pregnant woman. The mortality rate is higher for pregnant women and women who have given birth within a month. The mortality rate is 50% to 92%. Recovery occurs within 7 to 31 days after becoming symptomatic or death may ensue. Evidence suggests that the placenta may be a preferred site for viral replication, which may explain why illness and death increase during the third trimester (Jamieson, Theiler, & Rasmussen, 2006). Uterine evacuation may reduce maternal mortality. Most pregnant women will lose the fetus. Human cases of Lassa fever probably result from contamination of food with rodent urine, but human-to-human transmission can occur via urine, feces, saliva, vomitus, or blood.

Lassa fever begins with a viral prodrome, followed by unexplained disease in any organ system except the CNS. When following laboratory test results, the provider may notice massive proteinuria and elevated liver functions studies such as aspartate aminotransferase (AST), alanine aminotransferase (ALT), and lactate dehydrogenase (LDH) levels, which may be 10 times the normal level. Cell cultures are not routine and must be handled in a biosafety level IV laboratory. Lassa IgM antibodies or a 4-fold rise in the IgG antibody titer may be detected using an indirect fluorescent antibody technique. Polymerase chain reaction (PCR) is the most rapid test. Chest x-rays may show basilar pneumonitis and pleural effusions (May, 2009).

Diagnosis and treatment within the first six days may reduce the mortality by up to 10-fold. Supportive treatment includes correction of fluid and electrolyte imbalances. Anti-Lassa fever plasma is helpful as an adjunctive therapy in very ill patients. Antibiotic treatment recommendations can be found in Exhibit 21.2 (Mays, 2009).

EBOLA HEMORRHAGIC FEVER

Ebola virus (Filoviridae group) is transmitted by direct contact with blood, secretions, or contaminated objects and is associated with high fatality rates.

The Ebola virus begins to multiply within the body with symptoms beginning four to six days after infection. The incubation period can be as short as 2 days or as long as 21 days.

Presenting symptoms include the sudden onset of flu-like symptoms, such as sore throat, dry, hacking cough, fever, weakness, and severe headache, joint and muscle aches. Diarrhea, dehydration, stomach pain, vomiting may also occur, accompanied by a rash, hiccups, red eyes, and internal and external bleeding. In dark-skinned women, the rash may not be recognized until it begins to peel. Laboratory findings show low counts of white blood cells and platelets, and elevated liver enzymes (WHO, 2008).

When Ebola exposure has been documented, any woman presenting with fever, together with acute clinical symptoms, signs of hemorrhage such as bleeding of the gums or nose, conjunctival injection, red spots on the body, bloody stools and/or melena, or vomiting blood must be evaluated for possible Ebola. Pregnant women infected with Ebola more often have serious complications, such as hemorrhagic and neurologic sequelae. The risk for death from Ebola is similar among all trimesters of pregnancy, 50% to 90% (Jamieson, Theiler, & Rasmussen, 2006). Death usually occurs during the second week of symptoms from massive blood loss. The possibility of Ebola must be considered in the differential as a possible primary cause of bleeding (WHO, 2008).

Diagnosis is based on the enzyme-linked immunoassay (ELISA), or specific IgG and IgM antibodies or Ebola specific antigen detection. These tests are not commercially available and must be sent to specially equipped regional laboratories or WHO collaborating centers. There is no recommended treatment or prophylaxis, and management is supportive therapies with antibiotics used for secondary infections (WHO, 2008).

PLAGUE

Human plague in the United States occurs in scattered cases in rural areas (an average of 10 to 15 persons each year). Most human cases in the United States occur in two regions: a) northern New Mexico, northern Arizona, and southern Colorado; and b) California, southern Oregon, and far western Nevada (CDC, 2005). During pregnancy, infection with *Yersinia pestis,* the bacteria causing plague, can result in spontaneous abortion. More favorable outcomes have been reported due to the increased availability of treatment. Plague bacillus enters the skin from the site of a flea bite and travels through the lymphatic system to the nearest lymph node, resulting in the most prominent sign of human plague, a swollen and very painful lymph gland. Left untreated, plague bacteria invade the bloodstream. As the plague bacteria multiply, they spread rapidly throughout the body causing a severe and often fatal condition. Infection of the lungs causes the pneumonic form of plague. Untreated, the disease can progress rapidly to death. About 14% (one in seven) of all plague cases in the United States are fatal (CDC/NCID, 2001).

Presenting symptoms include the sudden appearance of fever, cough, shortness of breath, hemoptysis, tachypnea, and chest pain. These may be accompanied by nausea, vomiting, abdominal pain, and diarrhea. As the disease continues, the woman will progress to sepsis, shock, organ failure, purpuric skin lesions and necrotic digits (CDC/NCID, 2001; Inglesby et al., 2000; WHO, 2008).

EXHIBIT 21.3

Plague: Treatment for Pregnant Women[a]

- Doxycycline, 100 mg orally twice daily[b]
- Ciprofloxacin, 500 mg orally twice daily

Alternative choices
- Chloramphenicol, 25 mg/kg orally 4 times daily[c]

[a] Gentamicin is the recommended treatment for breastfeeding women (CDC, 2002; Inglesby et al, 2000).
[b] Tetracycline could be substituted for doxycycline
[c] Concentration should be maintained between 5 and 20 mcg/mL. Concentrations greater than 25 mcg/mL can cause reversible bone marrow suppression
Source: Adapted from CDC NCID (2001); Inglesby et al. (2000); WHO (2008).

Diagnostic laboratory studies include sputum, blood, or lymph node aspirate with gram-negative bacilli with bipolar staining on Wright, Giemsa, or Wayson stain. X-rays may reveal pulmonary infiltrates or consolidation. Rapid diagnostic tests are available at select health departments, the CDC and military laboratories (CDC NCID, 2001; Inglesby et al., 2000; WHO, 2008). Treatment recommendations are included in Exhibit 21.3.

ANTHRAX

When compared to other biologic agents, there is little research available about a pregnancy complicated by an anthrax infection. Anthrax affects the lungs, skin, gastrointestinal system or oropharynx. Diagnosis is classed as suspected, probable, or confirmed. A woman presenting with an illness suggestive of known anthrax clinical forms without definitive, presumptive, or suggestive laboratory evidence of *Bacillus anthracis*, or epidemiologic evidence related to anthrax, would be grouped as *suspected* anthrax (CDC, 2006a).

A woman would be classified as *probable* anthrax when the presentation consists of a clinically compatible illness that does not meet the confirmed case definition, but includes one of four clinical signs. The clinical signs are a documented anthrax environmental exposure; evidence of *B. anthracis* DNA in a clinical specimen collected from a normally sterile site (i.e. blood, cerebral spinal fluid); a lesion of other affected tissue (skin, pulmonary, reticuloendothelial, or gastrointestinal); or a positive result in serum specimens using Quick ELISA Anthrax-PA kit (CDC, 2006a). A diagnosis is *confirmed* with any one of the criteria summarized in Exhibit 21.4.

Recommended treatment for any type of Anthrax involves supportive care and antibiotics. Tetracyclines or ciprofloxacin are not recommended during pregnancy but they may be indicated for life-threatening illness. Adverse effects on developing teeth and bones are dose-related and may be used for a short time (7–14 days) before 6 months' gestation (CDC NCID, 2001; Inglesby et al., 2000; WHO, 2008). Additional symptomology and treatment recommendations are included in Table 21.1.

EXHIBIT 21.4

Criteria for Confirmed Diagnosis of Anthrax

- Identification of *B. anthracis* by Laboratory Response Network (LRN)
- Demonstration of *B. anthracis* antigens in tissues by immunohistochemical staining using both *B. anthracis* cell wall and capsule monoclonal antibodies
- Evidence of a 4 x rise in antibodies to protective antigen between acute and convalescent sera or a 4 x change in antibodies to protective antigen in paired convalescent sera using CDC quantitative anti-PA IgG ELISA testing
- Documented anthrax environmental exposure and evidence of *B. anthracis* DNA in clinical specimens collected from a normally sterile site or lesion of other affected tissue (skin, pulmonary, reticuloendothelial, or gastrointestinal)

Source: Adapted from CDC (2006a).

BIOTERRORISM

CLINICAL MANAGEMENT AND FOLLOW-UP DURING OR FOLLOWING A BIOTERRORISM EVENT

The Federal Emergency Management Agency (FEMA) suggests minimizing negative effects from any biologic agent by quickly moving away from unusual or suspicious substances in the environment, contacting the authorities and listening to the media for official instructions, washing with soap and water, and ensuring that others do the same. In addition, following a known exposure to a biologic agent, individuals should remove and bag clothing and personal items, follow official instructions for disposal of contaminated items, wash with soap and water and put on clean clothes, seek medical assistance, and follow directions to stay away from others or remain in quarantine (FEMA, 2007).

High-efficiency particulate air (HEPA) filters are useful in biological attacks. If there is a central heating and cooling system with a HEPA filter, leaving it running or turning on the fan will cause movement of the air in the house through the filter and will help to remove the agents from the air. If there is a portable HEPA filter, the recommendation is to turn it on and place it in an interior room. Apartments or office buildings with a modern central heating and cooling system often have a filtration system capable of providing a relatively safe level of protection from outside biological contaminants (FEMA, 2010).

It is important that health care providers are knowledgeable about the diagnosis and treatment of possible biohazard threats during pregnancy. They must remain vigilant, take safety precautions and actions and avail themselves of resources to protect women and themselves.

TABLE 21.1 Diagnostic Symptoms and Treatment Recommendations: Anthrax (*Bacillus anthracis*)

TYPE	DESCRIPTION	TREATMENT
Cutaneous:[a] Most common[b]	• Painless skin lesion developing over 2 to 6 days from papular to vesicular stage to depressed black eschar with surrounding edema • Fever, malaise, lymphadenopathy	• Ciprofloxacin 500 mg BID or Doxycycline 100 mg BID x 60 days
Inhalation:[a] Rare[b]	• Viral respiratory prodrome • Hypoxia, dyspnea or acute RDS with cyanosis/shock • Mediastinal widening or pleural effusion (x-ray)	• Ciprofloxacin 400 mg q 12 hr or doxycycline or doxycycline 100 mg q 12 hr. and 1 to 2 additional antimicrobials, that is rifampin, vancomycin, penicillin, ampicillin, chloramphenicol, imipenem, clindamycin and clarithromycin • Supportive care including controlling pleural effusions
GI:[a] Rare[b]	• Severe abdominal pain and tenderness, nausea, vomiting, hematemesis • Bloody diarrhea, anorexia, fever, abdominal swelling, septicemia	• Same as Inhalation anthrax • IV initially. Switch to oral when clinically appropriate
Oropharyngeal: Least common[b]	• Painless mucosal lesion in mouth or oropharynx • Cervical adenopathy, edema, pharyngitis, fever, septicemia	• Same as Inhalation anthrax • IV initially. Switch to oral when clinically appropriate

[a] Do **NOT** use extended-spectrum cephalosporins or trimethoprim/sulfamethoxazole because anthrax may be resistant to these drugs.

[b] Breastfeeding women should be offered prophylaxis with the same medications. All of these medications are excreted in breast milk. The babies should be treated with an antibiotic that is safe for the prophylactic treatment of the infant.

Source: Adapted from CSTE Position Statement Number: 09-ID-10; CDC (2002); CDC (2006a).

REFERENCES

Centers for Disease Control and Prevention (CDC). (2003a). Women with smallpox vaccine exposure during pregnancy reported to the National Smallpox Vaccine in Pregnancy Registry–United States, 2003). *MMWR, 52*(17), 386–388.

Centers for Disease Control & Prevention (CDC). (2003b). Smallpox vaccination information for women who are pregnant or breastfeeding. Retrieved from. www.bt.cdc.gov/agent/smallpox/vaccination/preg-factsheet.asp

Centers for Disease Control and Prevention (CDC). (2005). Plague: Epidemiology. Retrieved from www.cdc.gov/ncidod/dvbid/plague/epi.htm

Centers for Disease Control & Prevention (CDC). (2006a). Fact sheet: Anthrax information for health care providers. Retrieved from http://emergency.cdc.gov/agent/anthrax/anthrax-hcp-factsheet.asp

Centers for Disease Control & Prevention (CDC). (2006b). Emerging infections and pregnancy. Retrieved from wwwnc.cdc.gov/eid/article/12/11/06–0152_article.htm

Centers for Disease Control & Prevention (CDC). (2007). Evaluate a rash illness suspicious for smallpox–interactive tool. Retrieved from http://emergency.cdc.gov/agent/smallpox/diagnosis/riskalgorithm

Centers for Disease Control & Prevention (CDC). (2009). Questions and answers about smallpox vaccination while pregnant or breastfeeding. Retrieved from http://emergency.cdc.gov/agent/smallpox/faq/pregnancy.asp

Centers for Disease Control & Prevention (CDC) and National Center for Infectious Disease (NCID). (2001). A quick guide to plague. Retrieved from www.cdc.gov/nczved/divisions/dvbid/resources/plague_job.pdf

Cono, J., Cragan, J. D., Jamieson, J. D., & Rasmussen, S. A., (2006). Prophylaxis and treatment of pregnant women for emerging infections and bioterrorism emergencies. *Emerging Infectious Disease, 12*(11) Retrieved from wwwnc.cdc.gov/eid/article/12/11/06-0618_article.htm#suggestedcitation

Constantin, C., Martinelli, A., & Strickland, O. L. (2003). Smallpox: A disease of the past?: Considerations for midwives. *Journal of Midwifery Women's Health, 48*(4). Retrieved from www.medscape.com/viewarticle/458968

Federal Emergency Management Agency (FEMA). (2007). Fact sheet: Biological. (#570). Retrieved from www.fema.gov/library/irlSearchFemaNumber.do;jsessionid=57338CD3286BA10C6CC12CDC1F16B3B0.WorkerLibrary

Hogan, C. J., Harchelroad, F., & McGovern, T. W. (2010). Small pox. Retrieved from www.emedicinehealth.com/smallpox-health/article_em.htm

Inglesby, T. V., Dennis, D. T., Henderson, D. A., Bartlett, J. G., Ascher, M. S., Eitzen, E.,…Tonat, K. (2000). Plague as a biological weapon: Medical and public health management. *Journal of the American Medical Association, 283*(17), 2281–2290.

Jamieson, D. J., Theiler, R. N., & Rasmussen, S. A. (2006). Emerging infections and pregnancy. *Emerging Infectious Disease, 12(11)*. Retrieved from wwwnc.cdc.gov/eid/article/12/11/06–0152_article.htm#suggestedcitation

Mays, K. M. (2009). *Lassa fever, Merck manual*. Retrieved from www.merckmanuals.com/professional/infectious_diseases/arboviridae_arenaviridae_and_filoviridae/lassa_fever.html

Rao, A. R., Prahlad, I., Swaminathan, M., & Lakshmi, A. (1963). Pregnancy and smallpox. *Journal of Indian Medical Association, (40)*, 353–563.

Ryan, M. A., & Seward, J. F. (2008). Pregnancy, birth, and infant health outcomes from the National Smallpox Vaccine in Pregnancy Registry, 2003–2006.*Clinical Infectious Disease, 47* (Suppl. 3), S221–S226.

Suarez, V. R., & Hankins, G. D. (2002). Smallpox and pregnancy: From eradicated disease to bioterrorist threat. *Obstetrics and Gynecology, 1*, 878–893.

White, S. R., Henretig, F. M., & Dukes, R. G. (2002). Medical management of vulnerable populations and co-morbid conditions of victims of bioterrorism. *Emergency Medical Clinics of North America, 20*(2), 365–392.

World Health Organization (WHO). (2008). Communicable disease toolkit for Burundi: Case definitions. Retrieved from www.who.int/mediacentre/factsheets/fs103/en

22 Infections in Pregnant Women

Julie M. Johnson and Brenna Anderson

Infectious diseases commonly manifest during pregnancy, ranging from benign to life-threatening conditions. Many of these women will present in the acute care setting. Occasionally, symptoms of pregnancy and disease may overlap, making it difficult to accurately diagnose gravid women. In addition, pregnancy is an immune altering state, which in certain circumstances, affects the management of pregnant women versus their nonpregnant counterparts. It is crucial that in obstetric triage units and emergency room settings, providers are able to diagnose and appropriately treat pregnant women.

INTRA-AMNIOTIC INFECTION

Clinical intra-amniotic infection (IAI) or chorioamnionitis complicates 1% to 4% of all births (Gibbs & Duff, 1991). The major risk factor for IAI in the obstetric triage setting will be prolonged rupture of membranes. While intact chorioamnionitis does occur, it is less common and may be due to *Listeria monocytogenes*, group B streptococcus (GBS), or recent obstetric procedures such as cerclage or amniocentesis (Creasy, Resnik, Iams, Lockwood, & Moore, 2009; Tita & Andrews, 2010). While IAI is more commonly seen during labor, women with chorioamnionitis may still present to the obstetric or emergency room. In pregnant women with fever and other supporting symptomatology, IAI must be considered until proven otherwise.

PRESENTING SYMPTOMATOLOGY

The presenting symptoms of chorioamnionitis may overlap with other diagnoses seen more commonly in the emergency setting, such as pyelonephritis. Most women with chorioamnionitis will have ruptured membranes; therefore, leakage of fluid and contractions may be frequent complaints. To differentiate from normal labor, fever, constant abdominal pain, foul smelling discharge, general malaise, and/or body aches should be noted. In rare circumstances, IAI can be present in women with intact membranes. To make the diagnoses of IAI in a pregnant woman, a high index of suspicion is necessary with signs of infection and abdominal pain.

HISTORY AND DATA COLLECTION

A thorough history is recommended. A focus on pregnancy symptoms such as leakage of fluid and contractions, any recent procedures, or exposure to foodborne pathogens, such as *L. monocytogenes* can be elicited. Listeriosis is 18 times more common in the pregnant population versus the nonpregnant population, and transmission is through ingestion of contaminated foods such as unpasteurized milk and soft cheeses, unwashed meat and vegetables, and processed foods such as deli meat and hot dogs (Lamont et al., 2011). Tips for preventing listeriosis are listed in Exhibit 22.1.

PHYSICAL EXAMINATION

The diagnosis of IAI is usually clinical. Chorioamnionitis is diagnosed by the presence of fever (>100.4°F) and one or more of the following: uterine tenderness, maternal or fetal tachycardia, and foul smelling/purulent discharge (Tita & Andrews, 2010).

LABORATORY AND IMAGING STUDIES

Amniotic fluid testing, using rapid markers (Gram's stain, cell count, glucose, and leukocyte esterase), may be used when considering delivery of a preterm or nonviable fetus in whom the diagnosis of chorioamnionitis is unclear. A positive Gram's stain, low glucose (<15 mg/dL), or elevated white blood cell (WBC) count (>30/cubic mm) may be indicative of infection (Tita & Andrews, 2010). Amniotic fluid culture would be of low yield, due to the time it takes for results.

DIFFERENTIAL DIAGNOSIS

Chorioamnionitis may present with a wide range of symptoms. It varies from vague symptoms, such as abdominal pain or malaise, to acute pain with signs of peritoneal irritation. The differential diagnoses include pyelonephritis, gastroenteritis, appendicitis, and preterm labor.

EXHIBIT 22.1

Tips for Preventing Listeriosis

- Thoroughly wash all raw fruits and vegetables
- Thoroughly cook all meat and poultry
- Do not ingest unpasteurized milk or soft cheeses made from unpasteurized milk
- Do not eat deli meats or hot dogs or unless they are steaming hot prior to serving
- Do not eat smoked seafood unless it is canned or served as part of a cooked dish or casserole
- Keep kitchen and refrigerator clean, with special attention given to the above foods

Source: CDC (2011a).

CLINICAL MANAGEMENT AND FOLLOW-UP

The mainstay of treatment in the setting of chorioamnionitis is immediate antibiotic therapy and delivery. Antepartum treatment with antibiotics decreases the risk of neonatal sepsis and mortality, so it must be initiated without delay. Chorioamnionitis alone is not an indication for cesarean delivery. IAI is usually polymicrobial in nature, and a broad spectrum antibiotic is recommended, but the optimal regimen is not well established. A commonly used regimen is ampicillin every 6 hours and gentamicin every 8 hours until delivery. The optimal length of antibiotic treatment postpartum is unknown and varies from one dose of antibiotics after delivery to treatment for 24 to 48 postpartum hours (Hopkins & Smaill, 2002). If a cesarean delivery is performed, clindamycin 900 mg every 8 hours may be added for additional anaerobic coverage. Acetaminophen for fever may also be administered, not to exceed the maximum dose of 4 g/d.

INFLUENZA

During seasonal influenza outbreaks and influenza pandemics, most recently the H1N1 pandemic of 2009 and 2010, pregnant women are at a greater risk of hospitalization and death from complications of influenza (Siston et al., 2010). The influenza virus is an RNA virus with three main types: A (most common), B, and C. It is easily transmitted through respiratory droplets with an incubation period of 2 to 4 days (Cox & Subbarao, 1999). Once a woman is infected, she will remain infectious from about 1 day prior to the start of symptoms until approximately 1 week after becoming sick (Centers for Disease Control [CDC], 2011b).

PRESENTING SYMPTOMATOLOGY

Pregnant women presenting with influenza may have a fever (>100.4F), cough, dyspnea, sore throat, runny nose, body aches, headache, fatigue, vomiting, or diarrhea. All or some of the symptoms may be present, and not all women will have a fever.

HISTORY AND DATA COLLECTION

A complete history includes the length, type, and severity of symptoms. A vaccination history, infectious contacts, and history of comorbidities including asthma, diabetes, and hypertension are also critical to assist in diagnosis. Pregnant women with asthma or chronic hypertension are more likely to be admitted to an intensive care unit with influenza complications, so these women must be clearly identified (Siston et al., 2010; Varner et al., 2011).

PHYSICAL EXAMINATION

A complete physical examination must be performed with attention to the presenting symptoms. Findings may include throat erythema, runny nose, wheezing, rales/rhonchi, tachypnea, and tachycardia. Fetal tachycardia may also be present with maternal fever.

LABORATORY AND IMAGING STUDIES

A rapid influenza test (types A and B) is recommended in pregnant women if influenza is suspected. However, due to low sensitivity of the rapid tests, confirmation of negative tests may be performed with viral culture or reverse transcription polymerase chain reaction (RT-PCR; Harper et al., 2009). Treatment should not be withheld in the absence of a positive test if clinical suspicion is high. If there is uncertainty in the diagnosis, a complete blood count with a differential may help to determine if a bacterial infection is present versus influenza. A chest radiograph is indicated if there are respiratory symptoms, such as dyspnea and findings consistent with pneumonia.

DIFFERENTIAL DIAGNOSIS

The differential diagnoses include a variety of other respiratory illnesses. Pneumonia, pharyngitis, the common cold, sinusitis, or bronchitis must all be considered.

CLINICAL MANAGEMENT AND FOLLOW-UP

Pregnant women who are suspected of having influenza in the obstetric triage setting are offered treatment with antivirals and acetaminophen if febrile or in the presence of myalgias (Morbidity and Mortality Weekly Report, 2011). Oseltamivir (Tamiflu) is recommended by the CDC for use in pregnant women at a dose of 75 mg twice daily for 5 days. Ideally, to improve maternal outcomes, treatment should start within 48 hours of symptom onset. Bed rest and hydration are recommended as well. For women who respond to antipyretics and have no respiratory compromise, outpatient management may be appropriate. A follow-up visit with a care provider is recommended within 24 to 48 hours.

Hospitalization is recommended for pregnant women who are unable to tolerate oral intake, have fever unresponsive to acetaminophen, or respiratory compromise. If a superimposed bacterial pneumonia is suspected, the most common organisms are *Streptococcus pneumonia*, *Staphylococcus aureus*, *Haemophilus influenza*, and group A streptococci. Empiric therapy with ceftriaxone and azithromycin, for example, may be appropriate (Mandell et al., 2007).

SEPSIS

Sepsis is rarely diagnosed in pregnancy, complicating 1 in 8,000 deliveries (Martin & Foley, 2006). In 2001, the International Sepsis Definitions Conference defined sepsis as a systemic inflammatory response syndrome (SIRS) in the presence of infection. Of note, there are no established criteria for pregnancy. Lappen et al. (2010) demonstrated that neither the SIRS nor Modified Early Warning score (MEWS) were able to identify patients at risk of sepsis or death in the setting of IAI. There are varying degrees of sepsis, which are defined clinically and described in Table 22.1 (Levy et al., 2003).

PRESENTING SYMPTOMATOLOGY

The presenting symptoms will vary based on the underlying cause. The most common cause of sepsis in the obstetric population is genital tract infection

TABLE 22.1 Definitions of Sepsis

	DEFINITIONS
SIRS	At least two of the following findings: • Temperature <36°C or >38°C • Heart rate >110 bpm[a] • Respiratory rate >20/min • WBC >14,000/mcl[a]
Sepsis	SIRS + infection
Severe sepsis	Sepsis + organ dysfunction, may see: • Lactic acidosis (≥4 mmol/L) • Oliguria (<0.5 mL/kg/hr) • Altered mental status
Septic shock	Sepsis + hypotension (systolic blood pressure (SBP) <90 mmHg, MAP <60, or reduction in SBP by >40 mmHg from baseline despite fluid resuscitation

[a] Heart rate and WBC modified to reflect physiologic changes of pregnancy.

Source: Adapted from Levy et al. (2003) and Dellinger et al. (2008).

(chorioamnionitis, endometritis, and septic abortion); other nonobstetric causes are urosepsis, pneumonia, appendicitis, meningitis, bowel perforation, and cholecystitis (Kramer et al., 2009; Mabie, Barton, & Sibai, 1997). In the setting of obstetric-related infection, symptoms may include, fever, abdominal pain, general malaise, bleeding, foul smelling discharge, and contractions. Other symptoms may include dysuria, hematuria, cough, chest pain, shortness of breath, nausea/vomiting, headache, and neck or back pain.

HISTORY AND DATA COLLECTION

A quick but thorough history is obtained with a focus on possible causes of infection. It must be kept in mind that the presenting symptoms may overlap with other disease processes. The gestational age or days postpartum, presenting complaints, risk factors (preexisiting medical conditions or immunosuppression), recent medications, allergies, and recent activities and/or travel history all need to be carefully documented (Belfort, Saade, Foley, Phelan, & Dildy, 2010).

PHYSICAL EXAMINATION

Physical examination findings will depend upon the underlying cause of infection. It is critical to recognize that cardiovascular changes in pregnancy result in physiologically normal increases in heart rate and cardiac output and a decrease in blood pressure (Yeomans & Gilstrap, 2005). Significant findings will vary with the etiology. General findings associated with sepsis include fever, tachycardia, tachypnea, hypotension, warm extremities (early septic shock), cool extremities (late septic shock), fetal tachycardia, and fetal heart rate abnormalities such as variable or late decelerations. Pain with neck flexion or headache may be seen with meningitis. Lung findings such as rales, rhonchi, and decreased breath sounds may be present in the setting of pneumonia or acute respiratory distress syndrome (ARDS). Flank pain, costovertebral angle tenderness, and suprapubic pain are associated with urosepsis. Finally, women with sepsis from IAI may have uterine tenderness, contractions, purulent discharge, cervical motion tenderness, and pain with bimanual examination.

LABORATORY AND IMAGING STUDIES

When pregnant women present with symptoms and physical examination findings consistent with sepsis, the initial laboratory evaluation may be broad in an attempt to narrow the diagnosis. These women are usually ill-appearing with abnormal vital signs. To expedite treatment, complete blood count with differential, basic metabolic profile, liver function tests, lactic acid, arterial blood gas, and blood cultures should be obtained during the initial evaluation. As the history and physical progresses, a more tailored approach may be taken. Further testing may include urine, endometrial, or sputum cultures, rapid influenza, and lumbar puncture (LP).

If the pregnant woman has respiratory symptoms, a chest radiograph is recommended. If there are symptoms consistent with an acute abdomen, a pelvic ultrasound, pelvic and abdominal magnetic resonance imaging (MRI), or computed tomography (CT) is necessary.

DIFFERENTIAL DIAGNOSIS

The differential diagnosis for sepsis is extensive. Some potential entities include pulmonary embolus, amniotic fluid embolus, adverse drug reactions, and acute adrenal insufficiency.

CLINICAL MANAGEMENT AND FOLLOW-UP

Recognizing sepsis is critical to the initial management of pregnant women presenting for treatment. Early goal-directed therapy has been shown to improve survival in nonobstetric women (Rivers et al., 2001) and consists of fluid resuscitation, vasopressors, packed red cells, and inotropic agents aimed at normalizing clinical parameters (as listed below). The optimal goals for therapy in pregnant women are not known, but the same principles can be applied using these goals or frequent clinical assessment. The initial focus is largely on maternal stabilization because fetal compromise is often due to maternal disease (Fernandez-Perez, Salman, Pendem, & Farmer, 2005).

The following sepsis guidelines are largely derived from the Surviving Sepsis Campaign (Dellinger et al., 2008). Upon presentation, with sepsis, hypotension, and a lactate of ≥4 mmol/L, early and aggressive fluid resuscitation is recommended. The goal for adequate resuscitation is a central venous pressure (CVP) of 8 to 12 mmHg or urine output of 0.5 mL/kg/hr. A foley may be placed if necessary. If the mean arterial pressure (MAP) is not maintained above 65 mmHg with fluid, vasopressors are needed. If the hematocrit is less than 30%, packed red cells are recommended. Rapid identification of the infectious source and infection control (e.g., wound debridement) is paramount. Prior to obtaining cultures, empiric antibiotics with broad-spectrum coverage are administered, ideally within an hour of presentation. Antibiotic coverage is chosen with the possible source, common organisms, community resistance patterns, and fetus in mind.

TABLE 22.2 Suspected Sources of Sepsis and Recommended Antibiotic Treatment

SEPSIS WITHOUT A SOURCE	MEROPENEM
Endometritis	Gentamicin plus clindamycin
Chorioamnionitis	Ampicillin plus gentamicin
Pyelonephritis	Ceftriaxone
Pneumonia	Ceftriaxone plus azithromycin
Appendicitis	Cefoxitin
Bowel perforation	Cefoxitin (if severe infection, may use meropenem)
Cholecystitis	Ceftriaxone or cefazolin

Note: Antibiotic regimens should be chosen with community resistance patterns in mind.

Source: French & Smaill (2004); Hopkins & Smaill (2002); Wing, Hendershott, Debuque, & Millar (1998); Mandell et al. (2007); and Solomkin et al. (2010).

See Table 22.2 for suggested antibiotic regimens with specific suspected sources. A commonly used antibiotic in the setting of sepsis and no source is meropenem. Fetal monitoring of a viable fetus is recommended. Tocolysis is contraindicated. Delivery is recommended only for obstetric indications and must be balanced with the maternal status if a cesarean delivery is necessary (Fernandez-Perez et al., 2005).

The recognition and prompt treatment of sepsis in the obstetric triage setting is imperative, as early treatment may improve survival. Consultation of maternal-fetal medicine and hospital intensivists is recommended for further management. After stabilization, the pregnant woman can be admitted to the appropriate medical unit for ongoing care.

MENINGITIS

While meningitis is a relatively rare event, with an estimated incidence of 1.38 cases of bacterial meningitis per 100,000 in the United States, it is a life-threatening emergency that must be recognized promptly in the emergency setting (Thigpen et al., 2011). Meningitis is defined as inflammation of the meninges surrounding the brain and spinal cord. The main causes of bacterial meningitis are *Neisseria meningitides, S. pneumoniae, H. influenzae* serotype B, and GBS, and the primary causes of viral meningitis are enteroviruses, influenza, mumps, and herpesvirus (CDC, 2011c).

Women will present with sudden onset of fever, headache, and a stiff neck. They may also have photophobia, mental status changes, nausea, and emesis. If there is a suspicion of bacterial meningitis, a LP should be performed. Blood cultures and empiric antibiotic therapy must be initiated promptly. If the woman is immunocompromised, has a history of central nervous system disease, has a new onset seizure, papilledema, abnormal level of consciousness, or a focal neurologic deficit, a CT scan of the head should be performed prior to the LP (Hasbun, Abrahams, Jekel, & Quagliarello, 2001). In this case, if the LP is delayed, blood cultures must be obtained and empiric antibiotic therapy must be administered prior to imaging. Dexamethasone should also be given at the same time as antibiotic therapy because glucocorticoids may decrease the risk of death and neurologic complications in certain settings (Tunkel et al., 2004). Fetal monitoring of a viable fetus is recommended; however, one must consider the maternal risk of a cesarean delivery if it is warranted.

The cerebrospinal fluid (CSF) obtained on LP should be sent for Gram's stain, culture, glucose, protein, and cell count. In bacterial meningitis, the Gram's stain is 60% to 90% sensitive and depends on the bacterial concentration (Tunkel et al., 2004). The WBC count is usually elevated and the protein level may be high. The diagnosis of bacterial versus viral meningitis, however, depends on the Gram's stain and culture.

After the LP, when the pregnant woman is stabilized with empiric antibiotics, admission is appropriate if there is a strong suspicion of bacterial meningitis. Further antibiotic treatment is tailored to the microbiology results.

REFERENCES

Belfort, M. A., Saade, G. R., Foley, M. R., Phelan, J. P., & Dildy, G. A. (2010). *Critical Care Obstetrics* (5th ed.). Malden, MA: Wiley-Blackwell.

Centers for Disease Control and Prevention (CDC). (2011a). *Listeriosis.* Retrieved from http://www.cdc.gov/listeria/prevention.html.

Centers for Disease Control and Prevention (CDC). (2011b). *Influenza: Flu Basics.* Retrieved from http://www.cdc.gov/flu/keyfacts.htm

Centers for Disease Control and Prevention (CDC). (2011c). *Meningitis.* Retrieved from http://www.cdc.gov/meningitis/clinical-resources.html

Cox, N. J., & Subbarao, K., (1999). Influenza. *Lancet, 354(9186)*, 1277–1282.

Creasy, R. K., Resnik, R., Iams, J. D., Lockwood, C. J., & Moore, T. R. (2009). *Creasy and Resnik's maternal-fetal medicine: Principles and practice* (6th ed.). Philadelphia, PA: Saunders/Elsevier.

Dellinger, R. P., Levy, M. M., Carlet, J. M., Bion, J., Parker, M. M., Jaeschke, R.... Vincent, J. (2008). Surviving Sepsis Campaign: International guidelines for management of severe sepsis and septic shock: 2008. *Critical Care Medicine, 36*, 296–327.

Fernandez-Perez, E. R., Salman, S., Pendem, S., & Farmer, C. (2005). Sepsis during pregnancy. *Critical Care Medicine, 33(Supp)*, 286–293.

French, L. M., & Smaill, F. M. (2004). Antibiotic regimens for endometritis after delivery. *Cochrane Database of Systematic Reviews, 4*, CD001067.

Gibbs, R. S., & Duff, P. (1991). Progress in pathogenesis and management of clinical intraamniotic infection. *American Journal of Obstetrics and Gynecology, 164*, 1317–1326.

Harper, S. A., Bradley, J. S., Englund, J. A., File, T. M., Gravenstein, S., Hayden, F. G.... Zimmerman, R. K. (2009). Seasonal influenza in adults and children-diagnosis, treatment, chemoprophylaxis, and institutional outbreak management: Clinical practice guidelines of the Infectious Diseases Society of America. *Clinical Infectious Diseases, 48*, 1003–1032.

Hasbun, R., Abrahams, J., Jekel, J., & Quagliarello, V. J. (2001). Computed tomography of the head before lumbar puncture in adults with suspected meningitis. *New England Journal of Medicine, 345(24)*, 1727–1733.

Hopkins, L. & Smaill, F. (2002). Antibiotic regimens for management of intraamniotic infection. *Cochrane Database of Systematic Reviews, 3*, CD003254.

Kramer, H., Schutte, J. M., Zwart, J. J., Schuitemaker, N., Steegers, E., & van Roosmalen, J. (2009). Maternal mortality and severe morbidity from sepsis in the Netherlands. *Acta Obstetricia et Gynecologica, 88*, 647–653.

Lamont, R. F., Sobel, J., Mazaki-Tovi, S., Kusanovic, J. P., Vaisbuch, E., Kim, S. K.,... & Romero, R. (2011). Listeriosis in human pregnancy: A systematic review. *The Journal of Perinatal Medicine, 39(3)*, 227–236.

Lappen, J. R., Keene, M., Lore, M., Grobman, W. A., & Gossett, D. R. (2010). Existing models fail to predict sepsis in an obstetric population with intrauterine infection. *American Journal of Obstetrics and Gynecology, 203*(6), 573.e1–e5.

Levy, M. M., Fink, M. P., Marshall, J. C., Abraham, E., Angus, D., Cook, D.... Ramsay, G. (2003). 2001 SCCM/ESICM/ACCP/ATS/SIS international sepsis definitions conference. *Critical Care Medicine, 31*, 1250–1256.

Mabie, W. C., Barton, J. R., & Sibai, B. (1997). Septic shock in pregnancy. *Obstetrics & Gynecology, 90*, 553–561.

Mandell, L. A., Wunderink, R. G., Anzueto, A., Bartlett, J. G., Campbell, G. D., Dean, N. C.... Whitney, C. G. (2007). Infectious Diseases Society of America/ American Thoracic Society consensus guidelines on the management of community-acquired pneumonia in adults. *Clinical Infectious Diseases, 44*, S27–S72.

Martin, S. R., & Foley, M. R. (2006). Intensive care in obstetrics: An evidence-based review. *American Journal of Obstetrics and Gynecology, 195*, 673–689.

Morbidity and Mortality Weekly Report. (2011). Antiviral agents for the treatment and chemoprophylaxis of influenza. Retrieved from http://www.cdc.gov/mmwr/preview/mmwrhtml/rr6001a1.htm

Rivers, E., Nguyen, B., Havstad, S., Ressler, J., Muzzin, A., Knoblich, B.... Early Goal-Directed Therapy Collaborative Group (2001). Early goal-directed therapy in the treatment of severe sepsis and septic shock. *New England Journal of Medicine, 345*(19), 1368–1377.

Siston, A. M., Rasmussen, S. A., Honein, M. A., Fry, A. M., Seib, K., Callaghan, W. M.... Pandemic H1N1 Influenza in Pregnancy Working Group (2010). Pandemic 2009 influenza A(H1N1) virus among pregnant women in the United States. *Journal of the American Medical Association, 303*(15), 1517–1525.

Solomkin, J. S., Mazuski, J. E., Bradley, J. S., Rodvold, K. A., Goldstein, E. J., Baron, E. J.... Bartlett, J. G. (2010). Diagnosis and management of complicated intra-abdominal infection in adults and children: Guidelines by the Surgical Infection Society and the Infectious Diseases Society of America. *Clinical Infectious Diseases, 50*, 133–64.

Thigpen, M. C., Whitney, C. G., Messonnier, N. E., Zell, E. R., Lynfield, R., Hadler, J. L.... Schuchat, A. (2011) Bacterial meningitis in the United States, 1998–2007. *The New England Journal of Medicine, 364*, 2016–2025.

Tita, T. N., & Andrews, W. W. (2010). Diagnosis and management of clinical chroioamnionitis. *Clinical Perinatology, 37*(2), 339–354.

Tunkel, A. R., Hartman, B. J., Kaplan, S. L., Kaufman, B. A., Roos, K. L., Scheld, W. M., & Whitley, R. J. (2004). Practice guidelines for the management of bacterial meningitis. *Clinical Infectious Diseases, 39*(9), 1267–1284.

Varner, M. W., Rice, M. M., Anderson, B., Tolosa, J. E., Sheffield, J., Spong, C. Y.,... Van Dorsten, J. P. (2011). Influenza-like illness in hospitalized pregnant and postpartum women during the 2009–2010 H1N1 pandemic. *Obstetrics & Gynecology, 118*, 593–600.

Wing, D. A., Hendershott, C. M., Debuque, L., & Millar, L. K. (1998). A randomized trial of three antibiotic regimens for the treatment of pyelonephritis in pregnancy. *Obstetrics and Gynecology, 92*(2), 249–253.

Yeomans, E. R., & Gilstrap, L. C. (2005). Physiologic changes in pregnancy and their impact on critical care. *Critical Care Medicine, 33*(10), S256–S258.

Intimate Partner Violence and Sexual Assault in Pregnancy

23

Donna LaFontaine

Intimate partner violence (IPV) and sexual assault are common violent crimes perpetrated on women. Accurate statistics are difficult to obtain because these crimes are significantly underreported to both law officers and medical personnel. Sadly, pregnant women are not exempt from becoming victims of these crimes. When a woman is in a dysfunctional relationship, pregnancy may function as a stressor leading to increased episodes of violence (Jasinski, 2001). Depending on the patient population, up to 20.1% of pregnant women are victims of physical abuse (Gazmararian et al., 1996). In one trauma center, 31.5% of pregnant trauma patients suffered injuries as a direct result of IPV (Poole et al., 1996). Violent actions perpetrated on a pregnant woman can cause significant psychological trauma in addition to physical injury. Obstetric (OB) complications associated with trauma include miscarriage, preterm labor and placental abruption. All women who present to an OB triage unit or an emergency department (not just those who present with an injury or complication) must be screened for IPV. An organized plan for providing the victim with resources must be readily available when a screen is positive.

PRESENTING SYMPTOMATOLOGY

If a woman has sustained obvious or major trauma, it is likely the patient will first be taken to a general emergency room or a regional trauma center. The emergency room physician will stabilize the woman and likely call for an OB consultation. If a woman identifies herself as a victim of partner violence or sexual assault at the point of entry, the waiting time should be minimized. The victim ought to be brought immediately to a private room for evaluation. If a woman does not want to involve law enforcement, the medical provider is not obligated to report to the police unless she is a member of a vulnerable population, such as a child, or someone who is mentally or physically incapacitated. Mandated reporting is state specific, so it is important to know the requirements in the state where the medical provider practices.

Women who have sustained minor trauma may spontaneously present to an OB triage unit. Although complaints of preterm contractions, abdominal pain or vaginal bleeding may raise awareness to ask specifically about trauma events, all women who present to an OB triage unit must be screened for IPV.

Occasionally a woman presents to an OB triage, admits to trauma, and complains of head, neck, back, or neurological symptoms. If a normal fetal heart is obtained, strong consideration can be given to transfer the woman for an official trauma assessment by an emergency physician. More extensive fetal evaluation can be arranged in the trauma unit or after the mother is stabilized. Often, the victim will not admit to trauma and the complaints will be vague.

When a woman presents late in gestation with little or no prenatal care, the provider must consider that she may be a victim of IPV and the partner did not allow the woman to seek prenatal care early on. There are several IPV screening tools currently available, and most hospitals have policies for screening. An example of a quick and effective screening tool is presented in Exhibit 23.1.

It is crucial to be able to screen the woman alone. Many times a perpetrator will exert significant control over a victim and even when asked, will not leave the room. A simple diversion may be attempted once, but if the triage staff feels threatened at any time, it is crucial to have security alerted and available. In recent years, there has been a significant rise in violence perpetrated against health care workers in emergency room settings (Gates, Ross, & Mcqueen, 2006).

PHYSICAL EXAMINATION

A complete physical is performed on all women, especially noting any bruises, lacerations, reddened areas or evidence of bleeding. If the victim is pursuing charges against her perpetrator, with the victim's consent, photographic documentation of any findings will be helpful. Emergency rooms typically have policies regarding photographing injuries and a similar policy should be established in OB triage units. If the victim has already been photographed by police, repeating the process will not be necessary. A detailed description of any injuries should be thoroughly documented in the medical record.

LABORATORY TESTING AND IMAGING STUDIES

Blood type and a Kleihauer Betke (KB) test will need to be obtained. If trauma and/or bleeding have occurred in an Rh negative woman, there is a risk of feto-maternal hemorrhage with subsequent Rh D sensitization. All women with a history of trauma need to receive Rh D immunoglobulin within

EXHIBIT 23.1

Screening Tool for Domestic Violence

Patients are screened for domestic violence with the following questions:

- Is anyone close to you threatening or hurting you?
- Is anyone hitting, kicking, choking, or hurting you physically?
- Is anyone forcing you to do something sexually that you do not want to do?

Source: Courtesy of Women & Infants' Hospital, Providence, RI.

72 hours of the incident, but a KB test is necessary in order to determine the correct dose of Rh D immunoglobulin. The KB test is a measure of fetal blood cells in the maternal circulation. If more than 30 ml of fetomaternal hemorrhage is determined, then it will be necessary to administer more than the standard 300 mcg dose of Rh D immunoglobulin.

Injuries that cause tenderness and swelling can be x-rayed for evidence of fractures, and the pregnant uterus will need to be shielded. In the case of head injuries or other severe injuries, if computer tomography is indicated, this test must be performed. If the woman is not safe, neither is the fetus. A complete ultrasound examination is indicated if gestational age is unclear or there is vaginal bleeding. If a fetal nonstress test is nonreactive, a biophysical profile can be performed to further evaluate the fetal condition.

CLINICAL MANAGEMENT

The gestational age of the fetus must be carefully obtained and any fetus that is viable should undergo prolonged fetal monitoring. Monitoring is used to assess for contractions which will be present in cases of preterm labor or placental abruptio. The presence of late decelerations is frequently seen with a significant abruption. Delivery may be indicated, in the case of suspected abruption and a non-reassuring fetal status. In a previable gestation, auscultation of the fetal heart rate or real time ultrasonography, if available, is reassuring to the woman who has sustained an episode of violent trauma.

Anyone who is identified as a victim of interpersonal violence must receive caring, emotional support from the medical providers working in an OB triage unit or emergency care setting. When a victim is identified, social services, behavioral health or psychiatry are frequently helpful and can thoroughly assess a woman's needs. A safety assessment must be performed for each victim, specifically asking if the perpetrator has a weapon, does the victim own a cell phone, where will the victim go after release from the hospital and who will be available for support. The pregnant woman may also need assistance in obtaining shelter. Occasionally, a victim will express suicidal or homicidal ideation, which must be evaluated by a behavioral health professional.

Interpersonal violence leading to trauma of a pregnant woman is common and potentially life threatening to both the woman and fetus. The well-being of both the mother and the fetus must be ascertained when a woman presents with a history of trauma. Often, the medical staff will suspect IPV, but the woman will deny being subjected to violence. Asking the screening questions will allow the pregnant victim to know she can turn to an OB triage unit if she becomes ready to reveal her secret. The triage unit should be prepared with an organized plan when an IPV screen yields a positive result. A checklist is included in Exhibit 23.2. This list contains some of the information and resources needed in the event of a positive IPV screen.

SEXUAL ASSAULT

PRESENTING SYMPTOMS, HISTORY, AND PHYSICAL EXAMINATION

Most victims of sexual assault will not report the crime, either to medical professionals or law enforcement. Women who are already pregnant

EXHIBIT 23.2

Information and Checklist of Resources Needed When a Violence Screen Is Positive

1. The pregnant woman must first be medically stabilized. If there is a history of significant trauma, especially if the patient has head, neck, back, neurological symptoms, or mental status changes, consider consulting or transferring patient to a trauma center.
2. Once the pregnant woman is stable, ascertain if there is any danger of the perpetrator presenting to the OB triage. Contact security or local police if there is a possibility of this happening.
3. If the patient would like to report to the police, call the police office in the town where the violent episode occurred. Do not call the police without the patient's permission.
4. Know your state's laws on mandated reporting, especially in the case of an adolescent. If there are questions, contact your risk manager.
5. Perform an assessment of the pregnant woman and her fetus. Thoroughly document. Consider
   - Photography of bruises, lacerations, marks
   - X-rays or CT scans, if necessary for a complete evaluation
   - Fetal evaluation with ultrasound, NST, prolonged fetal heart monitoring, or biophysical profile as determined by fetal age.
   - Administer tetanus vaccine or Rh immune globulin when appropriate.
6. Perform a safety assessment:
   - Does the perpetrator have a weapon?
   - Does the victim have a cell phone?
   - Has the victim ever thought of hurting herself or others?
     If the pregnant woman expresses suicidal or homicidal ideation, this is an emergency and she should never be left alone. Behavioral health or psychiatry and nursing management must be contacted.
   - Where will the victim go?
     Maintain a list of local domestic violence advocacy centers. The national domestic violence hotline can be reached at 1-800-799-7233 or on the Internet at www.ncadv.org.
     Contact your hospital social worker for assistance in arranging discharge planning and shelters. A list of women's shelters that accept pregnant patients should be maintained.
   - Does the victim have support systems?
7. Make certain the patient has access to follow up prenatal care.
8. Make posters, cards, or brochures with local IPV resources easily available for patients in your triage unit.

comprise a small percentage of victims who present for a sexual assault evaluation. Unless it is the local protocol to care for victims in an OB triage unit, it is likely the victim will be directed to an emergency department or a rape crisis center. Immediate medical needs must be assessed and treated prior to evidence collection. Most sexual assault victims are not severely injured (Linden, 2011), but there are occasions where substantial trauma has occurred. In these cases, it is likely the OB care provider will be called to an emergency trauma room and if fetal monitoring is appropriate it would be performed on site. Calls to an OB triage unit from a rape crisis center or a general emergency room will likely question the need for fetal monitoring, the safety of radiographic imaging, or the safety of the prophylactic medications. Hospitals need policies regarding under what conditions fetal monitoring is indicated.

In the instances where physical trauma to the victim has been minimal and the woman has no complaints of vaginal bleeding or pelvic pain, it may be appropriate to have the emergency department document a normal fetal heart rate (110–160 beats per minute), perform any necessary evidence collection, and then transfer the victim to OB triage for prolonged fetal monitoring. If the victim wants an evidence collection kit performed, usually time limits are in effect. These time limits differ by state, but they typically range between 72 and 96 hours. The numerous steps that need to be performed to complete the forensic exam are beyond the scope of this text. Best practices in evidence collection and prophylaxis are seen when the examiner has received specific training, such as a sexual assault nurse examiner (SANE) or a sexual assault forensic examiner (SAFE) (Campbell, 2005; Sievers, 2003). These examiners have received extensive education regarding how to obtain the history, perform and document the physical exam, collect forensic evidence, provide appropriate prophylaxis against sexually transmitted infections (STIs), and arrange for any counseling and follow-up care that may be needed. For complete and comprehensive care of a pregnant woman presenting for evaluation of sexual assault, the steps that must be completed are outlined in Exhibit 23.3.

If a woman describes a loss of memory or motor skills, or suspects she was given something that affected mental capabilities, drug-facilitated sexual assault (DFSA) should be suspected. Special consent needs to be obtained before blood and urine can be collected to examine for those drugs associated with DFSA. A special drug screen needs to be performed and the chain of evidence needs to be maintained, so if there is concern for DFSA a forensic examiner will need to be contacted to collect the samples.

Fetal Monitoring

In the previable fetus, no fetal monitoring is necessary other than documentation of the fetal heart rate. It is often reassuring for the pregnant woman to see the fetus on ultrasound, if available. If the woman is reporting painful contractions and is beyond 20 weeks' gestation, there may be some utility in monitoring for contractions only. If regular contractions are identified, prolonged observation may be indicated, so she will not leave only to experience a complication shortly after discharge. Once a viable gestation (typically beyond 24 weeks) has been reached, prolonged monitoring may be indicated. If there has been trauma to the pregnant abdomen, the woman needs to be evaluated for preterm labor or placental abruption.

Prophylaxis for Sexually Transmitted Infections (STIs)

Once the maternal physical exam, a forensic exam (if requested), and fetal evaluation have been completed, there needs to be a thorough discussion with regards to the risk of contracting STIs. Transmission risks are difficult to ascertain and depend on the prevalence of the STI and the exact history

EXHIBIT 23.3

Steps in the Complete Assessment of a Pregnant Sexual Assault Victim

1. Prompt assessment of the maternal and fetal medical conditions. Treatment as necessary. Location and order to be determined based on the stability of patient and fetal condition, as well as local protocols. The initially contacted provider needs to coordinate care promptly.
2. Sexual assault evidence collection, if desired by the victim. As soon as indicated, based on the medical condition, contact a SANE, SAFE, or an emergency room physician. Findings should be clearly documented and chain of evidence must be maintained.
3. Contact police in the town where the assault occurred if desired by the victim. Know local and state mandatory reporting requirements, typically when the assault has been perpetrated on a minor, or a member of another vulnerable population.
4. Offer to call an advocate who can assist the patient with the exam and during the post discharge period. Contact local sexual assault advocacy services if desired.
5. Arrange for social service referral, behavioral health or psychiatry evaluation if needed based on the victim's situation and social condition.
6. Assess the need for STI and HIV prophylaxis and administer those medications which are safe for the pregnancy (see Exhibit 23.4).
7. Post discharge follow up can be quite lengthy to arrange. As needed, the victim may need assistance with:
   - Safe shelter
   - Prenatal follow-up appointments. With the victim's permission, contact her obstetrician, if she has one.
   - Medical follow-up is recommended for 2 weeks, 6 weeks, 3 months, and 6 months post assault.
   - Consider follow-up with maternal fetal medicine or an infectious disease specialist, if taking HIV prophylactic medications
   - Counseling
   - Legal advocacy

of the sexual assault. The estimated risks of infection transmission are below 20% for gonorrhea, chlamydia, and syphilis (Reynolds & Peipert, 2000). Even in pregnancy, appropriate STI prophylaxis is safe and effective. The Center for Disease Control (CDC) publishes guidelines every 4 years for medications that are recommended for STI prophylaxis following a sexual assault. Exhibit 23.4 lists medications from the 2010 CDC published guidelines that are safe for use in pregnancy.

The discussion for potential HIV transmission following a sexual assault is complicated. The incidence of HIV transmission to a woman after a single incidence of unprotected penile-vaginal sex (without injury) is estimated at 1 in 1,000 even if the male is known to be HIV positive (Varghese, Maher, & Peterman, 2002). Since no randomized trials are available, this estimate was extrapolated from studies involving health care workers exposed to blood

EXHIBIT 23.4

Recommendations for Sexually Transmitted Infections in Pregnancy

Recommended regimen for chlamydia, gonorrhea and trichomonas prophylaxis

Ceftriaxone 250 mg IM in a single dose

OR

Cefixime 400 mg orally in a single dose

PLUS

Metronidazole 2 g orally in a single dose

PLUS

Azithromycin 1 g orally in a single dose

*If patient is penicillin allergic with a history of a serious adverse reaction, the small but significant cross reaction with cephalosporins must be weighed against the likelihood of acquiring gonorrhea.

** Quinolones and Doxycycline are NOT used in pregnancy

Other recommendations to be considered and safe in pregnancy under special circumstances

- Tetanus toxoid, if patient has lacerations and has not received a vaccination within 10 years
- Hepatitis B vaccination: The first in the series of three to be given, if patient not immune
- If the patient is not immune and the perpetrator is known to be hepatitis B positive consider hepatitis B immune globulin

Source: Adapted from Centers for Disease Control and Prevention Sexually Transmitted Guidelines (2010).

and maternal-fetal transfer studies (Connor Sperling, & Gerber, 1994; Cardo, Culver, & Ciesielski, 1997). There are several factors which may relatively increase or decrease the incidence of HIV transmission and these are listed in Table 23.1.

For HIV prophylaxis to be effective, it must be administered within 72 hours of exposure. Other issues complicating HIV prophylaxis include the high cost of medications and the common incidence of side effects which often lead to discontinuance of the medication. In one study of nonpregnant patients, even when provided with a complete course of medication, only 33.6 % of patients who requested HIV prophylaxis completed the recommended 28 days of prophylaxis (Dumont, Hyer, & Hassan, 2008; Dumont, Myhr, Husson, et al., 2008). An incomplete course of HIV prophylaxis may lead to viral resistance to the medication used. Another important consideration is the laboratory testing which needs to be followed in women taking HIV prophylaxis. Tests to be monitored include a complete blood count, chemistries and liver functions. Recommendations regarding HIV prophylaxis must be made on an individual basis, particularly when the HIV status of the perpetrator is unknown.

TABLE 23.1 Factors That May Decrease or Increase the Risk of Acquiring HIV After a Sexual Assault

DECREASE RISK	INCREASE RISK
No ejaculation	Blood exchange through traumatic injury
Condom use	Anal assault
Perpetrator known to victim	Gang rape
Oral assault without blood exchange	Assailant known to be from a high risk group such as an IV drug user

Source: Adapted from Reynolds & Peipert (2000).

The HIV prophylaxis regimens used in pregnancy may be different than those used in a nonpregnant patient. The basic regimen for HIV prophylaxis in the pregnant woman is lamivudine plus zidovudine (Combivir) one tablet orally twice a day. Emtricitabine (Truvada) is currently not recommended in pregnancy. Different medications might be added or recommended if the woman has multiple risk factors or if the antiviral medications used by the perpetrator are known. A general obstetrician may be unfamiliar or uncomfortable with the many factors that need to be taken into consideration in order to provide HIV prophylaxis. Therefore, a consultation to a maternal fetal medicine or an infectious disease specialist needs to be considered.

Follow up examinations after a sexual assault are rarely pursued by nonpregnant female victims. One study that listed follow-up rates, quotes figures below 50% (Ackerman, Sugar, Fine, & Eckert, 2006). There are no studies specifically identifying follow-up rates in pregnant women, but the fact that the patient receives regular prenatal care, at least provides an opportunity for closer follow-up. If the woman has declined prophylaxis for STIs, the initial post assault examination should be scheduled for 2 weeks later. Chlamydia and gonorrhea need to be retested. Ideally, the woman is evaluated at 6 weeks, 3 months, and 6 months to retest for HIV, HCV, Hepatitis B, and syphilis. If the series of Hepatitis B vaccinations was started at the time of the assault, the remaining doses are to be given at the 6th week and the 6th month visits. Currently there are no recommendations for prophylaxis of herpes infections following a sexual assault. The patient must be educated regarding the symptoms of herpes and instructed to present for an examination if any lesions develop. There are special considerations for the pregnancy if herpes is contracted as a result of the assault.

Rape is a heinous violent crime and has significant potential to cause the victim to experience acute as well as prolonged emotional and behavioral symptoms. Prior to discharge, there should be a thorough assessment of the woman's emotional state and safety. A social services or psychiatric evaluation is indicated if there are expressions of suicidal or homicidal thoughts, the woman has limited supports, displays mental status or behavioral changes, is unwilling to communicate, or is inconsolable. The hospital social worker or the local sexual assault advocacy group can assist in arranging follow up counseling. There is a 30% risk that a victim of sexual assault will experience symptoms of post traumatic stress disorder known as rape trauma disorder. Symptoms may include anxiety, depression disorders, or substance abuse. These issues, in addition to the stressors of a having a new infant, require that the pregnant sexual assault victim receive substantial support.

Sexual assault occurs in the pregnant population and a victim deserves compassionate, supportive, and competent care from the medical personnel. Maternal injuries must first be addressed and if severe, are best treated in a trauma center. Once a fetus has reached a viable gestation, fetal monitoring is indicated to rule out preterm labor or abruption. Forensic evidence collection is best performed by a medical provider who has had specific training, such as a SANE or SAFE. Prophylactic medications, which are safe in pregnancy, are available to prevent STIs. Follow-up post assault can be complicated. Social workers and advocates can be of tremendous assistance in arranging safe discharge plans and counseling.

REFERENCES

Ackerman, D., Sugar, N., Fine, D., & Eckert, L. (2006). Sexual assault victims: Factors associated with follow-up care. *American Journal of Obstetrics and Gynecology, 194*(6), 1653–1659.

Campbell, R. (2005). The effectiveness of sexual assault nurse examiner (SANE) programs: A review of psychological, medical, legal, and community outcomes. *Trauma, Violence, & Abuse, 6*(4), 313–329.

Cardo, D. M., Culver, D. H., & Ciesielski, C. A. (1997). A Case-control study of HIV seroconversion in health care workers after percutaneous exposure. *New England Journal of Medicine, 337*, 1485–1490.

Centers for Disease Control and Prevention. (2005). Antiretroviral postexposure prophylaxis after sexual, injection-drug use, or other nonoccupational exposure to HIV in the United States: recommendations from the U.S. Department of Health and Human Services. *MMWR, 52,* (No.RR-2).

Centers for Disease Control and Prevention. (2010).Sexually transmitted diseases treatment guidelines, 2010. *MMWR*, 1–114.

Connor, E. M., Sperling, R. S., & Gerber, R. (1994). Reduction of maternal-infant transmission of human immunodeficiency virus type 1 with zidovudine treatment. *New England Journal of Medicine, 331*, 1173–1180.

Dumont, H., Hyher, T. L., & Hassan, J. (2008). HIV postexposure prophylaxis use among Ontario female adolescent sexual assault victims: A prospective analysis. *Sexually Transmitted Diseases, 35*, 973–978.

Dumont, J. L., Myhr, T. L., Husson, H., MacDonald, S., Rachlis, A., & Loutfy, M. R. (2008). HIV postexposure prophylaxis use among Ontario female adolescent sexual assault victims: a prospective analysis. *Sexually Transmitted Diseases, 35*, 973–978.

Gates, D., Ross, C., & Mcqueen, L. (2006). Violence against emergency department workers. *Journal of Emergency Medicine, 31*(3), 331–337.

Gazmararian, J. A., Lazorick, S., Spitz, A. M., Ballard, T. J., Saltzman, L. E., & Marks, J. S. (1996). Prevalence of violence against women. *Journal of the American Medical Association, 275*(24), 1915–1920.

Jasinski, J. L. (2001). Pregnancy and violence against women: An analysis of longitudinal data. *Journal of Interpersonal Violence, 16*(7), 712–733.

Linden, J. A. (2011). Care of the adult patient after sexual assault. *New England Journal of Medicine, 365*(9), 834–841.

Poole, G., Martinjr, J., Perryjr, K., Griswold, J., Lambert, C., & Rhodes, R. (1996). Trauma in pregnancy: The role of interpersonal violence. *American Journal of Obstetrics and Gynecology, 174*(6), 1873–1878.

Reynolds, M. R., & Peipert, J. F. (2000). Reducing the risk of sexual HIV transmission: quantifying the per-act risk for HIV on the basis of choice of partner, sex act, and condom use. *Obstetrical and Gynecological Survey, 55*(1), 51–57.

Sievers, V., Murphy, S., & Miller, J. J. (2003). Sexual assault evidence collection more accurate when completed by sexual assault nurse examiners: Colorado's experience. *Journal of Emergency Nursing*, *29*, 511–514.

Varghese, B., Maher, J. E., & Peterman, T. A. (2002). Reducing the risk of sexual HIV transmission: quantifying the per-act risk for HIV on the basis of choice of partner, sex act, and condom use. *Sexually Transmitted Diseases*, *29*, 38–43.

Substance Use and Psychiatric Disorders in Pregnancy

24

Catherine Friedman

Pregnancy is a unique time of convergence of internal and external motivators and mediators for change. This includes a pregnant woman's contact with social institutions, medical coverage and changes in family, social and interpersonal support systems. The issues of substance use and abuse in pregnancy as well as various other psychiatric disorders seen during pregnancy are the focus of this review. Substance use, including alcohol and drugs, specifically benzodiazepines and opioids, are presented in the first part of this review. Other preexisting or new psychiatric disorders that are often evaluated in an obstetric triage or emergency setting include depression, anxiety, panic attacks and insomnia. These topics encompass the remaining portion of the review.

SUBSTANCE USE

Women who use substances in pregnancy are women who are already using drugs and alcohol, get pregnant, and keep using. Almost no woman initiates an addictive behavior in pregnancy. Pregnant women are aware that certain substances are not healthy for fetuses. Substance use in pregnancy exists when reproduction and motherhood intersect with a pre-existing drug use problem. Even before substance use is identified by medical care providers as a problem, women will often employ a range of strategies to reduce or change substance intake and to reduce harm to the fetus. Such changes include decreasing or stopping usage, switching the drugs used, and entering prenatal care or a substance treatment program.

Substance use in pregnancy decreases for all substances both spontaneously and with treatment as pregnancy progresses. Muhuri and Gfroerer (2009) used epidemiological data to show that this is true for multiple substances. This change reverses during postpartum but does not return to preparenting levels. For example, in this sample, daily cigarette use was 20.1% in nonparenting and nonpregnant women and decreased to 12.4% in the first trimester and to 9.3% by the third trimester of pregnancy. Binge alcohol use decreased from 25.8% to 7.6% in the first trimester, and 1% in the third trimester of pregnancy.

Smoking nicotine cigarettes and alcohol use during pregnancy have well-defined risks. Smoking increases the risk of low birth weight and prematurity.

No amount of alcohol is considered safe in any stage of pregnancy, and there appear to be differences in fetal vulnerability to the toxic effects. Alcohol exposure in the first trimester is associated with low birth weight, decreased birth length and head circumference, minor physical abnormalities, and neurodevelopmental disorders. Second and third trimester exposure can lead to developmental abnormalities such as intellectual deficits and behavioral abnormalities. The full constellation of effects is called fetal alcohol syndrome (FAS). However, fetal alcohol spectrum disorders that do not meet full FAS criteria are common.

PRESENTING SYMPTOMATOLOGY

Etiology and Risk Factors

The etiology of substance misuse is both genetic and environmental. Associations with substance use in pregnancy include missed or inadequate prenatal care, recurrent somatic complaints (chronic pain, nausea, sleep, etc.), which may result in multiple visits to obstetric triage, past history of substance misuse and/or treatment, active psychiatric diagnosis, and a psychiatric history and/or history of trauma (including intimate partner violence), prior unexplained fetal death, and a previous child with alcohol-exposure related disorders.

HISTORY AND DATA COLLECTION

Screening Questions

Substance use screening questions developed for the general population are not as accurate among reproductive-aged and pregnant women. The screening tool for drug use, The 4 Ps Plus© (Chasnoff et al., 2007), Parents, Partner, Past and Pregnancy, has been validated for drug use (alcohol, cannabis, heroin, cocaine and methamphetamines) in pregnant women. T-ACE© (Sokol et al., 1989) and TWEAK© screening tools (Russell et al., 1994) have been validated for alcohol use in pregnant women. See Exhibit 24.1 for these screening tools. Women who screen positive require further assessment for current use.

ASSESSING CURRENT DRUG USE AND DRUG HISTORY

All questions must be asked in a nonjudgmental manner, including questions about drug usage in pregnancy. Each common and suspected substance needs to be questioned specifically, beginning with those perceived as the most common and least harmful and progressing to more stigmatized substances. For example, one can begin with caffeine or cigarettes and proceed through alcohol and marijuana, then nonprescribed pills and other drugs (cocaine, heroin, methamphetamine, etc.). Many people do not think of beer and wine as alcohol so it is important to ask about these specifically. Likewise, many people do not think about marijuana and nonprescribed pills when asked about drugs, so these need to be noted as well. The language women use to describe drug names and quantities can be unfamiliar, as shown in Table 24.1.

EXHIBIT 24.1

Screening Tools for Tobacco, Alcohol, and Drugs in Pregnancy

4 Ps Plus©

Parents: Did either of your parents have a problem with alcohol or drugs?
Partner: Does your partner have a problem with alcohol or drugs?
Past: Have you ever drunk beer, wine, or liquor?
Pregnancy: In the month before you knew you were pregnant, how many *cigarettes* did you smoke?
In the month before you knew you were pregnant, *how many beers/how much wine/how much liquor* did you drink?

Scoring: Women who acknowledge any use of tobacco or alcohol in the month prior to pregnancy have a positive screen, and need further assessment for current substance use.

T-ACE©

T **Tolerance:** How many drinks does it take to make you feel high?
A Have people **annoyed** you by criticizing your drinking or drug use?
C Have you ever felt you ought to **cut down** on your drinking or drug use?
E **Eye-opener:** Have you ever had a drink or drug first thing in the morning to steady your nerves or get rid of a hangover?

Scoring: A score of 2 or more is considered positive, and these patients need further assessment for current substance use.

A, C, E = Affirmative answers are 1 point each.
T = Reporting tolerance to more than 2 drinks = 2 points.

TWEAK©

T **Tolerance:** How many drinks can you hold? (positive if $\geq$ 6 drinks) *or* How many drinks does it take before you begin to feel the first effects of alcohol (positive if $\geq$ 3 drinks)
W Have close friends or relatives **worried** or complained about your drinking in the past year?
E **Eye-opener:** Do you sometimes take a drink in the morning when you first get up?
A **Amnesia:** Has a friend or a family member ever told you about things you said or did while drinking that you could not remember?
K Do you sometimes feel the need to **cut down** on your drinking?

Scoring: A score of more than 2 is positive; these women need further assessment for current substance use.

E, A, K = Affirmative answers are 1 point each.
T, W = Affirmative answers are 2 points each.

*Source:*Adapted from Chasnoff et al. (2007); Sokol et al. (1989); Russell et al. (1994); Reis et al. (2009).

TABLE 24.1 Determination of Drug Quantities

Nicotine	**Cigarettes:** 1 pack = 20 cigarettes, 1 carton = 10 packs **Cigars:** 1 pack or carton (5–10 cigars) **Snuff, "Dip," Chewing/Dipping Tobacco** comes in cans, tins, pouches and is often described by number of times/"dips"/"pinches" per day
Alcohol	**Beer:** cans, bottles, and drafts come in ounces. 12 oz., 16 oz. = a pint, 22 oz. = a double-deuce, 32 oz. = a quart, 40 oz. = a 40. 1 case is 24 cans of beer. **Wine:** A bottle is typically 750 mL = 25 oz. Wine also comes in other sizes and containers. **Hard Alcohol** "Miniature" = 1.6 oz., "Shorty" = 3.4 oz., Pint = 16 oz., Quart = 32 oz., "Fifth" = 25.6 oz., Liter = 33.8 oz., "Handle"=1.75 L. Mixed drinks often contain greater than 1.5 oz. of liquor
Marijuana	Measured in ounces Joints (small cigarette size), blunts (large joint, often in hollowed-out cigar or rolled in cigar paper, may use name of cigar), bowls (of a pipe or a "bong")
Heroin	$10 = a "dime" = 1 "bag" (also $6 & $20 bags) = 1 "pill" = 1 "cap." "Raw" (uncut; up to 90% pure) or "scramble" (cut; 5%–10% pure)
Cocaine	$10 (a "dime") "vials," "pills," "bags" Crack used in "rocks" Powder also bought in ½ oz., ¼ oz., ⅛ oz. ("eight ball")
Benzodiazepines	**"Benzos"** (the appearance of generic brands may vary but doses are the same) **Xanax** (alazopram) 0.25 mg = "white football," 0.5 mg = "peach football," 1mg = "blue football," 2 mg = white "bar" (4 segments) **Klonopin** (clonazepam) = "Pins"- round **Valium** (diazepam) = cut-out "V" in center
Pill Opioids	**Oxycontin ("Oxys")** = 10, 20, 30, 40, 60, 80, and 160 mg **Percocet ("Percs")** (oxycodone) = 2.5, 5, 7.5, 10 mg **Vicodin** (hydrocodone) = 5, 10, 15 mg

PHYSICAL EXAMINATION

Physical and behavioral indicators of possible substance misuse include a woman who smells of alcohol or chemicals, and inappropriate behavior such as quick or unfocused anger. Changes in mental status such as extreme mood liability and mood extremes, disorientation, somnolence, and loose associations can be due to intoxication and/or withdrawal.

Physical signs of substance abuse or withdrawal vary by substance, and include increased pulse and blood pressure, increased body temperature, low body weight (failure to gain weight in pregnancy), dilated or constricted pupils, rapid eye movements, nystagmus, inflamed or eroded nasal mucosa, nose bleeds, gum or periodontal disease (meth mouth), hair loss, track marks or abscesses or injection sites, abscesses, and skin sores.

Maternal-fetal obstetric and postpartum abnormalities associated with substance use in pregnancy include intrauterine growth restriction, failure to gain adequate weight, placenta abruptio, preterm labor, nonreassuring fetal status and both maternal and infant withdrawal symptoms in the peripartum period.

LABORATORY AND IMAGING STUDIES

Urine drug screening is the standard test for drug use in pregnancy. However, regulations on urine drug screening, and reimbursement for this test, vary from hospital to hospital and state to state. There are restrictions on ordering this test and most will need consent. Urine drug screens are immunoassays, and there are many limitations to this specificity and sensitivity of these tests. For example, urine drug testing will often not detect synthetic opioids including methadone, dilaudid, fentanyl, buprenorphine, and so on unless testing is ordered specifically. Many common cold preparations (e.g., pseudoephedrine) can cause false positives for amphetamines. Urine drug screens can also miss some common benzodiazepines like low-dose clonazepam. When in doubt of a result, a more specific confirmatory screen can be ordered generally performed with gas chromatography/mass spectrometry. Furthermore, there are variable time limits to the detection of use of each substance tested as noted in Exhibit 24.2. Alcohol use can only reliably be detected with a breathalyzer test for blood alcohol level. There are no other reliable means to determine recent or chronic use. In addition opiates and benzodiazepines are often administered for medical reasons in an obstetric triage setting before urine is obtained for drug screening.

CLINICAL MANAGEMENT

Generally drug intoxication and withdrawal are managed symptomatically in pregnant women with comfort measures and safety for mother and fetus paramount concerns. Alcohol and benzodiazepines, and opioids are exceptions.

Alcohol and Benzodiazepines

Although greater than 95% of alcohol withdrawal cases are uncomplicated and self-limited, intoxication and withdrawal can be fatal. Alcohol, benzodiazepine, and phenobarbital withdrawal are managed similarly. Management options include a standing protocol or a symptom-triggered protocol that is linked to a standardized assessment such as the Alcohol Withdrawal Scale (AWS) or Clinical Institute Withdrawal Assessment (CIWA). For a symptom-triggered protocol, signs and symptoms of withdrawal are monitored regularly (q 10–60 min). Lorazepam is initiated (2–4 mg PO or IV) at the earliest sign of withdrawal. Benzodiazepine is given until sedated or signs and symptoms of withdrawal cease.

EXHIBIT 24.2

Urine Toxicology Screen: Time Limits for Positive

Heroin	1 to 3 days
Methadone	2 to 4 days
Cocaine	1 to 3 days
Benzodiazepines	Up to 30 days
Marijuana	1 to 3 days (occasional use) Up to 30 days (chronic use)

All women presenting with alcohol withdrawal, intoxication, or suspicion of heavy alcohol use and related malnutrition should receive 50 or 100 mg thiamine intramuscularly or intravenously at the time of presentation followed by daily oral supplementation to prevent development of Wernicke's encephalopathy and other complications.

Opioids

Opioid withdrawal can be objectively and subjectively measured with a withdrawal scale such as the Clinical Opioid Withdrawal Scale (COWS) (Wesson & Ling, 2003). This quantifies signs and symptoms of opioid withdrawal including resting pulse rate, sweating, restlessness, pupil size, joint and bone aches, running nose or eyes, gastrointestinal upset, tremor, yawning, gooseflesh skin, and anxiety/irritability.

Methadone maintenance treatment (MMT) is the recommended treatment for opioid dependence in pregnancy. The primary goal of treatment with methadone is to prevent relapse to illicit substance use. Even medically supervised withdrawal is not the standard of care due to poor outcomes and the potential catastrophic consequences of relapse (Jones et al., 2010). New data suggest that buprenorphine—a partial opioid agonist—may be appropriate and safe for many (but not all) pregnant women, with reduced incidence and severity of neonatal abstinence syndrome (Czerkes et al., 2010; Jones et al., 2010). Yet, buprenorphine is not the appropriate treatment for all women—women on high doses of opioids will not have withdrawal symptoms treated with buprenorphine, and many women with severe active dependency require the structured daily treatment setting of a methadone maintenance clinic for safe treatment.

Initiation of opioid replacement therapy in opioid dependent pregnant women varies from hospital to hospital across the country and is performed on an inpatient basis in some settings, and outpatient in others. There are also logistical issues regarding discharge after inpatient initiation of methadone for opioid dependence. One must have the ability to seamlessly transition the woman from inpatient to outpatient MMT—e.g., to go from inpatient methadone maintenance to entry into an outpatient methadone maintenance treatment program (MMTP) the day of or after discharge from an inpatient MMTP. Yet many MMTPs do not admit on a daily basis and many require an intake appointment a few days before they actually get admitted and dosed. One cannot write a prescription for methadone for opioid dependence; *this is illegal in the United States.* Methadone must be provided through a licensed facility when prescribed for opioid maintenance. Furthermore, outpatient pharmacies will not fill a methadone prescription unless it is written on the script that the indication is for pain.

CHILD SERVICES INVOLVEMENT

Reporting requirements vary by law from state to state, and they often vary in practice from institution to institution within a state. In some states drug use in pregnancy is not reported. In other states requirements for reporting vary by trimester. Each institution's social services and legal advisors can determine specific reporting requirements and processing. National Advocates for Pregnant Women (http://advocatesforpregnantwomen.org) provides resources on this topic.

FOLLOW-UP

Women using cigarettes, drugs and alcohol can be referred for appropriate treatment. Social services can assist with available local resources.

OTHER PSYCHIATRIC DISORDERS IN PREGNANCY

Acute treatments of many common psychiatric symptoms in the obstetric triage setting, which when necessary can be initiated while awaiting a psychiatric consultation, are listed in Table 24.2.

TABLE 24.2 Psychiatric Disorders: Symptoms and Triage Interventions

	ENVIRONMENTAL, BEHAVIORAL	PRN MEDICATIONS
Anxiety	Support and empathy Reassurance about signs and symptoms Education about the etiology and treatment of this disorder	Diphenhydramine (12.5–50 mg PO q 4 hr) *or* hydroxyzine (10–50 mg PO q 4hr) *or* lorazepam (0.25–1 mg PO q 8 hr) *or* clonazepam (0.25–1 mg PO q 8 hr)
Panic	Calm, quiet environment Support and empathy Reassurance about signs and symptoms Education about the etiology and treatment of this disorder	Lorazepam (0.25–1 mg PO or 0.25–1 mg IM) *or* clonazepam (0.25–1 mg PO)
Agitation	Calm, quiet environment When necessary, remove objects that could be used to hurt oneself or others	Lorazepam (0.25–1 mg PO or 0.25–1 mg IM) For psychotic agitation, or agitation refractory to lorazepam to haloperidol 0.5 to 1 mg PO or IM
Severe suicidality, with danger of attempt.	Remove all objects that could be used to harm oneself from the immediate environment Constant observation to ensure safety. STAT psychiatric consult or transfer to psychiatric emergency room for evaluation once medically stable	To calm thoughts, consider lorazepam (0.25–1 mg PO or 0.25–1 mg IM) *or* clonazepam (0.25–1 mg PO) For associated psychotic features, haloperidol 0.5 to 1 mg PO or IM
Psychosis	Calm, quiet environment Dimmer lighting When indicated remove objects that could be used to hurt oneself or others Constant observation to ensure safety	Haloperidol (0.5–1 mg PO or IM.) Atypical antipsychotics (such as risperidone, olanzapine, and ziprasidone) can be used in pregnancy. At this time little is known about the fetal safety profile; if they are known to work for an individual, and there are safety concerns, they should be used in preference to no treatment even in the triage setting

TABLE 24.3 Psychiatric Disorders by Pregnancy Status

	PAST-YEAR NONPREGNANT WOMEN % (SE) (N = 13 025)	PAST-YEAR PREGNANT WOMEN % (SE) (N = 1524)	ADJUSTED ODDS RATIO (95% CI)	POSTPARTUM WOMEN % (SE) (N = 994)	ADJUSTED ODDS RATIO (95% CI)
Any psych d/o	30.1 (0.8)	25.3 (1.3)	**0.75 (0.62–0.90)**	25.7 (1.8)	0.81 (0.65–1.02)
Any substance use d/o	19.9 (0.7)	14.6 (1.2)	**0.68 (0.57–0.82)**	12.0 (1.3)	**0.44 (0.33–0.59)**
Any mood disorder	13.7 (0.5)	13.3 (1.1)	1.04 (0.83–1.32)	15.2 (1.5)	1.28 (0.97–1.69)
MDD	8.1 (0.9)	8.4 (0.4)	1.24 (0.94–1.64)	9.3 (1.1)	**1.52 (1.07–2.15)**

Source: Adapted from Vesga-Lopez et al., (2008).

Contrary to popular belief, the incidence of many common psychiatric disorders actually decreases during pregnancy as seen in Table 24.3.

DEPRESSION

Depression can present with a depressed or sad mood, lack of enjoyment, and/or irritability. Other somatic complaints such as changes in appetite and sleep, concentration, energy, libido, and fatigue are common. Since many of these changes are common in pregnancy and the postpartum period, care must be taken to distinguish physical changes that are within normal limits for this time period and those that are unusual and associated with other symptoms of depression. Depression can be related to a medical disorder, substance use (including prescribed medications), or unipolar or bipolar depression. Medical causes and substance use must be assessed prior to assigning a psychiatric etiology to depression.

Pregnant women who present with depression require further assessment for suicidal ideation, thoughts and plans to harm others, and the ability to care for themselves and dependents. If there is any question, psychiatric consultation is sought; this may involve referral to an outside psychiatric emergency room once obstetric stability is ensured. If a pregnant woman who is at-risk to herself or others must be kept in obstetric triage or an emergency setting, she must be under constant observation. In less severe cases, outpatient referral can be made for further psychiatric evaluation and therapy and/or psychotropic medications.

Initiation of antidepressants in the obstetric triage setting or emergency setting needs to be done with care, and only in those pregnant women who are already established in prenatal and/or psychiatric care and who will have outpatient follow-up within a week of being started on medication. Screening is required for a history of mania, hypomania, and bipolar disorder prior to initiating an antidepressant. Initiating antidepressants in women with a history of mania can precipitate a manic episode. Recommendations as to the safest antidepressant in pregnancy change frequently as this is an area of active research. On-line databases such as Reprotox (available at many institutions through Micromedex) provide the most recent information as to known drug safety in pregnancy. If an antidepressant has worked in the past, and it is not a contraindicated medication in pregnancy, this is considered a first line treatment.

ANXIETY AND PANIC ATTACKS

Anxiety is characterized by combined physiological and psychological manifestations. Physiological signs frequently include those of autonomic hyperactivity: flushing and pallor, tachycardia, palpitations, sweating, dry mouth, cold hands, diarrhea and urinary frequency. Other signs are dizziness, increased startle response, muscular tension, physical pain such as headaches and body aches, shortness of breath, hyperventilation, trembling, and restlessness. Psychological manifestations include feelings of worry, feelings of doom, hopelessness, inability to concentrate, and hypervigilance. Physical symptoms often precipitate presentation to medical care, and many visits to obstetric triage with vague somatic complaints and unclear physical findings can be due to undiagnosed anxiety and/or depressive disorders. However, underlying and precipitating medical disorders must be ruled out prior to diagnosing a pure anxiety disorder.

Panic attacks occur or recur when the signs and symptoms of anxiety develop abruptly, peak within 10 minutes, and then decrease significantly. Women who experience a panic attack for the first time will often present to an emergency room because they are afraid they are having a heart attack or dying. Pregnant women are no exception, and may present with these concerns. Other conditions must be ruled out before a panic attack can be diagnosed including cardiac, endocrine, and pulmonary etiologies, and substance use/toxins. The specific medical evaluation is guided by the presenting physical and psychological signs and symptoms.

Panic attacks can occur without a clear acute precipitating stressor, or be associated with agoraphobia—the fear of and avoidance of situations from which one might not be able to escape such as crowds, public transportation, and being alone in open spaces. Panic attacks often occur/recur in places or situations that can cause panic to become a learned reaction. Agoraphobia can develop when a person with prior panic attacks begins to fear similar places and situations. A panic disorder is diagnosed when a person has had at least one panic attack and then develops at least 1 month of persistent worries about having another attack or associated changes in behavior. Panic disorder usually begins in the mid-twenties and is more common in women than in men.

Treatment for anxiety and panic involves support and empathy, including reassurance about their symptoms and education about the disorder. Benzodiazepines, particularly lorazepam (0.25–1 mg PO every 8 hr as needed for anxiety), are often the treatment of choice in the obstetric triage or emergency setting. These can both alleviate acute symptoms and facilitate the remainder of the evaluation (Petit, 2004; Stewart, 2011). Lorazepam can also be administered sublingually for faster onset of action. Low dose diphenhydramine (12.5–50 mg PO q 4 hr) and hydroxyzine (10–50 mg PO q 4hr) can also be utilized in women hesitant to take a prescription medication such as a benzodiazepine in pregnancy and for women with past or current substance abuse or dependency. Prescriptions for benzodiazepines in particular should

EXHIBIT 24.3

Online Resources

- The Marce Society for Perinatal Mental Health (**www.marcesociety.com**)
- Motherrisk (**www.motherisk.org/prof/index.jsp**)
- National Advocates for Pregnant Women (**advocatesforpregnantwomen.org**)
- Organization of Teratology Information Specialists (OTIS) (**www.otispregnancy.org**)
- Reprotox (**www.reprotox.org**) Subscription, but currently free for trainees. This may also be available through institutional subscription websites such as Micromedex
- Toxnet (**www.toxnet.nlm.nih.gov**) Medications in pregnancy and lactation. Select "Lactmed" for safety in lactation

only be written for a few days' worth of medication, with follow-up through the obstetric or psychiatric provider.

INSOMNIA

Disturbed sleep is often another symptom of psychiatric disorders. In all pregnant women presenting with psychiatric symptoms, sleep must be evaluated (initiation, quality, disturbance, etc.) as part of the assessment. Difficulty falling asleep can be treated symptomatically in the short term with diphenhydramine (12.5–50 mg nightly), trazodone (25–100 mg nightly) or zolpidem (2.5–10 mg nightly). A list of on-line resources is noted in Exhibit 24.3.

REFERENCES

Chasnoff, I. J., Wells A. M., McGourty, R. F., & Bailey, L. K. (2007). Validation of the 4 Ps plus screen for substance use in pregnancy. *Journal of Perinatology, 27*(12), 744–748.

Czerkes, M., Blackstone, J., & Pulvino, J. (2010). Buprenorphine vs. methadone treatment for opiate addiction in pregnancy: An evaluation of neonatal outcomes. *58th annual clinical meeting of The American College of Obstetricians and Gynecologists*. San Francisco, CA.

Jones, H. E., Kaltenbach, K., Heil, S. H., Stine, S. M., Coyle, M. G., Arria, A. M.,… Fischer, G. (2010) Neonatal abstinence syndrome after methadone or buprenorphine exposure. *The New England Journal of Medicine, 363*(24), 2320–2331.

Muhuri, P. K., & Gfroerer, J. C. (2009) Substance use among women: Associations with pregnancy, parenting, and race/ethnicity. *Maternal and Child Health Journal, 13*(3), 376–385.

Petit, J. R. (2004). *Handbook of emergency psychiatry*. Philadelphia, PA: Lippincott, Williams and Wilkins.

Reis, R. K., Fiellin, D. A., Miller, S. C., & Saitz, R. (2009). *Principles of addiction medicine* (4th ed.). Philadelphia, PA: Lippincott, Williams and Wilkins.

Russell, M., Martier, S. S., Sokol, R. J., Mudar, P., Bottoms, S., Jacobson, S., & Jacobson, J. (1994). Screening for pregnancy risk-drinking. *Alcoholism, Clinical and Experimental Research, 18*(5), 1156–1161.

Sokol, R. J., Martier, S. S., & Ager, J. W. (1989). The T-ACE questions: Practical prenatal detection of risk-drinking. *American Journal of Obstetrics and Gynecology, 160*, 863–868.

Stewart, D. E. (2011) Depression during pregnancy. *The New England Journal of Medicine, 365*(17), 1605–1611.

Vesga-Lopez, O., Blanco, C., Keyes, K., Olfson, M., Grant, B. F., & Hasin, D. S. (2008). Psychiatric disorders in pregnant and postpartum women in the United States. *Archives of General Psychiatry, 65*(7), 805–815.

Wesson, D. R., & Ling, W. (2003). The Clinical Opiate Withdrawal Scale (COWS). *Journal of Psychoactive Drugs, 35*(2), 253–259.

25 Sexually Transmitted Infections

Donna LaFontaine

Sexual intercourse is a risk factor for both pregnancy and the acquisition of a sexually transmitted infection (STI). Therefore, STIs represent a fairly common diagnosis in pregnant women. The Centers for Disease Control and Prevention (CDC) estimates that over 19 million cases of STIs are diagnosed annually in the United States (CDC, 2010). The 15- to 24-year age group has the highest reported rates of chlamydia and gonorrhea, and these years overlap age groups with high-pregnancy rates (CDC, 2011a). Since symptoms may be absent, vague, or generalized, a thorough history including a sexual history must be obtained on all pregnant women presenting for evaluation to an obstetric triage unit. Many STIs can cause fetal infections, which are contracted either in utero or during delivery as the infant passes through an infected birth canal. Pregnancy complications such as preterm labor are also associated with some STIs. Effective prenatal screening, diagnosis, and treatment of these infections will reduce most of the pregnancy complications that are attributable to STIs. The general clinical features of STIs in pregnancy are presented first, followed by more specific, detailed information regarding the most prevalent and clinically significant STIs.

The risk of acquiring an STI in pregnancy is related to the prevalence of STIs in the community. Information on the prevalence rates of STIs at the state level may be available at the state's department of health website or at the U.S. CDC website (www.cdc.gov). All treatment recommendations in this chapter are consistent with the CDC's *"Sexually transmitted diseases treatment guidelines, 2010"* and are considered safe in pregnancy (CDC, 2010).

PRESENTING SYMPTOMATOLOGY

Several of the STIs, including chlamydia and gonorrhea, frequently go unrecognized by women. The most effective key to diagnosis and treatment in the pregnant woman is to perform screening tests at the initial prenatal visit. STIs commonly screened for at the first prenatal visit include chlamydia, gonorrhea, hepatitis B, hepatitis C, human immunodeficiency virus (HIV), and syphilis. At this time, there are no recommendations for routine prenatal screening for bacterial vaginosis (BV) and herpes simplex virus (HSV).

If there are symptoms present, the woman's complaints typically will be dependent upon the specific infection. Symptoms of chlamydia and gonorrhea include vaginal discharge, irritation, vaginal spotting, cramping, discomfort, or pain. Herpetic lesions may present as itchy or painful ulcerations of the genital tract. Generalized symptoms of fevers, fatigue, and nausea can be seen with a HSV primary outbreak, hepatitis B, hepatitis C, or HIV infection. Skin lesions or rashes on the body can appear in syphilis, disseminated gonorrhea, HIV, and scabies. Warty vulvar or vaginal lesions can appear with human papilloma virus (HPV).

If a pregnant woman presents complaining of vaginal spotting, cramping, or preterm contractions, testing must be considered for STIs, since many STIs have been shown to increase the risk of miscarriage or preterm labor (Klein & Gibbs, 2004). Table 25.1 lists STIs that have been associated with increased risks for a pregnancy loss; causal relationships have not been proven. Note that treatment of these STIs in pregnancy has not been proven to lower risks of preterm delivery, as will be discussed below.

HISTORY AND PHYSICAL EXAMINATION

A complete sexual history will include any history of prior STIs and if there is an exposure to a new partner. The social history may reveal information about other risk factors, such as intravenous (IV) drug use or a partner with IV drug use. Women at high risk must be screened for hepatitis C. A recent immigration or travel history may be helpful because infections such as lymphogranuloma venereum (LGV) and chancroid are much more common in warmer, tropical countries.

In addition, prenatal records must be reviewed to verify what STI screening evaluations have already been performed. If the pregnant woman is late to prenatal care and has not been recently screened, screening for HIV, hepatitis B, syphilis, chlamydia, and gonorrhea will need to be performed. Ideally, STI screening is performed in the setting of continuous prenatal care, but if a woman is noncompliant, an obstetric triage or emergency setting visit might be the only contact point for screening.

A general physical examination should be performed. Many of the STIs are manifested in the form of skin lesions, so a thorough examination of the skin is indicated. Table 25.2 describes common skin findings associated with STIs.

In cases of hepatitis, jaundice or right upper quadrant tenderness may be recognized. A vulvar examination and a vaginal speculum examination are essential. Herpetic blisters and lymphogranuloma granulosum (LGV) classically present with painful vulvar lesions, while secondary syphilis can

TABLE 25.1 STIs Implicated in Increasing Risk of Pregnancy Loss

INCREASES RISK OF SPONTANEOUS ABORTION	INCREASES RISK OF PRETERM LABOR	INCREASES RISK OF PERINATAL DEATH
Primary herpes	BV Gonorrhea Chlamydia Syphilis Trichomonas Primary herpes	Primary herpes Syphilis

Source: Adapted from CDC (2011a) and Klein & Gibbs (2004).

TABLE 25.2 Cutaneous Manifestations of STIs

STI	FINDINGS ON SKIN EXAMINATION
BV	Occasionally may see mild vulvar irritation secondary to excessive moisture exposure
Chancroid	Start as small red bumps around the genitalia that fill with pus, ulcerate, and become painful; take weeks to heal Frequently associated with enlarged firm inguinal lymph nodes that become tender (buboes)
Chlamydia	No associated skin changes
Granuloma inguinale	Small beefy red nodules found in the genitalia, which are painless but persist and as the skin wears away, granulation tissue appears
Gonorrhea	Disseminated gonorrhea, which is rare, may be associated with septic emboli that start as reddened papules then turn into hemorrhagic lesions
Hepatitis B and C	With infections severe enough to raise liver function tests (LFTs) may see jaundice of sclera and skin
HIV	Initial infection may be associated with a rash typical of viral syndrome meaning a diffuse macular reddened rash, which may or may not be pruritic and associated with fevers, malaise, fatigue, usually start in head and neck Kaposi's sarcoma—seen in late stages, full blown AIDS, purple to red or brown flat or raised skin growths
HPV	White- or flesh-colored growths, typically cauliflower-like, usually seen around vaginal opening, anus, cervix, or within the vagina
HSV	Small reddened areas that at first may itch. They blister, then ulcerate, then crust over and heal over the course of 5 to 7 days. Typically painful and typically seen near the vaginal opening or anus May be associated with enlarged inguinal lymph nodes
LGV	Genital papules that ulcerate, lymphatics may be infected, and there may be significant vulvar swelling
Pubic lice	Reddened areas of the skin, which are pruritic and may have small spots of blood where the lice fed and/or can be visualized in pubic hair, armpits
Scabies	Mites burrow under the skin leaving a red brown wavy line visible on the skin, these burrows more commonly seen between fingers, the elbow crease, or the buttocks, itching intense especially at night Scattered itching reddened papules are allergic reaction to the mites and their feces
Syphilis	Primary—painless chancre typically in the genitals at the site of infections inoculation, classically described as punched out with rolled-up borders Secondary—rash-disseminated small macules, reddened or brown, may be seen in palms, soles, and oral mucosa, these represent the disseminated organisms Condyloma lata—painless grey white lesions in moist, warm sites
Trichomonas	Vulvar and vaginal redness and irritation

Source: Adapted from CDC (2011a).

present as a nonpainful vulvar lesion. Occasionally herpetic lesions can also be identified on the cervix. Abnormal discharge is a hallmark feature of gonorrhea, BV, and trichomonas. Of note, BV is not considered to be sexually transmitted in all cases. BV is typically identified as a creamy off-white discharge that is adherent to the vaginal walls. A potassium hydroxide (KOH) "whiff" test can be performed at the bedside. Discharge from BV typically releases an amine or "fishy" odor when exposed to KOH. Trichomonas is classically described as a frothy, grey to green discharge that may be malodorous. With trichomonas, the cervix may be irritated and covered with punctuate hemorrhages, a condition commonly referred to as a "strawberry cervix." Gonorrheal vaginal discharge is frequently yellow and referred to as mucopurulent.

DIAGNOSTIC TESTING

A saline wet mount microscopic examination of any vaginal discharge can be used to diagnose trichomonas and BV. Trichomonas will appear as a flagellated motile protozoan. However, microscopy is only 60% or less sensitive for trichomonas (van der Schee et al., 1999). The rapid antigen testing or direct hybridization techniques that are more sensitive and specific are becoming more widespread in their usage. BV is diagnosed when three out of four of Amstel's criteria are identified. These criteria include an off-white vaginal discharge adherent to the vaginal walls, an amine odor, or positive "whiff test," a pH > 4.5, and greater than 20% clue cells per high-powered field. A clue cell is an epithelial cell whose borders are completely obscured by bacteria.

Nucleic acid amplification tests (NAATs) identify specific deoxyribonucleic acid (DNA) sequences. NAATs have replaced cultures as the preferred test for chlamydia and gonorrhea in many institutions, as they are the most sensitive tests available. The Food and Drug Administration (FDA) has approved NAATs for use with urine, cervical, and urethral specimens. Herpetic lesions can be diagnosed with a viral culture or by polymerase chain reaction (PCR) testing. Viral cultures have a very high false negative rate especially with recurrent lesions, but more institutions are still using cultures over the more sensitive PCR tests (Geretti & Brown, 2005). Serologic testing for HSV is available. Often HSV I and II serotypes will be positive from unrecognized prior infections. IgM is present only in the first few weeks of an infection, so a new finding of IgM antibodies in the absence of IgG antibodies is indicative of a new infection. Blood work is necessary to test for HIV, hepatitis B and C, and syphilis antibodies.

MANAGEMENT

The treatment recommendations are disease specific. Exhibit 23.4 includes the 2010 CDC's "Sexually Transmitted Diseases Treatment Guidelines" (CDC, 2010) and is modified to include only those treatments that are safe in pregnancy.

States' departments of health may have reporting requirements for specific diseases and typically this information is available on their websites. Treatment of the sexual partner is critical to prevent reinfection. More than half of all state health departments have developed expedited partner therapy (EPT). EPT allows for treatment of the sex partners of patients with an STI, without a complete medical evaluation of the partner. Providers must contact the Department of Health website for an individual state, in order to clarify the particular EPT laws in effect for that state. A test of cure should be considered in the case of some STIs to minimize risks to the fetus. If NAAT is used, wait at least 3 weeks to retest, so there is opportunity to clear the DNA of the organism.

CONSIDERATIONS AND CONSEQUENCES SPECIFIC TO CERTAIN INFECTIONS

Chlamydia

Chlamydia is the most commonly transmitted bacterial STI in the United States. If an infant travels through a birth canal infected with chlamydia, the neonate can also become infected. Neonatal chlamydial infections are manifested in the form of pneumonias or conjunctivitis. Nearly half of all patients diagnosed with gonorrhea are concomitantly infected with chlamydia (Datta et al., 2007).

Bacterial Vaginosis (BV)

There is no consensus as to the exact significance of BV in the pregnant woman. When women with BV are exposed to gonorrhea, chlamydia, or HSV, they are more likely to become infected with STIs than women who do not have BV (Schwebke, 2003; Weisenfeld, Hillier, & Krohn, 2003). Pregnant women with BV have higher risks for spontaneous abortion, preterm delivery, and chorioamnionitis (Klein & Gibbs, 2004). There are, however, no interventional trials available to show that treatment of BV decreases these complications (MacDonald, Brocklehurst, & Gordon, 2007; Leitich et al., 2003). Therefore, there are no recommendations that necessitate treatment in asymptomatic pregnant women.

Genital Herpes Simplex Virus (HSV)

Genital HSV can cause devastating neonatal complications or mortality if there is an active infection at the time of the delivery, especially, in the case of a primary outbreak. The clinical manifestations of a primary outbreak are highly variable. The classic description of the primary outbreak includes fever, flu-like symptoms, inguinal lymphadenopathy, and multiple, painful genital ulcers. Up to one-third of primary infections, however, will be asymptomatic, or cause only mild symptoms. Between 1% and 2% of pregnant women will serologically convert to HSV positive, during their pregnancy, but only 36% of those gravidas recognized a clinical lesion (Brown & Selke, 1997). When patients have previously received the diagnosis of HSV, they may experience a prodrome of itching or irritation and a majority are able to identify a recurrent lesion. The differentiation between serotype 1 (HSV-1) and type 2 (HSV-2) is not clinically important at the time of delivery, as both serotypes cause neonatal sequella. Disseminated HSV in the neonate can cause lesions as well as encephalitis, which can lead to neonatal death or long-term diminished mental capacity.

If a pregnant woman presents to an obstetric triage or emergency setting complaining of symptoms of vulvar irritation, dysuria, or pain in the setting of a vulvar lesion, the woman must be tested for herpes virus. If available, polymerase chain reaction (PCR) is obtained, as viral cultures have a low sensitivity. Serologic testing is typically unhelpful in a triage setting as the results may be negative in a primary infection. If serologies are obtained and are negative, follow-up will be necessary at a future prenatal visit approximately 6 weeks from the obstetric triage visit. A genital herpes outbreak diagnosed during pregnancy can be treated with acyclovir during any trimester. A study based on over 1,000 pregnant women followed in a registry found no increased risk in birth defects above the baseline risk of the general population (Stone, Reiff-Eldridge, & White, 2004). The data regarding safe use of famciclovir and valacyclovir are more limited.

When a woman with a history of HSV presents with contractions, a thorough examination of the vulva, vagina, and cervix must be performed. When an active lesion is present in the genital tract at the time of delivery, a cesarean delivery is currently indicated. Cesarean deliveries will not eliminate the risk of neonatal transmission completely. In diagnosed cases of neonatal herpes, approximately 25% were delivered by cesarean (Brown et al., 2003). Although primary outbreaks at the time of delivery carry the highest risk of infection for the neonate, recurrent outbreaks at the time of delivery also carry significant risk. If the woman has a history of herpes but no active lesions, a cesarean delivery is not recommended. A completely crusted over lesion is not considered to be active. When a recurrent herpetic lesion appears on the thigh or buttocks, there have been cases where these have been covered, and a vaginal delivery has been pursued without neonatal complications.

If a pregnant woman presents with preterm rupture of membranes at term and an identifiable herpetic lesion is present, a cesarean section is indicated. In the case of premature preterm rupture of membranes without labor, a maternal fetal medicine consultation may be helpful in planning the optimal delivery time. If the lesion is primary or recurrent, a cesarean delivery is indicated in patients over 32 weeks, even if the patient is not in labor. In those cases, the risk of neonatal herpes is greater than the risk of major morbidity due to prematurity. In patients less than 28 weeks gestation with an active lesion, the risk of sequellae due to prematurity typically outweighs the risks of neonatal infection (Major, Towers, Lewis, & Garite, 2003). In cases where expectant management is chosen, IV glucocorticoids to assist in lung development and IV acyclovir 8 mg/kg every 8 hours should be given.

Pregnant women between 28 and 32 weeks are particularly challenging, and since outcomes may depend on access to neonatal intensive care, the choice between expectant management and delivery by cesarean is likely made with input from maternal fetal medicine and the neonatologists. The American College of Obstetrics and Gynecology (ACOG) supports daily prophylaxis with acyclovir starting at 36 weeks, as there are research studies available showing a lower incidence of herpetic lesions at the time of delivery when compared with women without prophylaxis (Scott, Hollier, & McIntire, 2002; Sheffield, Hollier, & Hill, 2003; Watts, Brown, & Money, 2003).

Gonorrhea

Continually evolving antibiotic resistance to *Neisseria gonorrhoeae* is a growing U.S. public health concern. The CDC (as of July 2011) recommends that adults receive dual therapy with ceftriaxone and azithromycin. The dual therapy is recommended to account for strains of the bacteria that have been found to be less susceptible to either of the two antibiotics alone (CDC, 2011b). The CDC continues to have surveillance systems in place to continue to monitor for gonorrheal strains resistant to antibiotics and up to date information is available on their website.

Optimal treatment of HIV infection in the pregnant woman can be complicated and research is still evolving very rapidly. Ideally, an HIV screen will be obtained at the first prenatal visit. ACOG supports universal HIV testing of all pregnant women using an "opt-out" approach. Most states have laws in place regulating HIV and these are available at the state's department of health website. The HIV screen may be repeated at the 36-week appointment, especially if the patient is in a high-risk category. Women at high risk include IV drug users, sexual partners of male IV drug users, sexual partners of men diagnosed with HIV, and sex workers.

Pregnant women diagnosed with HIV may need treatment with antiviral agents, for improvement or maintenance of maternal health. The HIV transmission rate from mothers to neonates is highest for mothers with high viral loads (>30,000 copies/mL)—23% compared with only 1% for women with a nondetectable viral load (<400 copies/mL; Cooper et al., 2004). In high-resource areas, multidrug combination therapy is the gold standard for viral suppression and immune recovery (NIH, 2011). Certain antiviral agents have been identified as safe in pregnancy, while others may be toxic to the developing fetus. A maternal fetal medicine or infectious disease consultation may be advised to create a prenatal care plan that will treat the mother, as well as lower the perinatal transmission risk to the child. A key resource is the National Institute of Health (NIH), which frequently updates its recommendations for use of antiretroviral drugs in pregnant HIV-1-infected women for maternal health, as well as up to date interventions to reduce perinatal HIV transmission. Recommendations are continually updated on the AIDsinfo website (http://AIDSinfo.nih.gov). The NIH also maintains the National Perinatal HIV Hotline (1–888-448-8765), which provides free clinical consultation on all aspects of perinatal HIV, including infant care.

Even if HIV has not been screened prenatally, there is tremendous value in obtaining a rapid HIV screening test at the time of a late gestation obstetric triage visit, especially if it appears that the woman will be delivering. Antiretroviral prophylaxis is indicated in all HIV positive women at the time of labor and delivery, regardless of whether the maternal viral load is known. Currently, zidovudine (AZT) is the recommended drug to be administered intravenously in labor but recommendations are still evolving. In addition, elective cesarean deliveries alone have been shown to lower risks of maternal-to-child transmission (European Collaborative Study, 2005). Finally, the infant can receive antiviral prophylaxis, which has been proven to lower infection risks for the infant. For the woman with HIV infection identified at the time of labor, maternal prophylaxis with antivirals together with 6 weeks of prophylaxis of the infant reduces the risk of maternal-child transmission by 60% (Wade et al., 1998).

PELVIC INFLAMMATORY DISEASE

The diagnosis of pelvic inflammatory disease (PID) in pregnancy is controversial. The hormonal changes in pregnancy cause thickening of cervical mucus, theoretically making it difficult for STIs to ascend to the uterus and adnexa. If chronic PID exists prior to pregnancy, successful implantation of the embryo should be very rare, due to the inflammatory changes affecting the

TABLE 25.3 Sexually Transmitted Disease and Recommended Treatments in Pregnancy

INFECTION	COMMON SYMPTOMS OR FINDINGS	DIAGNOSIS	RECOMMENDED TREATMENT	SPECIAL CONSIDERATIONS
Bacterial vaginosis	Asymptomatic Vaginal discharge with an odor	Vaginal swab for DNA probe identification of *Gardnerella vaginalis* Amstel's criteria (3 of 4): pH ≥ 4.5; creamy, off-white discharge adheres to vaginal walls; ≥ 20% clue cells; fishy odor	Asymptomatic infections—the only efficacy in treatment decreasing PTL is in patients with previous preterm delivery Treat all symptomatic patients with choice of: Metronidazole 500 mg PO BID x 7 days, *OR* Metronidazole 250 mg PO TID x 7 days, *OR* Clindamycin 300 mg PO BID x 7 days	Strictly not considered a STI, but more prevalent in women with multiple partners
Chancroid (*H. ducreyi*)	Painful genital ulcer and enlarged inguinal lymph nodes	Special culture or PCR testing	Azithromycin 1 g PO once, *OR* Ceftriaxone 250 mg PO once, *OR* Erythromycin base 500 mg PO TID x 7 days	Typically seen in the Caribbean, Africa No adverse effects on pregnancy have been reported
Chlamydia	Asymptomatic Spotting, cramping	Nucleic acid amplification testing (NAAT): vaginal swab or urine Test of cure should be obtained 4 to 6 weeks posttreatment	Azithromycin 1g PO once Amoxicillin 500 mg PO TID x 7 days Erythromycin base 500 mg po QID x 7 days	Can cause conjunctivitis or pneumonia in infant
Genital herpes simplex virus	Asymptomatic Vulvar itching, irritation, painful lesions or blisters Primary outbreaks may also be associated with generalized flu-like symptoms	PCR (polymerase chain reaction) Viral cultures (poor sensitivity; only 50% positive) Tzanck prep	First lesion: Acyclovir 200 mg PO 5 x for 7–10 days *OR* Acyclovir 400 mg PO TID for 7 to 10 days Recurrence: Acyclovir 400 mg PO TID for 5 days Prophylaxis: Acyclovir 400 mg PO BID	Cesarean indicated for active lesion at the time of delivery If lesion has completely crusted *OR* if lesion is nongenital; cover with barrier dressing and cesarean not necessarily recommended

Granuloma inguinale	Large painless ulcers or buboes	Donovan bodies seen on dark field prep	Azithromycin 1 g PO q wk for 3 wks or until healed, *OR* Erythromycin base 500 mg PO QID for 3 wks or until healed	Seen in the Caribbean, Africa, Australia, India
Gonorrhea	Asymptomatic Yellow discharge, spotting Disseminated infection arthralgia, rash, meningitis	NAAT–vaginal swab or urine Culture	Ceftriaxone 250 mg IM, *OR* Cefixime 400 mg PO, *OR* Azithromycin 1g PO once Disseminated ceftriaxone 250 mg IM q day, *OR* IV q day until better, then Cefixime 400 mg PO BID for 1 week	Can cause conjunctivitis in neonate Can cause rectal/pharyngeal infection Check with local Dept. of Health regarding resistance
Hepatitis B	Nausea, jaundice, pain	Hep B s AG	Supportive	Cesarean not absolutely recommended at this time, but since theoretically can be transmitted during delivery, consider C-section
Hepatitis C	Nausea, jaundice, pain		Supportive	Cesarean not absolutely recommended at this time, but since theoretically can be transmitted during delivery, consider C-section
Human papilloma virus	Asymptomatic, Warty lesion Vulvar irritation	Clinical exam or biopsy	Delay treatment postdelivery or surgical removal	Cesarean may be considered if massive infection; can cause laryngeal papillomas in infant
Lymphogranuloma venereum			Erythromycin base 500 mg PO QID for 21 days	

Continued

TABLE 25.3 Sexually Transmitted Disease and Recommended Treatments in Pregnancy *Continued*

INFECTION	COMMON SYMPTOMS OR FINDINGS	DIAGNOSIS	RECOMMENDED TREATMENT	SPECIAL CONSIDERATIONS
Pediculosis pubis (pubic lice)	Itching	Lice visualized	Permethrin 1% cream rinse applied to affected areas and washed off after 10 min	
Scabies	Itching, rashes	Scrape lesion and identify under microscope	Permethrin cream (5%) applied to all areas of the body from the neck down and washed off after 8–14 hr	Wash bedding with hot water
Syphilis	Chancres Rashes Neurological symptoms Early latent (<1 yr)	RPR VDRL Treptonemal testing	Benzathine penicillin G 2.4 million units IM for primary and secondary or early latent phase Benzathine penicillin G 2.4 million units IM once a week for 3 weeks for late latent phase or unknown duration or tertiary Aqueous crystalline penicillin G 4 million units IV q 4 hr for 10 days Pregnant women with a penicillin allergy should be desensitized	Treatment with penicillin may initiate a Jerric Herxheimer reaction—fever, which can lead to fetal distress
Trichomonas	Asymptomatic Yellow green foul-smelling discharge, spotting or cramping	Rapid diagnostic kits using DNA probes Microscopy only identifies 60% of cases	Asymptomatic infections—treatment shows does not prevent PTL; may increased PTL Symptomatic infections treat with: Metronidazole 2 g PO once, *OR* Metronidazole 500 mg PO BID for 7 days	Neonates who travel through an infected birth canal can obtain fever, nasal, or vaginal discharge

Source: 2010 CDC STD Treatment Guidelines.

endometrium. However, the literature does contain case reports of tubo-ovarian abscesses diagnosed in pregnancy (Navada & Bhat, 2011; Yalcin, Tanir, & Eakalen, 2002). More common infectious processes like appendicitis and inflammatory bowel syndrome must first be ruled out before a diagnosis of PID in pregnancy is considered.

SYPHILIS

The incidence of syphilis in the United States has been slowly rising since 2001, but most of the increase is attributable to infections in men having sex with men. There were 377 cases of congenital syphilis in the United States in 2010 (CDC, 2010). Untreated syphilis infections in pregnant women can result in stillbirth, neonatal death, or can result in infants living with congenital syphilis.

The primary stage of syphilis is marked by a small, round painless genital lesion referred to as a chancre. The chancre typically lasts up to 6 weeks and if untreated, progresses into secondary syphilis, which is marked by a rough, brown red rash on the palms and feet. Symptoms of the rash may be mild. Constitutional symptoms of fever and fatigue may be present. If still untreated, syphilis will next proceed into a latent phase. If the syphilitic treponema enters the neurological system, neurosyphilis with seizures and headaches can result.

Penicillin is used for the treatment of syphilis, but the forms and the dosage change depending on the stage at the time of diagnosis. Specific penicillin doses are noted in Table 25.3. The CDC's *"Sexually transmitted disease treatment guidelines, 2010"* recommend desensitization in penicillin-allergic pregnant women, followed by treatment with penicillin.

REFERENCES

Brown, Z. A., & Selke, S. (1997). The acquisition of herpes simplex virus during pregnancy. *New England Journal of Medicine, 337*, 509.

Brown, Z. A., Wald, A, Morrow, R. A., Selke, S., Zeh, J., & Corey, L., (2003). Effect of serologic status and cesarean delivery on transmission rates of herpes simplex virus from mother to infant, *Journal of American Medical Association, 289*, 203–209.

Centers for Disease Control and Prevention (CDC). (2010). Recommendations and reports: Sexually transmitted diseases treatment guidelines, 2010. *MMWR, 59(RR-12)*, 1–114.

Centers for Disease Control and Prevention (CDC). (2011a). *Sexually transmitted diseases surveillance, 2010*. Atlanta, GA: U.S. Department of Health and Human Services.

Centers for Disease Control and Prevention (CDC). (2011b).Cephalosporin susceptibility among *Neisseria Gonorrheoeae* isolates—United States, 2000–2010. *MMWR, 60(RR-26)*, 873–877.

Cooper, E. R., Charurat, M., Mofenson, L., Hanson, I. C., Pitt, J., Diaz, C.... Women and Infants' Transmission Study Group. (2002). Combination antiretroviral strategies for the treatment of pregnant HIV-1-infected women and prevention of perinatal HIV-1 transmission. *Journal of Acquired Immune Deficiency Syndromes, 29(5)*, 484–494.

Datta, S. D., Sternberg, M., Johnson, R. E., Berman, S., Papp, J. R., McQullin, G., & Weinstock, H. (2007). Gonorrhea and chlamydia in the United States among persons 14 to 39 years of age, 1999 to 2002. *Annals of Internal Medicine, 147*, 89–96.

European Collaborative Study. (2005). Mother-to-child transmission of HIV infection in the era of highly active antiretroviral therapy. *Clinical Infectious Disease, 40*, 458–465.

Geretti, A. M., & Brown D. W. (2005). National survey of diagnostic services for genital herpes. *Sexually Transmitted Infections, 81*, 316–317.

Klein, L. L, & Gibbs, R. S. (2004). Use of microbial cultures and antibiotics in the prevention of infection-associated preterm birth. *American Journal of Obstetrics and Gynecology, 190*, 1493–1502.

Leitich, H., Brunbauer, M., Bodner-Adler, B., Kaider, A., Egarter, C., & Husslein, P. (2003). Antibiotics for treatment of bacterial vaginosis in pregnancy: A meta-analysis. *American Journal of Obstetrics and Gynecology, 188*(3), 752–758.

MacDonald, H., Brocklehurst, P., & Gordon, A. (2007). Antibiotics for treating bacterial vaginosis in pregnancy. *Cochrane Database Systemic Review,* (1), CDC000262.

Major, C. A., Towers, C. V., Lewis, D. F., & Garite, T. J. (2003). Expectant management of preterm premature rupture of membranes complicated by active recurrent genital herpes. *American Journal of Obstetrics and Gynecology, 188*, 1551–1554.

Navada, H. M., & Bhat, P. R. (2011). Pelvic inflammatory disease in the form of peritoneal abscess complicating late pregnancy. *Case Reports in Obstetrics and Gynecology, 2011*, 3.

NIH. (2011, September 14). *Panel of Treatment of HIV-Infected Pregnant Women and Prevention of Perinatal Transmission. Recommendations for use of antiretroviral drugs in pregnant HIV-1-infected women for maternal health and interventions to reduce perinatal HIV transmission in the United States.* Retrieved January 11, 2012, from http://aidsinfo.nih.gov/contentfi les/PerinatalGL.pdf

Schwebke, J. R. (2003). Gynecologic consequences of bacterial vaginosis. *Obstetrics and Gynecology Clinics of North America, 30*(4), 685–694.

Scott, L. L., Hollier, L. M., & McIntire, D. (2002). Acyclovir suppression to Prevent Recurrent Genital Herpes at Delivery. *Infectious Diseases in Obstetrics and Gynecology, 10*, 71.

Sheffield, J. S., Hollier, L. M., & Hill, J. B. (2003). Acyclovir prophylaxis to prevent herpes simplex virus recurrence at delivery: A systematic review. *Obstetrics and Gynecology, 102*, 1396.

Stone, K. M., Reiff-Eldridge, R., & White, A. D. (2004). Pregnancy outcomes following systemic prenatal acyclovir exposure: June 1984–1993. *Birth Defects Research, Part A. Clinical and Molecular Teratology, 70*, 201–207.

van der Schee, C., van Belkum, A., Zwijgers, L., van der Brugge, E., O'Neill, E. L., Luijendijk, A. . . . Sluiters, H. J. F. (1999). Improved diagnosis of *Trichomonas vaginalis* infection by PCR using vaginal swabs and urine specimens compared to diagnosis by wet-mount microscopy, culture and fluorescent staining. *Journal of Clinical Microbiology, 27*, 4127–4130.

Watts, D. H., Brown, Z. A., & Money, D. (2003). A double-blind, randomized, placebo-controlled trial of acyclovir in late pregnancy for the reduction of herpes simples virus shedding and cesarean delivery. *British Journal of Obstetrics and Gynaecology, 188*, 836.

Wade, N. A., Birkhead, G. S., Warren, B. L., Charbonneau, T. T., French, P. T., Wang, L. . . . Savicki, R. (1998). Abbreviated regimens of zidovudine prophylaxis and perinatal transmission of the human immunodeficiency virus. *New England Journal of Medicine, 339*(20), 1409–1414.

Weisenfeld, H. C., Hillier, S. L., & Krohn, M. A. (2003). Neisseria gonorrhoeae and Chlamydia trachomatis infection. *Clinical Infectious Diseases, 37*, 319–325.

Yalcin, O. T., Tanir, H. M., & Eakalen, M. (2002). Unruptured pelvic abscesses in pregnancy: A report of the two cases. *Gynecological and Obstetric Investigation, 53*, 133–134.

26 Postpartum Preeclampsia Complications

Mollie A. McDonnold

Hypertensive disorders are common in pregnancy, occurring in 5% to 10% of all cases (Graeber, Vanderwal, Stiller, & Werdmann, 2005). Of these, 30% are due to chronic disease, while 70% are due to the spectrum of gestational hypertension to preeclampsia (Matthys, Coppage, Lambers, Barton, & Sibai, 2004). Eclampsia is one of the most concerning complications of hypertensive disorders of pregnancy and contributes significantly to maternal mortality. In Canada, a case fatality rate of 3.4 per 1,000 deliveries was noted from 2003 to 2009, making the risk of death from eclampsia 26.8 times greater than those who do not experience eclampsia (Liu et al., 2011). In addition, eclampsia is associated with increased risk of morbidity including the need for assisted ventilation, adult respiratory distress syndrome, acute renal failure, and cardiac arrest (Liu et al., 2011). Significant research and resources have been devoted to the problem, leading to a marked reduction of eclampsia in the antenatal period. However, women with hypertensive disorders postpartum have been excluded from this research (Sibai, 2011). As women will frequently manifest problems due to postpartum hypertension after discharge from the hospital, they are often initially managed in an obstetric triage or emergency room setting.

Rates of eclampsia have been declining. In Canada, the rate of eclampsia was noted to fall from 12.4 per 10,000 deliveries in 2003 to 5.9 in 2009 (Liu et al., 2011). While there has been reduction in the incidence of antenatal eclampsia due to improved prenatal care, screening, and prophylactic treatment with magnesium sulfate, in the last 6 decades there has been no decrease in the incidence of postpartum eclampsia, with 14% to 26% of eclamptic seizures noted to occur greater than 48 hours after delivery (Chames, Livingston, Ivester, Barton, Sibai, 2002; Liu et al., 2011; Yancey, Withers, Bakes, & Abbot, 2011).

It is difficult to define the incidence of hypertensive disorders of pregnancy presenting in the postpartum period. Traditionally, this time period has been considered to extend into the fourth postpartum week (Yancey et al., 2011). After discharge, many women are not seen in follow-up until 6 weeks and may not present earlier unless they experience symptoms. Women with the antenatal diagnosis of pregnancy-induced hypertensive disorders do not normalize blood pressure immediately following delivery. In one study of 62 patients, 81% had normalized by 3 months postpartum and required a mean of 5.4 weeks to reach normal blood pressures (Podymow & August, 2010).

However, there may be a brief 48-hour window following delivery of normal blood pressures followed by an increase in blood pressure between postpartum days 3 to 6, likely due to physiologic volume expansion and fluid mobilization (Ghuman, Rheiner, Tendler, & White, 2009; Podymow & August, 2010). As most women are discharged home prior to the fifth postpartum day in which blood pressure has been shown to reach peak values, the need for possible postpartum blood pressure treatment may not be identified (Podymow & August, 2010).

Of women who presented with seizure in the postpartum period, more than 90% presented within 7 days of their original hospital discharge (Al-Safi et al., 2011). While women with mild preeclampsia are 25 times more likely to experience hypertension during the postpartum period than normal controls, hypertensive disorders, including eclampsia, may onset in the postpartum period (Cruz, Gao, & Hibbard, 2011). Overall, the incidence of new-onset hypertensive disorders in the postpartum period ranges from 0.3%–27.5% (Sibai, 2011).

In a 10 year review of 3,899 cases of preeclampsia, 5.7% were initially diagnosed in the postpartum period, 66% after original discharge (Matthys et al., 2004). Chames et al. (2002) noted that 79.3% of women with eclampsia in the postpartum period presented late (>48 hours after delivery), and of these, only 22% had a history of preeclampsia in the index pregnancy. Similarly, Al-Safi found 63% of women with postpartum preeclampsia and 77.3% of those with eclampsia had no antecedent history of hypertensive disorder of pregnancy (Al-Safi et al., 2011).

Women in the postpartum period often present initially to the emergency room rather than directly to an obstetric provider. It is critical to quickly evaluate and treat those who present with elevated blood pressure, especially if associated with prodromal symptoms such as headache. This was the most common presenting symptom in women with delayed postpartum preeclampsia in Al-Safi's series, present in 69.1% (Al-Safi et al., 2011). In Chames's series, 91% of women with postpartum eclampsia were noted to have prodromal symptoms. Only seven sought care prior to onset of seizure activity, but six of these women were deemed to have had a preventable seizure due to failure to consider a diagnosis of preeclampsia in the postpartum setting (Chames et al., 2002). Since the differential diagnosis of postpartum hypertension is broad, a careful history and physical examination must elucidate the etiology and appropriate management.

PRESENTING SYMPTOMATOLOGY

Although it is unclear how many women with elevated blood pressure are not evaluated postpartum due to lack of symptoms, it is clear that those with postpartum eclampsia will likely experience symptoms. 91% to 100% of women with postpartum eclampsia are noted to have prodromal symptoms (Al-Safi et al., 2011; Chames et al., 2002). In multiple studies, headache has been shown to be the most common symptom (Al-Safi et al., 2011; Chames et al., 2002; Matthys et al., 2004; Yancey et al., 2011). Other common symptoms are displayed in Table 26.1.

It is essential to note that while headache is the most common presenting symptom, and headache with associated elevated blood pressure should prompt evaluation for preeclampsia, headache itself is nonspecific and is associated with a broad differential. Hypertensive disorders of pregnancy

TABLE 26.1 Common Symptoms Associated With Postpartum Preeclampsia

SYMPTOM	PERCENTAGE IN WOMEN (%)
Headache	62–82
Visual changes	19–31
Shortness of breath/chest pain	13–30
Nausea	12.5–18
Vomiting	11.2–14
Abdominal pain	7–14
Edema	9–10.5
Neurologic deficits	5.3

Source: Al-Safi et al. (2011), Matthys et al. (2004), and Yancey et al. (2011).

represent 24% of postpartum headaches, second most common behind tension-type headaches (Stella, Jodicke, How, Harkness, & Sibai, 2007).

HISTORY AND DATA COLLECTION

Given the broad differential associated with postpartum hypertension, a thorough history is critical. This includes the determination of the interval between delivery and presentation, a thorough medical and pregnancy history, determination of associated symptoms, family history with particular attention to cerebrovascular accidents, and confirmation of medication usage.

The time course of postpartum hypertensive disorders has classically been defined to extend into the fourth postpartum week (Yancey et al., 2011). After 6 weeks' postpartum, an alternative diagnosis, especially essential hypertension, should be considered. While it is critical to know about the antenatal history, many cases of hypertension postpartum, especially eclampsia, have not been previously diagnosed. In a series of 152 cases readmitted for delayed postpartum preeclampsia or eclampsia, 96 (63.2%) had no antecedent diagnosis (Al-Safi et al., 2011).

Although some studies have noted that African American women are more at risk for the development of eclampsia, specific risk factors have not been well established for the development of postpartum preeclampsia or eclampsia, as they have been for the antepartum period (Al-Safi et al., 2011; Matthys et al., 2004). Even chronic hypertension itself does not appear to be a risk factor for postpartum eclampsia. Of 543 women with superimposed preeclampsia on chronic hypertension, only 5.2% were readmitted postpartum and none developed eclampsia (Al-Safi et al., 2011). In the same study that found women with mild preeclampsia had 25 times the risk of having elevated pressures postpartum, women with chronic hypertension were only seven times more likely than women without hypertensive disorders to have elevated blood pressure postpartum (Cruz et al., 2011). However, while women with chronic hypertension were six times more likely to have a seizure as compared with normal controls, those with preeclampsia had only four times the risk (Cruz et al., 2011). Ultimately, knowledge of any underlying history may help to distinguish worsening essential hypertension from developing preeclampsia.

Other associated symptoms may be clues that an alternative diagnosis is present. Hyperthyroidism, either Grave's disease or the hyperthyroid phase of postpartum thyroiditis may present with palpitations and heat intolerance. Shortness of breath and chest pain are associated with peripartum cardiomyopathy, of which 23% to 46% of cases have associated hypertension (Sibai, 2011). Symptoms of other cerebrovascular complications often overlap with those of preeclampsia and include refractory or thunder clap headache (a sudden onset pain often described as the worst headache a woman has ever experienced), visual disturbances, or neurologic deficits (Stella et al., 2007). Pheochromocytoma, although a rare entity, is associated with high morbidity and symptoms such as palpitations, excessive sweating, chest pain, and dizziness (Sibai, 2011).

Medication usage is an essential part of the history. The use of nonsteroidal anti-inflammatory medications like ibuprofen is common practice. These medications have been shown to lead to hypertension by reducing compensatory renal prostaglandin synthesis in hypertensive patients while concomitantly increasing renal synthesis of vasoconstricting agents (Makris, Thronton, & Hennessy, 2004). They may also inhibit salt and water loss postpartum as well as decrease the effectiveness of many antihypertensive drugs including beta blockers, angiotensin-converting enzyme inhibitors, and thiazide diuretics (Ghuman et al., 2009). Anticongestants such as ephedrine and phenylpropanolamine are other commonly used medications associated with exacerbation of hypertension. Ergot alkaloids like methylergonovine, administered for uterine atony in the postpartum period, cause vasoconstriction by acting on alpha adrenergic receptors and therefore add to the hypertensive issues (Sibai, 2011).

PHYSICAL EXAMINATION

Potential life-threatening complications of postpartum hypertension include cerebral infarction or hemorrhage, congestive heart failure of pulmonary edema, or renal failure (Sibai, 2011). Signs of these processes may be detected while performing a thorough physical examination. Vital signs alone may provide clues as to the etiology of the hypertension. Widened pulse pressure and tachycardia may be seen with hyperthyroidism, postural hypotension with pheochromocytoma, and decreased oxygen saturation with congestive heart failure or pulmonary edema (Sibai, 2011).

A thorough neurologic examination including evaluation of cranial nerves, visual fields, motor strength, sensation, cerebellar function, reflexes, and presence of clonus must be performed. Brisk reflexes, especially if associated with clonus, are classically associated with a preeclamptic state. Forty seven percent of women presenting with postpartum hypertension or eclampsia were noted to have hyperreflexia (Yancey et al., 2011). It is critical to urgently evaluate any neurologic deficits as they are indicative of possible serious intracranial abnormalities.

Cardiovascular and respiratory examination may reveal possible fluid overload associated with pulmonary edema noted with both preeclampsia and peripartum cardiomyopathy. Abdominal examination may reveal right-upper-quadrant tenderness. In Yancey's study of women presenting with postpartum preeclampsia or eclampsia, 18% were noted to have this finding

(Yancey et al., 2011). Although a very common finding seen in as high as 84% of women presenting with postpartum hypertension, edema is a nonspecific finding (Yancey et al., 2011). The presence may be noted but may not help elucidate etiology.

LABORATORY AND IMAGING STUDIES

A complete laboratory panel upon presentation consists of measurement of urine protein, either measured qualitatively with a urine dip or quantitatively on a urinalysis or with urine protein to creatinine ratio, complete blood count, liver enzymes, serum creatinine, and electrolytes. As normal postpartum lochia may influence the presence of proteinuria, it is necessary to obtain the sample by catheterization.

Although the antepartum diagnosis requires the presence of 300 mg/dL of protein in a 24-hour urine sample, it is seen in only 29% to 79% of postpartum eclampsia, less often than when seen in the antepartum period (Yancey et al., 2011). While the presence of proteinuria strongly suggests preeclampsia as an etiology, its absence does not rule out preeclampsia and possible impending eclampsia.

Hemolysis, elevated liver enzymes, and low platelets, or HELLP syndrome, another serious complication of preeclampsia, has also been noted to initially present in 30% of women who develop this syndrome from postpartum days 1 through 7 (Sibai, 2011). In Yancey's study, of 22 women with postpartum hypertension or eclampsia, 41% had noted elevated liver enzymes, 24% had anemia, but none were noted to have thrombocytopenia (Yancey et al., 2011).

As with physical examination findings, other laboratory findings may help to identify alternative etiologies of hypertension. For example, serum potassium levels less than 3 mEq/L with associated metabolic acidosis are indicative of hyperadlosteronism. Confirmation of adrenal tumor may then be made with either computed tomography (CT) or magnetic resonance imaging (MRI) of the abdomen (Sibai, 2011). Low serum creatinine is suggestive of volume overload (Sibai, 2011).

Presenting symptoms and physical examination concerning for pheochromocytoma, such as paroxysmal hypertension associated with headache, profuse sweating, palpitation, tachycardia, pallor, and possible fever, measurement of 24-hour urine epinephrine, norepinephrine, and their metabolites (metanephrine and normetanephrine) can lead to the diagnosis, which is then confirmed with either CT or MRI of the abdomen (Sibai, 2011). Symptoms and physical examination findings that point to pulmonary edema necessitate further evaluation with chest x-ray and possible echocardiography (Sibai, 2011).

In the antepartum evaluation of hypertensive disorders of pregnancy, neurodiagnostic imaging is rarely indicated. However, in the postpartum period, the differential diagnosis is wider, especially as distinguishing laboratory findings, such as proteinuria, are not always present. Different studies have examined the utility of neurodiagnostic imaging. Chames and his coworkers studied 23 women with late-onset postpartum preeclampsia and noted only one with significant findings on neurodiagnostic imaging, a transverse sinus thrombosis (Chames et al., 2002). In Yancey's series of 22 women with postpartum hypertension or eclampsia, 40.9% underwent head CT, and of these, three had significant findings including diffuse edema, cerebellar hypodensities, and small white matter hypodensities (Yancey et al., 2011). In the evaluation of postpartum headache, Stella found normal imaging in only 32% by employing indications including focal neurologic deficits, new-onset seizures, recurrent seizures despite prophylactic magnesium sulfate, persistent visual changes, or persistent refractory headache (Stella et al., 2007).

Abnormal findings included pituitary hemorrhage, posterior reversible encephalopathy syndrome, cerebral venous thrombosis, inflammatory changes, thalamic lesions, and subarachnoid hemorrhage (Stella et al., 2007). Ultimately, neurodiagnostic imaging studies aimed at evaluating the cerebral vasculature—MRI and arterial and venous angiography—will need to be obtained if these findings are present.

Posterior reversible encephalopathy syndrome, or PRES, is commonly associated with eclampsia and is clinically characterized by acute onset headache, altered mental status, cortical blindness, and seizures with parietooccipital involvement (Stella et al., 2007). Primarily occurring in the setting of preeclampsia, the syndrome is likely caused by large changes in blood pressure that result in an imbalance of pressure between the capillaries and interstitial spaces. In preeclampsia, endothelial cells are damaged and this pressure imbalance leads to vasogenic edema (Bushnell & Chireau, 2011). Classic findings of edema in the parietooccipital white matter are seen in Figure 26.1, which shows extensive areas of subcortical increased T2 signal with enhanced diffusivity involving posterior parietal and occipital white matter.

Reversible cerebral vasoconstrictive syndrome is a similar condition, classically presenting with a thunderclap headache, which is more severe and sudden than that associated with PRES. Although the pathophysiology is unclear, it is likely due to a disturbance in the control of cerebral vascular tone

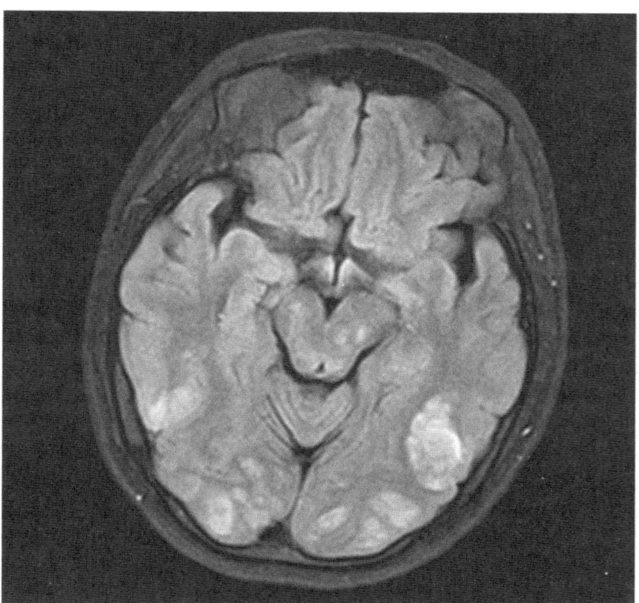

FIGURE 26.1 MRI findings in posterior reversible encephalopathy syndrome (PRES).

Source: Courtesy of Department of Radiology, Women & Infants Hospital, Providence, RI.

(Bushnell & Chireau, 2011). Other possible intracranial etiologies and associated radiographic findings are displayed in Table 26.2.

DIFFERENTIAL DIAGNOSIS

The most common etiology of postpartum hypertension remains the hypertensive disorders of pregnancy, including gestational hypertension and preeclampsia, whether diagnosed originally in the antepartum period or newly onset postpartum. Although the blood pressure may initially appear controlled in the first 48 hours, prompting discharge from the hospital following delivery, it will rise again between postpartum days 3 and 6 (Sibai, 2011). Prior to discharge, women with known hypertensive disorders need to be advised to have blood pressure checked in 2 to 3 days and receive counseling to seek care for severe headaches, which do not respond to pain medications, visual changes, shortness of breath, or chest pain. Women may either present to an emergency facility due to routine blood pressure checks at home or due to associated symptoms and may require antihypertensive therapy in the postpartum period. Possible etiologies of postpartum hypertension are reviewed in Table 26.3.

Other medical causes of hypertension need to be considered and evaluated if the clinical situation is suspicious. These conditions are usually associated with hypertension refractory to treatment, as is the case with renal artery stenosis, and also with associated findings on evaluation. For example, in hyperaldosteronism, the elevated progesterone of pregnancy simulates spironolactone and reverses hypokalemia and hypertension. With the rapid decrease of progesterone postpartum, exacerbations of hypertension and severe hypokalemia may occur (Sibai, 2011). Graves' disease or postpartum

TABLE 26.2 Possible Neurologic Etiologies of Postpartum Hypertension

ETIOLOGY	CLINICAL PRESENTATION	RADIOGRAPHIC FINDINGS
Posterior reversible encephalopathy syndrome (PRES)	Acute onset headache, altered mental status, cortical blindness, and seizures	MRI shows edema in the white matter of the parietooccipital areas of the cerebral hemisphere
Cerebral vasoconstriction syndrome	Thunderclap headache, visual changes, neurologic deficits, onset postpartum days 3–14	Similar to PRES but with the presence of segmental vasoconstriction on MRI or angiography, areas of T2/FLAIR hyperintensity especially in watershed areas
Cerebral venous thrombosis/stroke	Gradual or acute headache, neurologic deficits, seizures, onset postpartum days 3–7	Evidence of thrombus on cerebral venography, possible associated cerebral hemorrhage, magnetic resonance (MR) angiography may show reversible vasospasm of large and medium vessels

Source: Del Zotto et al. (2011), Stella et al. (2007), and Sibai (2011).

TABLE 26.3 Differential Diagnosis of Postpartum Hypertension

ETIOLOGY	POSSIBLE CONDITIONS
Pregnancy related	Gestational hypertension/preeclampsia (prior antepartum diagnosis or denovo postpartum) Volume overload postdelivery HELLP syndrome Postpartum eclampsia
Medical conditions	Chronic hypertension Preexisting renal disease Hyperthyroidism Cardiomyopathy Lupus nephritis Primary hyperaldosteronism Renal artery stenosis Pheochromocytoma Thrombotic thrombocytopenic purpura/hemolytic uremic syndrome (TTP/HUS)
Intercranial	Posterior reversible encepalopathy syndrome Cerebral vasoconstriction syndrome Cerebral venous thrombosis/stroke Hypertensive encephalopathy
Medications	Nonsteroidal anti-inflammatories Anticongestants (phenylpropanolamine, ephedrine) Ergotamine, methylergonovine

Source: Sibai (2011), Ghuman et al. (2009), and Graeber et al. (2005).

thyroiditis may present with palpitations, tachycardia, sweating, dry skin, and associated heart failure.

When seizures are present, the differential is wide and includes eclampsia, cerebral venous thrombosis, intracerebral hemorrhage, cerebral vasoconstriction syndrome, PRES, hypertensive encephalopathy, space occupying lesions of the brain, and metabolic disorders such as hypoglycemia or hyponatremia (Graeber et al., 2005). A stroke, either due to cerebral hemorrhage or cerebral venous thrombus may initially present with hypertension due to increased intracranial pressure with increased peripheral vascular tone (Sibai, 2011). In addition, stroke shares many other presenting symptoms with postpartum preeclampsia. A series of 27 women with hemorrhagic or ischemic stroke found that 96% experienced headache, 63% had nausea and vomiting, 71% had focal neurologic changes, and 37.5% had visual changes (Bushnell & Chireau, 2011).

Although it remains rare, stroke incidence in pregnancy, either hemorrhagic or ischemic, has increased. Analysis of the Nationwide Inpatient Sample, the largest nationwide hospital inpatient care database in the United States, showed a rise in all stroke types by 47% in antenatal hospitalizations (0.15–0.22 per 1,000 deliveries) and 83% in postpartum hospitalizations (0.12–0.22/1,000 deliveries) from 1994 to 2006 (Kuklina, Tong, Bansil, George, & Callaghan, 2011). A similar rise in pregnant women with heart disease and hypertensive disorders, strong risk factors for stroke, were also seen during this time period, a likely contributor to increased stroke events (Kuklina et al., 2011).

Pregnancy itself is a hypercoagulable state associated with venous stasis. These procoagulant changes are highest in the immediate postpartum period and do not return to normal until 3 weeks after delivery (Del Zotto et al., 2011). Data from the Nationwide Inpatient Sample demonstrate that the highest incidence of stroke occurs in the postpartum period (Bushnell & Chireau, 2011). A separate study found a 0.7 relative risk of cerebral infarction during pregnancy increased to 5.4 in the first 6 postpartum weeks (Del Zotto et al., 2011). While 28% to 46% of stroke cases in pregnancy have no determined etiology, preeclampsia and cardioembolic events are frequently responsible (Del Zotto et al., 2011). Stroke and preeclampsia share many common risk factors including endothelial dysfunction, dyslipidemia, hypertension, hypercoagulability, and abnormal cerebral vasomotor reactivity, and preeclampsia is seen with 6% to 47% of stroke events, placing women at four times the risk of stroke as compared to women without preeclampsia (Bushnell & Chireau, 2011; Del Zotto et al., 2011). Prompt diagnosis with neuroimaging, especially in women with neurologic changes, is necessary to initiate proper treatment.

CLINICAL MANAGEMENT AND FOLLOW-UP

As the presentation of postpartum hypertension has been largely excluded from studies examining the management of pregnancy-associated hypertension, there are no clear guidelines for management. Appropriate blood pressure control and prevention of seizures are the key management steps. In cases of isolated hypertension, it is appropriate to initiate antihypertensive medications if the systolic blood pressure is persistently above 150 mmHg or the diastolic blood pressure is persistently above 100 mmHg (Podymow & August, 2010). Women with severely elevated blood pressures upon presentation (>160 mmHg systolic or >105 mmHg diastolic) may receive initial treatment with intravenous injections of labetalol or hydralazine, then followed by an oral regimen (Sibai, 2011). Hypertensive regimens are displayed in Table 26.4.

It is necessary to continue treatment until the blood pressure remains below hypertensive levels for at least 48 hours, possibly several weeks postpartum. In those women requiring antihypertensives prior to pregnancy or with comorbid conditions such as diabetes or heart disease, it is reasonable to restart the pregestational medication regimen (Sibai, 2011). Nearly all antihypertensive medications are secreted into breast milk, but given the unlikelihood of large placebo-controlled trials being performed in the future, data will always be limited regarding outcomes. However, overall, antihypertensive medications are safe during lactation and require a dialogue between woman and physician regarding risks and benefits (Ghuman et al., 2009). Of note, while thiazide diuretics are rated as compatible with breast-feeding by the American Academy of Pediatrics, the drug class has been shown to decrease milk production and can be used in large doses to suppress lactation, making this option less ideal for breast-feeding women (Ghanem & Movahed, 2008; Ghuman et al., 2009).

The treatment of women diagnosed with severe preeclampsia postpartum based on severe pressures, possible proteinuria, and possible associated symptoms includes magnesium sulfate for seizure prophylaxis. This is the preferred management in the antepartum period and its use has been continued in postpartum patients. In Al-Safi's study, 84.9% of patients received

TABLE 26.4 Postpartum Antihypertensive Regimens

MEDICATION	DOSAGE	BENEFITS	METHOD OF ACTION	SIDE EFFECTS	BREAST-FEEDING CLASS
ACUTE INTRAVENOUS TREATMENT					
Labetalol	10–20 mg followed by 20 mg incremental increased doses up to 80 mg every 10 min, total cumulative dose 300 mg	Response within 5–10 min, lasts 3–6 hr	Combined alpha-beta blocker, vasodilatory effects	Nausea, vomiting, bronchoconstriction, dizziness, heart block, orthostatic hypotension, avoid in heart failure	Secretion into breastmilk, concentration varies, compatible with breastfeeding
Hydralazine	5 mg followed by additional 5–10 mg in 20 min, maximum bolus 20 mg, total cumulative dose 30 mg	Response within 10–30 min, lasts 2–4 hr	Direct acting arteriolar vasodilator	Reflex tachycardia, hypotension, flushing, headache, aggravation of angina, lupus- like syndrome	Relatively low concentration in breastmilk, compatible with breastfeeding
MAINTENANCE ORAL TREATMENT					
Labetalol	200–400 mg every 8–12 hr, maximum 2.4 g/d	Lack of associated flushing, tachycardia noted with Nifedipine	Combined alpha-beta blocker, vasodilatory effects	Nausea, vomiting, bronchoconstriction, dizziness, heart block, orthostatic hypotension, avoid in heart failure	Secreted into breastmilk, concentration varies, compatible with breast-feeding
Nifedipine	10–20 mg every 4–6 hr, maximum 180 mg/d	Improved renal blood flow with resultant diuresis as compared with labetalol	Calcium channel blocker, dihydropyridine type, decreases vascular smooth muscle contractility	Tachycardia, headache, flushing	Secreted into breastmilk, relatively high concentration, compatible with breast-feeding
Nifedipine XL	30–90 mg every 24 hr, maximum 120 mg/d	Once daily dosing	Extended release calcium channel blocker, decreases vascular smooth muscle contractility	Tachycardia, headache, flushing, symptoms may be less than with rapid release	Secreted into breast milk, compatible with breast-feeding

Note: All ratings are compatible with breast-feeding as per the American Academy of Pediatrics.

Source: Ghanem & Movahed (2008), Ghuman et al. (2009), and Sibai (2011).

magnesium sulfate during their postpartum admission (Al-Safi et al., 2011). A 4 to 6 g loading dose over 20 minutes followed by a maintenance dose of 2 g/hr for at least 24 hours is the recommended regimen (Sibai, 2011). When other etiologies are suspected, a multidisciplinary approach based on the most likely diagnosis is recommended.

REFERENCES

Al-Safi, Z., Imudia, A., Filetti, L., Hobson, D., Bahado-Singh, R., & Awonuga, A. (2011). Delayed postpartum preeclampsia and eclampsia. *Obstetrics and Gynecology, 118*(5), 1102–1107.

Bushnell, C., & Chireau, M. (2011). Preeclampsia and stroke: Risks during and after pregnancy. *Stroke Research and Treatment, 2011*, DOI: 10.4061/2011/858134.

Chames, M., Livingston, J., Ivester, T., Barton, J., Sibai, B. (2002). Late postpartum eclampsia: A preventable disease? *American Journal of Obstetrics and Gynecology, 186*, 1174–1177.

Cruz, M., Gao, W., & Hibbard, J. (2011). Obstetrical and perinatal outcomes among women with gestational hypertension, mild preeclampsia, and mild chronic hypertension. *American Journal of Obstetrics and Gynecology, 205*, 260.e1–e9.

Del Zotto, E., Giossi, A., Volonghi, I., Costa, P., Padovani, A., & Pezzini, A. (2011). Ischemic stroke during pregnancy and puerperium. *Stroke Research and Treatment, 2011.*

Ghanem, F., & Movahed, A. (2008). Use of antihypertensive drugs during pregnancy and lactation. *Cardiovascular Therapeutics, 26*, 38–49.

Ghuman, N., Rheiner, J., Tendler, B., & White, W. (2009). Hypertension in the postpartum woman: Clinical update for the hypertension specialist. *Journal of Clinical Hypertension, 11*, 726–733.

Graeber, B., Vanderwal, T., Stiller, R., & Werdmann, M. (2005). Late postpartum eclampsia as an obstetric complication seen in the ED. *The American Journal of Emergency Medicine, 23*, 168–170.

Kuklina, E., Tong, X., Bansil, P., George, M., & Callaghan, W. (2011). Trends in pregnancy hospitalizations that included a stroke in the United States from 1994 to 2007. Reasons for concern? *Stroke, 42*, 2564–2570.

Liu, S., Joseph, K., Liston, R, Bartholomew, S., Walker, M., León, J. A. . . . Maternal Health Study Group of Canadian Perinatal Surveillance System (Public Health Agency of Canada). (2011). Incidence, risk factors, and associated complications of preeclampsia. *Obstetrics and Gynecology, 118*, 987–994.

Makris, A., Thronton, C., & Hennessy, A. (2004). Postpartum hypertension and nonsteroidal analgesia. *American Journal of Obstetrics and Gynecology, 190*, 577–578.

Matthys, L., Coppage, K., Lambers, D., Barton, J., & Sibai, B. (2004). Delayed postpartum preeclampsia: An experience of 151 cases. *American Journal of Obstetrics and Gynecology, 190*, 1464–1466.

Podymow, T., & August, P. (2010). Postpartum course of gestational hypertension and preeclampsia. *Hypertension in Pregnancy, 29*, 294–300.

Sibai, B. (2011). Etiology and management of postpartum hypertension-preeclampsia. *American Journal of Obstetrics and Gynecology.* DOI: 10.1016/j.ajog.2011.09.002

Stella, C., Jodicke, C., How, H., Harkness, U., & Sibai, B. (2007). Postpartum headache: Is your work-up complete? *American Journal of Obstetrics and Gynecology, 196*, 318e1–318e7.

Yancey, L., Withers, E., Bakes, K., & Abbot, J. (2011). Postpartum preeclampsia: Emergency department presentation and management. *The Journal of Emergency Medicine, 40*, 380–384.

Postpartum Breast Complications 27

Chelsy Caren and David A. Edmonson

Women commonly present to the obstetric (OB) triage/emergency department during the postpartum period with breastfeeding concerns and complications. Breastfeeding has become increasingly popular secondary to worldwide research that has consistently demonstrated significant benefits to both infant and mother. Whereas only 24.7% of women in the United States initiated breastfeeding in 1971, 75.5% did so in 2007 (ACOG, 2007).

The most common difficulties encountered by breastfeeding women are generalized engorgement of the breasts, plugged ducts, and nipple trauma. These conditions generally respond well to supportive care and continued attempts at feeding, and will be discussed briefly. Postpartum inflammatory breast disease, including puerperal, or lactational, mastitis and breast abscess are less common. It has been estimated that 2% to 33% of breastfeeding women experience mastitis (Jahanfar, Ng, & Teng, 2009), while only 0.1% (Kvist & Rydhstroem, 2005) to 0.4% (Amir, Forster, McLachlan, & Lumley, 2004) develop abscesses. These latter disorders are infectious in nature and require more intensive treatment, including antibiotics and possibly surgery, which will be addressed.

COMMON BREASTFEEDING DIFFICULTIES

Engorgement and Plugged ducts

Breast engorgement is the swelling of the breasts resulting from incomplete emptying of milk. Early engorgement occurs with the onset of increased milk production that characterizes the first few days postpartum, when the breasts swell secondary to edema and inflammation in addition to milk accumulation. The lactating mother will commonly report distinct tenderness, firmness, and warmth of the breasts. These findings are usually bilateral and generalized, and erythema tends to be absent. Late engorgement is generally due to milk stasis alone and can be either localized or generalized, though swelling is often not as pronounced. It is uncommon for women with either type of engorgement to report systemic symptoms such as fever or malaise. Both types are generally attributable to incorrect or inconsistent breastfeeding technique, prohibiting efficient drainage of milk from the breasts.

Plugged ducts are also commonly seen in women who report suboptimal breastfeeding technique or who have increased milk supply relative to demand due to a change in feeding frequency or intensity. Localized distension of breast tissue occurs as a result of inadequate drainage in a single duct, and can be palpable by the breastfeeding woman as a distinct, tender mass. As with engorgement, systemic symptoms are absent. If unrelieved, a galactocele, or milk retention cyst, may form. Although these are full of milk initially, the contents can become thicker over time. Tenderness usually resolves as well. A soft cystic mass, with no evidence of infection, is often the sole finding on clinical examination. Ultrasound imaging of a galactocele may show a well-defined mass with internal complexity, as shown in Figure 27.1.

The key to the management of generalized breast engorgement without infection, as well as plugged ducts, is prevention. This is accomplished by frequent emptying of the breasts, and is most efficiently achieved by breastfeeding the infant directly. A satisfactory latch-on is essential, which proves difficult for many nursing women to establish. Proper positioning of the infant, consistency in feeding techniques, and an environment that is conducive to breastfeeding are all instrumental in allowing the infant to latch on successfully. Lactation consultants can be called upon when needed to advise and demonstrate to women how best to optimize these factors.

If the latch-on is not sufficient for relief of engorgement or a plugged duct, the use of a breast pump to drain the breasts is recommended. Manual expression and massage can also be helpful. While cold compresses are preferred to address the swelling that accompanies early engorgement, heat is more useful in cases of late engorgement and plugged ducts, both for symptom relief and to encourage milk flow. Galactoceles may resolve spontaneously or may be treated with aspiration or surgical removal.

Nipple Trauma

Nipple trauma, including abrasions, cracking, blistering, or bruising, can be the cause or result of a poor latch-on, thereby discouraging ongoing efforts to

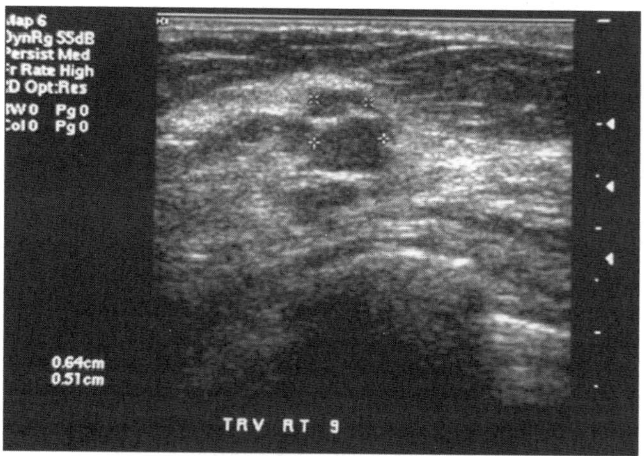

FIGURE 27.1 Ultrasound appearance of a galactocele.

Source: Courtesy of Department of Radiology, Women & Infants Hospital, Providence, RI.

breastfeed. The best preventative measure is proper positioning of the infant to ensure optimal latch-on. When this is complicated by an anatomic abnormality of the woman's nipples or the infant's mouth, a lactation consultation is recommended.

Once present, various treatments are available that can be used to decrease soreness and heal traumatized nipples. These include purified lanolin ointments, hydrogel dressings, or the combination of antibiotic, antifungal, and mild steroid therapy known as "all-purpose nipple ointment." In addition, breast shields may be utilized to prevent friction to nipples between feedings as needed. Since infections of the skin and breast, most commonly with *Candida albicans* or *Staphylococcus aureus* (see below), occur more frequently in women with injured nipples (Lawrence RA & Lawrence RM, 2005), it is crucial to address nipple trauma early in its course.

Resources

Women presenting with the above generalized breastfeeding difficulties may be experiencing a great deal of distress and anxiety. The ability to provide information and guidance to these nursing mothers can help to reassure them that such challenges are not uncommon and encourage them to continue breastfeeding. Some popular resources are listed in Exhibit 27.1 and can assist in providing lactation support or verifying the compatibility of a certain recommended treatment with breastfeeding.

POSTPARTUM INFLAMMATORY BREAST DISEASE

The term "postpartum inflammatory breast disease" includes both lactational mastitis and breast abscesses. Mastitis is caused when bacteria, commonly skin flora and/or oral flora from the infant, have access to stagnant milk in the breast, generally via the nipple. If left untreated, the infection may progress to abscess formation, which is estimated to occur approximately 3% to 11% of the time (Amir et al., 2004).

The most common etiologic organism in postpartum inflammatory breast disease is *Staphylococcus aureus*. *Streptococcus pyogenes*, *Escherichia Coli*, *Bacteroides* species, coagulase negative staphylococci, *Proteus*, and *Corynebacterium* species are also found in some milk cultures. *Candidal* breast infections will be discussed separately in the differential diagnosis section below. Methicillin-resistant *S. aureus* (MRSA) is gaining increasing importance as a causative organism of mastitis as well as skin infections in general

EXHIBIT 27.1

Lactation Resources

La Leche League	www.llli.org
The Academy of Breastfeeding medicine	www.bfmed.org
Medications and Mother's Milk	www.medsmilk.com/menu.html

Source: Briggs, Freeman, & Yaffe (2011); The Academy of Breastfeeding Medicine (2012).

(Schoenfeld & McKay, 2010). Risk factors for the presence of MRSA include recent hospitalization, positive culture results confirming colonization by MRSA in the past (personal or close family member), chronic illness or non-healing wounds, or failure of treatment directed toward MRSA. In one study of milk cultures from women who required hospitalization for treatment of mastitis, MRSA was the most common organism isolated, 44% (24 of 54) for women with mastitis alone, and 67% (18 of 27) in women with abscess formation (Reddy, Qi, Zembower, Noskin, & Bolon, 2007).

PRESENTING SYMPTOMATOLOGY

The most common complaints reported by a breastfeeding woman with mastitis include pain and tenderness in the affected breast. Warmth and/or redness of the breast and nipple discomfort, cracking, or excoriation are often noted as well. Fever and flu-like symptoms including malaise and myalgias are common. Axillary pain due to reactive swelling of the lymph nodes on the affected side may also occur. Finally, when a breast abscess is present, the breastfeeding woman may report the presence of a painful mass in the affected breast. Septic shock is rare.

HISTORY AND DATA COLLECTION

The postpartum woman with the above symptoms will typically describe a history of difficulty with breastfeeding. Reports of poor milk production or a sensation of incomplete emptying of the affected breast are common, as is a history of prolonged engorgement, a blocked duct, or nipple trauma. Weaning may be in progress. Any factor that increases the likelihood that stagnant milk is present increases the risk of postpartum inflammatory breast disease. A prior episode of mastitis and/or breast abscess while breastfeeding either the current or a previous infant increases this risk as well.

A woman who presents with worsening symptoms despite standard treatment for mastitis is at increased risk for having either less common or resistant organisms such as MRSA present in the breast milk. A breast abscess is more likely under these circumstances as well. Breast abscesses are more frequently seen in primigravidas, women over the age of 30, and women who delivered at 41 weeks' gestation or more (Kvist & Rydhstroem, 2005). Smokers, obese women, and African Americans are at higher risk of both lactational and nonlactational abscesses (Bharat et al., 2009).

PHYSICAL EXAMINATION

Examination of the affected breast of a woman with postpartum inflammatory breast disease usually reveals erythema and swelling. Early in the course of the infection, subtle streaks of light pink in a single region of the breast may be the only visible abnormality. In later stages, a firm, red, swollen area of the breast, exquisitely tender to palpation or to ongoing attempts to breast-feed, may develop. Classically, these findings are limited to one region of the breast, extending from the nipple outward in a wedge-shaped pattern. However, either localized or generalized engorgement may be found as well. A fluctuant mass is often palpable when an abscess is present. Fever may be documented, and, if so, tachycardia may present as well. Hypotension is uncommon except in rare cases of systemic inflammatory response syndrome (SIRS) or sepsis related to an ongoing or inadequately treated infection.

LABORATORY AND IMAGING STUDIES

Lactational mastitis can be diagnosed by clinical examination alone, and empiric antibiotic therapy may be initiated without laboratory testing or culture results. If a complete blood count (CBC) is drawn, however, the white blood cell count may be elevated. Breast milk can and often should be cultured, especially with a severe or recurrent infection, or with one that is persistent despite prior antibiotic treatment. The results can then be used to tailor the ultimate antibiotic selection, since mixed flora, anaerobes and *Proteus* are found more commonly in these cases (Bharat et al., 2009). Blood cultures are recommended only if the breastfeeding mother appears septic.

Imaging studies are not required for the diagnosis of lactational mastitis, nor are they necessary to make a diagnosis of a lactational abscess if a fluctuant mass is found on clinical breast examination. However, ultrasound is often used to confirm an uncertain diagnosis, as well as to perform direct aspiration of a fluid collection. Figure 27.2 shows the typical appearance of a breast abscess on ultrasound.

DIFFERENTIAL DIAGNOSIS

Lactational mastitis is the most common, benign, inflammatory breast disorder (Pearlman & Griffin, 2010). The differential diagnoses for postpartum inflammatory breast disease include conditions similarly unique to breastfeeding women, such as generalized engorgement and plugged ducts (discussed above) and infections with *Candida albicans*. Several additional nonpuerperal inflammatory skin conditions and breast disorders are included as well, the most common of which are discussed here.

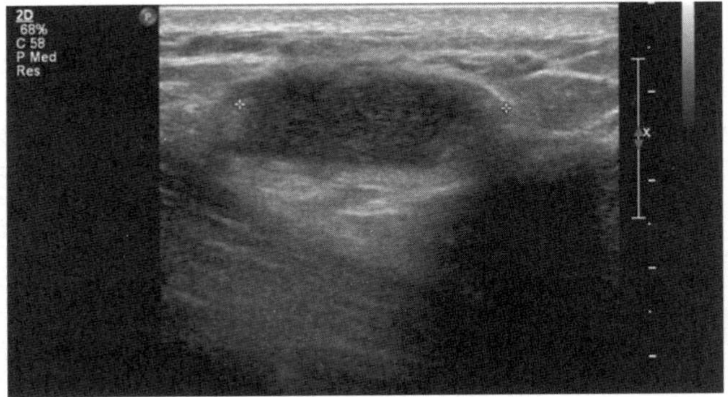

FIGURE 27.2 Ultrasound appearance of breast abscess.

Source: Courtesy of Department of Radiology, Women & Infants Hospital, Providence, RI.

Candidal Breast Infections

The lactating woman with a candidal infection of the breast will often present complaining of "shooting pains" in the breast along with redness and nipple discomfort. A history of a recent diagnosis of or treatment for oral thrush in the infant may also be reported. The inflammation seen with *Candida* of the breast, as elsewhere, is typically a localized erythema with satellite lesions, consistent with but not essential for the diagnosis. Systemic findings are generally absent. Candidal infections are treated with the topical or oral antifungal agents listed in Table 27.1 (Pearlman & Griffin, 2010). Of note, unlike the ointments used for the treatment of nipple trauma mentioned above, topical preparations of nystatin should be washed off prior to breastfeeding.

TABLE 27.1 Presentation and Treatment of Common Postpartum Breast Complications

COMPLICATION	BREAST ENGORGEMENT	PLUGGED DUCTS	CANDIDA
Symptoms/signs	Pain, fullness/firmness, warmth and tenderness of breasts Bilateral and generalized Absence of erythema Absence of systemic symptoms	Distinct, painful breast mass Absence of erythema Absence of systemic symptoms	"Shooting pains" in the breast Erythema often localized with satellite lesions Nipple discomfort
Management	Frequent emptying of the affected breast Cold compresses with early presentation Warm compresses with late presentation Treatment of nipple trauma Pain management (ibuprofen and other NSAIDs)	Frequent emptying of affected breast Warm compresses Pain management (ibuprofen and other NSAIDs)	**First Line:** Topical Nystatin 100,000 mcg; apply BID-TID after breastfeeding and wash off prior to next feeding **Second Line:** Fluconazole 100 mg PO daily for 10–14 days

COMPLICATION	LACTATIONAL MASTITIS	LACTATIONAL ABSCESS	INFLAMMATORY BREAST CANCER
Symptoms/ signs	Pain and tenderness of the affected breast Erythema and warmth of one region of the affected breast Usually unilateral Fever and flu-like symptoms are common	Same as for mastitis **Plus:** Distinct, painful breast mass Systemic symptoms are common	Same as for mastitis and abscess **Possible:** Skin thickening and/ or edema "Peau d'orange" Persistence of symptoms and signs despite appropriate treatment for mastitis and/or abscess

Continued

TABLE 27.1 Presentation and Treatment of Common Postpartum Breast Complications *Continued*

COMPLICATION	BREAST ENGORGEMENT	PLUGGED DUCTS	CANDIDA
Management	Dicloxacillin, 500 mg PO QID *or* Cephalexin, 500 mg PO QID **If beta-lactam hypersensitive:** Clindamycin, 300 mg PO QID **If MRSA suspected:** Trimethoprim-sulfamethoxizole, 1–2 tablets PO BID *or* clindamycin, 300 mg PO QID (All of the above for 10–14 days) **If severe:** Vancomycin 30 mg/kg IV in two divided doses daily	Antibiotics as for mastitis General surgery consultation Needle aspiration or Incision and drainage	Imaging Breast surgery consultation

Source: ACOG (2007), Jahanafar et al. (2009), Lawrence & Lawrence (2011), and Pearlman & Griffin (2010).

Superficial Skin Conditions

Additional skin conditions such as eczema and contact dermatitis may be part of the differential diagnosis in some breastfeeding mothers, as well. A thorough medical history including any possible exposures to substances that may cause such skin conditions will assist in making an accurate diagnosis. These conditions often respond to conventional therapies. Of note, recurrent scaling/crusting of the nipple is seen in Paget's disease. If this diagnosis is entertained, evaluation with a breast specialist for a biopsy should be arranged, to investigate the possibility of an underlying inflammatory breast cancer, as noted below.

Periductal Mastitis

Squamous metaplasia of the breast duct lining along with keratin plugging of the ducts is thought to lead to a condition known as periductal mastitis, or "mammary duct-associated inflammatory disease syndrome" (MDAIDS). This is a focal, often recurrent, benign inflammation specifically of the periareolar area of the affected breast. It can be accompanied by abscess formation or mammary duct fistula, can occur at any age, and is particularly common in smokers (70% of affected women are active smokers; Degnim, 2012). Empiric antibiotic therapy is broad-spectrum, to include for anaerobes as well as for *Staphylococcus* species. In addition to cultures, prompt imaging evaluation and biopsies are advocated to exclude inflammatory breast cancer, especially when worrisome skin findings (see below) or nipple retraction are present.

With the rate of recurrence and/or chronic fistula formation estimated to be as high as 80% and 90%, definitive surgical treatment is often warranted (Bland & Klimberg, 2011).

Inflammatory Breast Cancer

As previously mentioned, inflammatory breast cancer has many characteristics in common with postpartum breast disease. It is crucial to consider this diagnosis in cases where a presumed mastitis does not respond to the usual treatments. It is also more likely with nipple retraction, skin thickening, edema, or a "peau d'orange" appearance, as shown in Figure 27.3. Imaging and referral to a breast surgeon for definitive diagnosis are recommended in such cases. Of note, while ultrasound and/or mammogram are usually performed initially, magnetic resonance imaging (MRI) of the affected breast can be helpful in distinguishing between mastitis and inflammatory breast cancer (Renz et al., 2008). However, it is generally reserved for cases in which the latter is suspected, as in Figure 27.4.

Postoperative and Postirradiation Mastitis

In established breast cancer patients, surgical site infections as well as radiation changes can mimic puerperal disease, but the clinical history and treatment will differ accordingly. Postoperative or postirradiation mastitis is a delayed cellulitis found in women who have undergone prior surgery or radiation for breast cancer, commonly 3 months to several years posttreatment. It is recommended that these women be referred to their oncologists for evaluation, as this may be a sign of altered lymphatic or venous circulation.

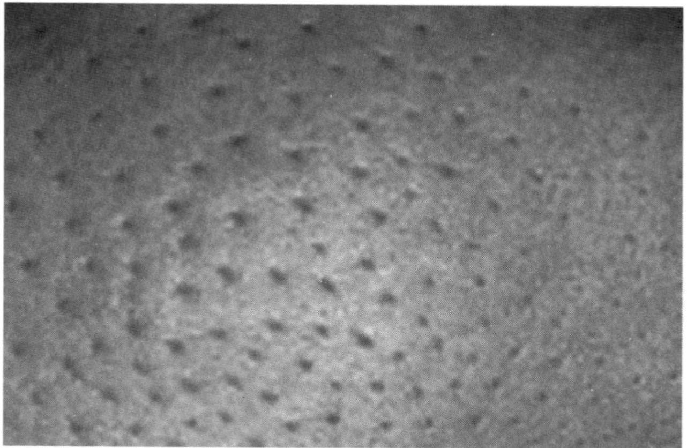

FIGURE 27.3 Photograph of "peau d'orange."

Source: Courtesy of David Edmonson, MD, Department of Obstetrics and Gynecology, Women & Infants Hospital, Providence, RI.

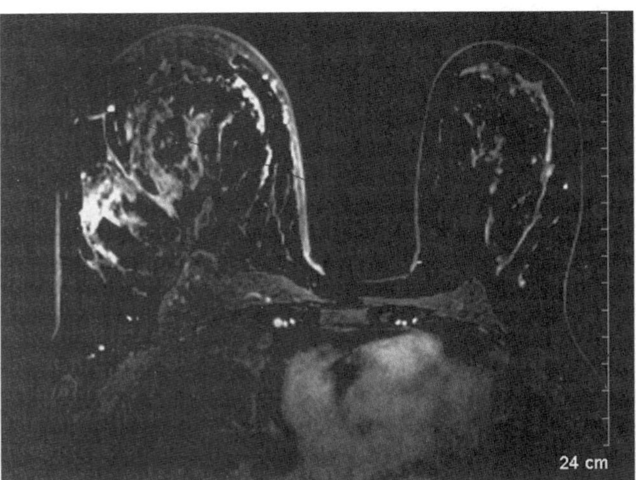

FIGURE 27.4 Magnetic resonance imaging of inflammatory breast cancer.
Source: Courtesy of Department of Radiology, Women & Infants' Hospital, Providence, RI.

CLINICAL MANAGEMENT AND FOLLOW-UP OF POSTPARTUM INFLAMMATORY BREAST DISEASE

The management of a breastfeeding woman with mastitis includes empiric antibiotic therapy as well as supportive care intended not only to provide relief of symptoms, but also to promote continued breastfeeding during treatment. Although one study showed that probiotics may be a useful alternative to antibiotics in the management of women with lactational mastitis (Arroyo et al., 2010), antibiotics remain the standard of care at present. In the absence of severe infection, abscess, or risk factors for MRSA, outpatient therapy is directed primarily against *S. aureus*. A 10 to 14 day course of dicloxacillin or cephalexin is first-line, with clindamycin preferred for women with beta-lactam hypersensitivity. If there is concern for MRSA infection, either trimethoprim-sulfamethoxizole or clindamycin is recommended. Table 27.1 lists the recommended antibiotic regimens. Reevaluation is recommended if improvement is not noted within a few days of initiating therapy, or if full resolution is not present upon completion of therapy. In severe cases, defined as such by progressive erythema despite empiric therapy or hemodynamic instability indicative of sepsis, hospitalization, and intravenous vancomycin are recommended. In such cases, culture and sensitivity results from a midstream milk culture can be used to direct the ultimate antibiotic regimen/therapy.

Continued breastfeeding throughout treatment for mastitis is strongly recommended. Regular emptying of the breast, by preventing engorgement and milk stasis, can significantly decrease duration of symptoms as well as prevent abscess formation (Jahanafar et al., 2009). Cold compresses/ice packs and anti-inflammatory agents such as ibuprofen can provide symptomatic relief of pain and swelling and may increase the ability to comply with this recommendation. Improved breastfeeding techniques can also be helpful, as can treatment of traumatized nipples, as mentioned above.

If, despite all of these measures, breastfeeding is too difficult or painful, breast pumps or hand expression may facilitate emptying and maintain milk supply until it can be resumed. Finally, rest and increased fluid intake are advised. Of note, bromocriptine, a dopamine agonist used in the past to suppress lactation in postpartum women, is no longer recommended due to reports of serious adverse reactions including stroke, myocardial infarction, seizures, and severe hypertension (DCAHD, 2000). If discontinuation of breastfeeding becomes necessary, natural suppression is endorsed as the best method.

When an abscess is present, standard management is drainage of the contents in addition to the antibiotic therapy described above (Stafford et al., 2008). Consultation with a surgeon with expertise in breast disease is recommended in these cases. Traditionally, drainage was by incision and drainage (I&D). More recently, however, needle aspiration has been shown to be equally effective (Erylimaz, Sahin, Hakan Tkelioglu, & Daldal, 2005). Particularly in the presence of normal-appearing overlying skin, aspiration with a medium-to-large bore needle under local anesthesia is now recommended as the initial approach. This results in decreased incisional prominence and pain, thereby optimizing the likelihood of ongoing lactation. Ultrasound guidance is advised to completely drain the contents of the abscess cavity, since the collection may not be detectable by physical examination alone, or more than one loculation may be present, as in Figure 27.5. Serial evaluations and aspirations are then performed, approximately every 2 to 3 days, until no further purulent material is obtained. It has been estimated that greater than 90% of lactational abscesses can be treated in this manner, thereby avoiding surgery (Bland & Kirby, 2011).

In cases where an abscess persists despite standard antibiotic regimens and serial aspirations, surgical drainage is indicated (Christensen et al., 2005). This is more common when there is a delay in initial treatment, when the infection is more severe, or when the abscess is greater than 5 cm in diameter (Eryilmaz et al., 2005). Skin changes such as thinning, excessive tension, and/or devascularization generally mandate I&D as well. If skin necrosis is present, the affected skin is excised and the cavity irrigated to drain the pus, and then the site is intervally reinspected to resolution. Packing and/or drains are

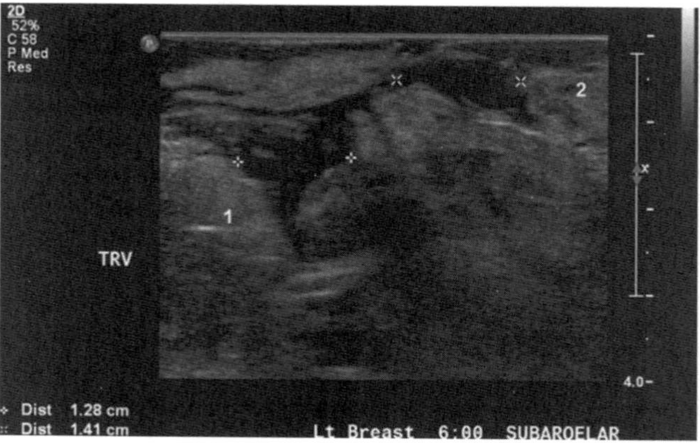

FIGURE 27.5 Ultrasound appearance of a multiloculated breast abscess.

Source: Courtesy of Department of Radiology, Women & Infants Hospital, Providence, RI

generally not implemented (Dixon, 2007), and may increase the risk of formation of a milk or a mammary duct fistula, a communication between the skin and a lactiferous duct or major subareolar duct, respectively. Both types result in milk draining through the skin of the breast. While a milk fistula generally resolves with cessation of breastfeeding, a mammary duct fistula requires additional surgical intervention for correction (Bland & Klimberg, 2011). Poor cosmetic outcome is rare, though may result from the initial I&D of a breast abscess or from the attempts to correct any subsequent complications. Diagnostic imaging is recommended approximately 3 months after resolution of any lactational abscess, to evaluate for any residual mass or signs of malignancy.

REFERENCES

American College of Obstetricians and Gynecologists (ACOG). (2007). Breastfeeding: Maternal and infant aspects. Special report from ACOG. *ACOG Clinical Review,12(suppl)*, 1S–16S.

Amir, L. H., Forster, D., McLachlan, H., & Lumley, J. (2004). Incidence of breast abscess in lactating women: Report from an Australian Cohort. *British Journal of Obstetrics and Gynecology, 111*, 1378–1381.

Arroyo, R., Martin, V., Maldonado, A., Jiménez, E., Fernández, L., & Rodríguez, J. M. (2010). Treatment of infectious mastitis during lactation: Antibiotics versus oral administration of Lactobacilli isolated from breast milk. *Clinical Infectious Disease, 50*, 1551–1558.

Bharat, A., Gao, F., Aft, R. L., Gillanders, W. E., Eberlein, T. J., & Margenthaler, J. A. (2009). Predictors of primary breast abscesses and recurrence. *World Journal of Surgery, 33*, 2582–2586.

Briggs, G., Freeman, R., & Yaffe, S. (2011). *Drugs in pregnancy and lactation* (9th ed.) Philadelphia, PA: Lippincott, Williams and Wilkins.

Christensen, A. F., AL-Suliman, N., Nielsen, K. R., Vejborg, I., Severance, N., Christensen, H., & Nielsen, M. B. (2005). Ultrasound-guided drainage of breast abscesses: Results in 151 patients. *British Journal of Radiology, 78*, 186–188.

Degnim, A. C. (2011). Drainage of breast cysts and abscesses. In K. Bland & V. Klimberg (eds.), *Breast surgery* (pp. 25–44). Philadelphia, PA: Lippincott, Williams and Wilkins.

Department of child and adolescent health and development (DHAHD). (2000). *Mastitis: Causes and management.* World Health Organization, 2000. Retrieved from http://whqlibdoc.who.int/hq/2000/WHO_FCH_CAH_00.13.pdf (accessed October 5, 2011).

Dixon, J. M. (2007). Breast abscess. *British Journal of Hospital Medicine (London), 68*, 315–320.

Erylimaz, R., Sahin, M., Hakan Tkelioglu, M., & Daldal, E. (2005). Management of lactational breast abscesses. *Breast, 14*, 375.

Jahanfar, S., Ng, C. J., & Teng, C. L. (2009). Antibiotics for mastitis in breastfeeding women. *Cochrane Database System Review,* CD005458.

Kvist, L. J., & Rydhstroem, H. (2005). Factors related to breast abscess after delivery: A population-based study. *British Journal of Obstetrics and Gynecology, 112*, 1070–1074.

Lawrence, R. A., & Lawrence, R. M. (2011). *Breastfeeding: A guide for the medical profession* (7th ed.), Maryland Heights, MO: Elsevier Mosby.

Pearlman, M. D., & Griffin, J. L. (2010). Benign breast disease. *Obstetrics and Gynecology, 116*, 747–758.

Renz, D. M., Baltzer, P. A., Bottcher, J., Thaher, F., Gajda, M., Camara, O.,... Kaiser, W. A. (2008). Magnetic resonance imaging of inflammatory breast carcinoma and acute mastitis. A comparative study. *European Radiology, 12*, 2370–2380.

Reddy, P., Qi, C., Zembower, T., Noskin, G. A., & Bolon, M. (2007). Postpartum mastitis and community-acquired methicillin-resistant Staphylococcus aureus. *Emergency Infectious Disease, 13*, 298–301.

Schoenfeld, E. M., & McKay, M. P. (2010). Mastitis and methicillin-resistant *Staphylococcus aureus* (MRSA): The calm before the storm? *Journal of Emergency Medicine, 38*, e31–e34.

Stafford, I., Hernandez, J., Laibl, V., Sheffield, J., Roberts, S., Wendel, G. Jr. (2008). Community-acquired methicillin-resistant Staphylococcus aureus among patients with puerperal mastitis requiring hospitalization. *Obstetrics and Gynecology, 112*, 533–537.

The Academy of Breastfeeding Medicine. Retrieved from www.bfmed.org (accessed November 5, 2011).

28 Secondary Postpartum Hemorrhage and Endometritis

Martha Pizzarello and Donna LaFontaine

In the postpartum period, secondary postpartum hemorrhage (SPPH) and endometritis are two conditions that frequently present to an obstetric (OB) triage unit. These complications frequently coexist and can occur from 24 hours postpartum to 6 weeks post delivery. SPPH is typically not as severe as a primary bleeding episode. Only 10% of the time will the hemorrhage be significant enough to cause a change in vital signs (Neil & Thorton, 2002). Likewise, postpartum women ultimately diagnosed with endometritis are generally stable but less commonly can present in septic shock. In the OB triage or emergency setting, continual monitoring of vital signs is essential as healthy, young women frequently maintain their vital signs, only to quickly decompensate as the hemorrhage or infection continues.

SECONDARY POSTPARTUM HEMORRHAGE

SPPH is diagnosed following 0.5%–2% of deliveries in developed countries (Lu et al., 2005). There are no randomized controlled trials to guide the evaluation and treatment as in primary postpartum hemorrhage but guiding principles for managing hemorrhage remain the same.

PRESENTING SYMPTOMATOLOGY

The postpartum woman often presents with a sudden increase in bleeding, after having experienced a tapering of normal lochia. Pain may or may not be present. Fever and uterine tenderness may be present if an infection coexists.

HISTORY AND DATA COLLECTION

The initial history includes quantifying the amount of bleeding. Symptoms of clinically significant anemia, such as shortness of breath, lightheadedness, heart racing, or syncope are solicited. A determination of the specific cause of the hemorrhage may assist in the treatment plans. Therefore, a thorough history is taken to include prior OB procedures, fertility treatments, and other surgeries that have been associated with specific conditions such as an intrauterine aneurysm or placental abnormalities (Kovo, Behar, Friedman, & Mailinger, 2007). Any history of bleeding in the initial postpartum period is significant since two-thirds of women with SPPH will have experienced a primary hemorrhage. In these cases, the pace of the evaluation must be prioritized, as significant anemia may already preexist the second bleeding episode. Details about bleeding disorders are solicited as one-third of women who experience a SPPH have Von Willebrand's disease (Barbarinsa, Hayman, & Draycott, 2011). The delivery record is reviewed and the following are noted: length of rupture of membranes, length of labor, augmentation of labor, and any chorioamnionitis and blood counts on discharge. Also, note how the placenta was delivered and if any abnormalities were observed on inspection. The mode of delivery is another key piece of history, since retained products as a cause for the hemorrhage is less likely with cesarean birth.

PHYSICAL EXAMINATION

In OB triage, vital signs need to be noted immediately. It is also critical to remember that in a healthy woman, over 1 L of estimated blood loss can occur before there is a significant change in vital signs. Therefore, the vitals will need to be trended regularly and monitored for increasing tachycardia, hypotension, and decreasing oxygen saturation. A fever would suggest a coexisting infection. Skin color and capillary refill are helpful physical indicators of hemoglobin levels. Abdominal palpation of the postpartum uterus for tenderness and size is informative. An enlarged uterus may suggest that retained products of conception are a factor in the bleeding. A pelvic examination is performed to examine the vagina and cervix for lacerations. The presence of foul smelling lochia in the vagina and whether or not the woman is still actively bleeding are additional key findings to note on pelvic examination.

LABORATORY AND IMAGING STUDIES

Essential lab tests include a complete blood count, coagulation profile, type and screen, and/or cross match if indicated. A radiology ultrasound is indicated if the woman is clinically stable. If there is hemodynamic instability, a bedside ultrasound can be useful in quickly determining a cause for the SPPH. If the uterine cavity is distended and full of heterogeneous material, especially if flow is seen when the color Doppler function is applied, retained products of conception is the likely diagnosis. Figure 28.1 represents a sonographic image of retained products of conception, subsequently confirmed at the time of dilation and curettage.

Fluid and mixed echogenicity can be seen in a normal involuting uterus postpartum, depending on how much time has elapsed since delivery. The maximum thickness of the intrauterine contents is noted. Hematometra and clots will typically not demonstrate flow. If flow to the intrauterine contents is noted, it is more likely to represent retained products of conception (Multic-Lutvica & Axelsson, 2006). Additional pathologic findings that can be diagnosed by ultrasound include fibroids or intrauterine vascular malformations.

DIFFERENTIAL DIAGNOSIS

The primary differential in SPPH is menses and secondarily postpartum bleeding that is within normal range, but bothersome to the woman. Rarely,

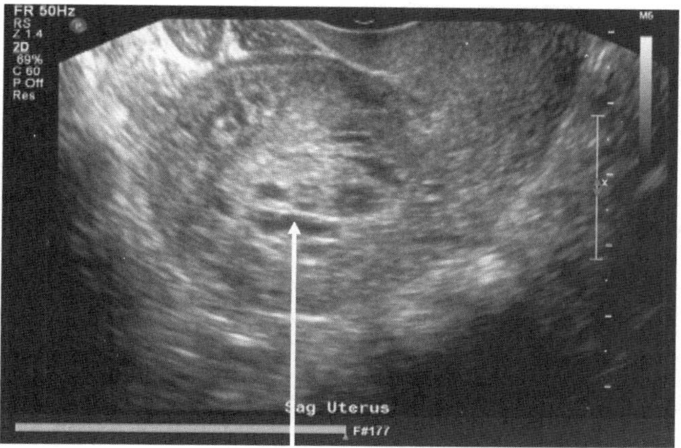

FIGURE 28.1 Retained products of conception.

Source: Courtesy of Department of Radiology, Women & Infants' Hospital, Providence, RI.

EXHIBIT 28.1

Causes of SPPH

- Idiopathic subinvolution of the uteroplacental vessels
- Retained placental tissue
- Endometritis
- Placenta accreta, increta, or percreta
- Von Willebrand's disease
- Fibroids
- Vascular malformation of the uterus including A-V malformations and uterine artery aneurysms

Source: Adapted from Barbarinsa et al. (2011).

cancers can present as late postpartum bleeding both with an acute bleed or persistent postpartum bleeding (Riggs, Zaghami, Najid, Haber, & Schreffler, 2010). If SPPH is diagnosed, the determination of the cause of the hemorrhage will assist in formulating an appropriate treatment plan. Exhibit 28.1 lists the causes of SPPH, appearing in order of decreasing incidence (Barbarinsa et al., 2011).

CLINICAL MANAGEMENT AND FOLLOW-UP

Clinical management is driven by the initial assessment. If vital signs are abnormal and there is active bleeding, stabilization is the primary goal. Clinical management is initially similar to primary postpartum hemorrhage. Intravenous access with two large bore lines and crystalloid fluid boluses will be the first step. Anesthesia assistance may be necessary to secure intravenous lines and the airway. Blood transfusions, intravenous antibiotics, and medical versus surgical treatment are the next decision points. A stat bedside ultrasound will reveal information to drive the next steps. Review of the literature indicates that there is no single management protocol that is proven to have better outcomes than any other (Alexander, Thomas, & Sanghera, 2002). Figure 28.2 outlines one management protocol based on evidence in the literature, but it remains unproven.

Surgical procedures performed for a woman who is experiencing significant postpartum hemorrhage carry increased risks. The woman must be made aware of these risks at the time of consent. If the uterus is atonic or infected, then the risk of uterine perforation and the time of dilatation and curettage are increased significantly. Disseminated intravascular coagulation (DIC) may result from an episode of massive hemorrhage or severely infected retained produces of infection. If DIC occurs, surgical attempts may be unsuccessful and a hysterectomy will need to be performed. Hysterectomy also will be indicated if a placenta accreta or percreta is diagnosed at the time of curettage.

Ninety percent of the time, the woman's condition will not be critical and there is time for more options to be considered. In a 2001 study of 132 women with SPPH, 75 (57%) women were initially treated with surgery, which was successful 90% of the time. Of the 57 women initially managed medically, treatment was successful in 41 (72%) women, but 12 of 16 women with continued symptoms ultimately required surgery. In the cases that submitted tissue for pathology, retained products of conception were documented in one-third of the women (Hoyveda & MacKenzie, 2001). So, if retained products are not identified on ultrasound, the literature indicates that surgery may still be helpful. If bleeding continues or if an arteriovenous malformation or pseudoaneurysm is considered, then embolization by interventional radiology may be indicated. Placement of a balloon tamponade may also be considered, as either a temporizing measure, or until interventional radiology can be summoned for definitive treatment of hemorrhage.

Medical management consists of intravenous antibiotics and uterotonic medications. Again, no specific uterotonic agent has proven more beneficial than any other. In the clinically stable patient without ultrasound findings of retained placental tissue, medical management may avoid the risks inherent to surgery. The Cochrane review on treatments for SSPH points out the need for a well-designed randomized controlled trial to compare the various therapies (Alexander et al., 2002).

POSTPARTUM ENDOMETRITIS

Postpartum endometritis refers to infection of the decidua or myometrium and parametrial tissues after the first 24 hours postpartum. Endometritis is most commonly a polymicrobial infection involving both aerobes and anaerobes from the female genital tract. Rare, but lethal causes of endometritis include group A *Streptococcus and Clostridium* leading to toxic shock-like syndrome. Group A *Streptococcus* typically presents with endometritis early in the postpartum period with high fever (Jorup-Ronstrom, Hofling, Lunberg, & Holm, 1996). Postpartum endometritis infections caused by *Clostridium sordellii* are likely to present during the first postpartum week, and are notable for rapid decompensation, leading to septic shock (Bitti et al., 1997).

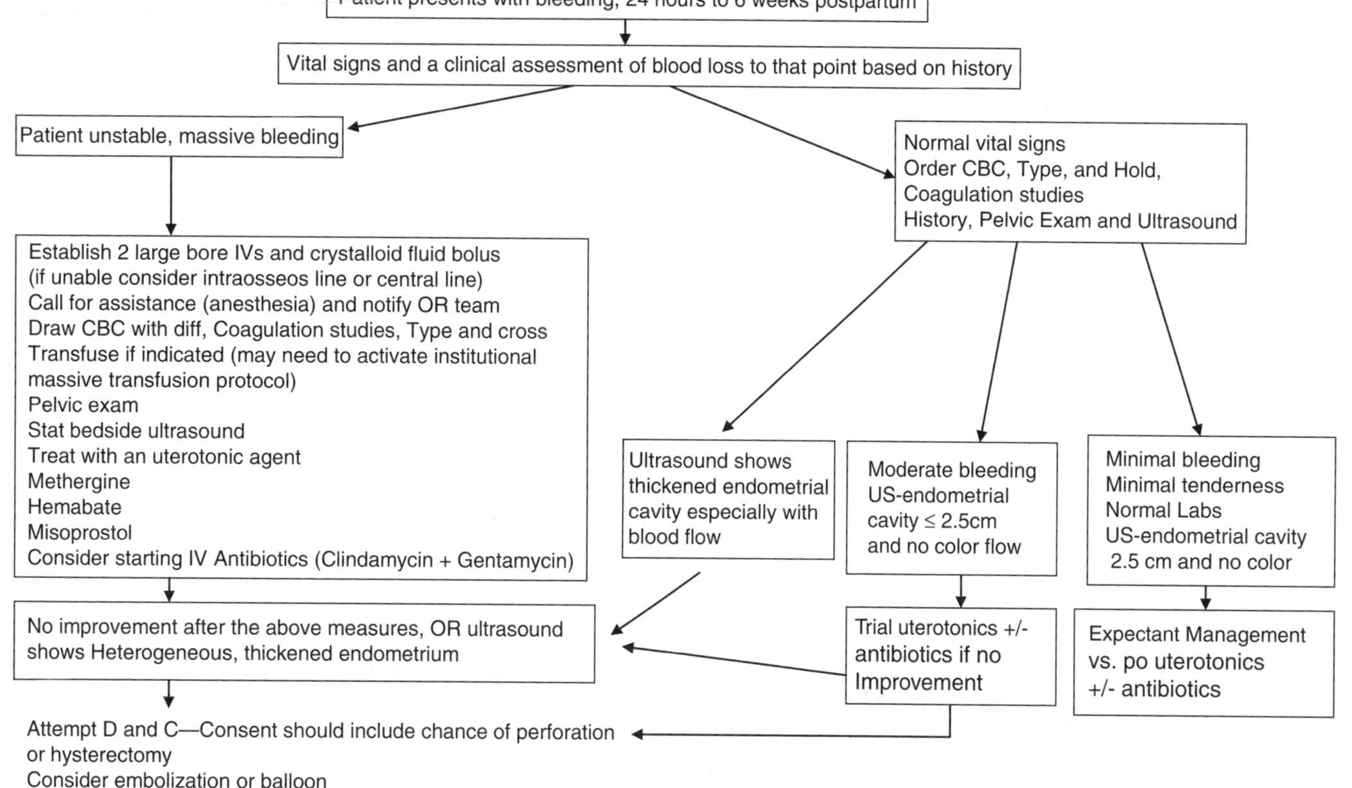

FIGURE 28.2 Management plan for SPPH.

PRESENTING SYMPTOMATOLOGY

The most common presenting symptom in cases of postpartum endometritis is fever, typically 38°C to 39°C. Abdominal pain is another common presenting symptom. The postpartum woman may also note a foul odor to the lochia or an increase in vaginal bleeding. The diagnosis is a clinical one and is based on the combination of abdominal pain and fever in the absence of other causes of pathology. To make a correct diagnosis of postpartum endometritis, the following conditions must be excluded: urinary tract infection, mastitis, wound infection, pulmonary embolism, viral illness, appendicitis, or other obvious infectious etiologies. Endometritis must be high in the differential of the postpartum patient who presents in septic shock.

HISTORY AND DATA COLLECTION

The mode of delivery is a key piece of information, since the single most important risk factor for endometritis is route of delivery (Burrows, Meyn, & Weber, 2004). The risk for endometritis following a surgical delivery is much higher than that of a vaginal delivery. Other risk factors are solicited during the history and these include prolonged labor, prolonged rupture of membranes, multiple cervical exams, internal monitoring, and manual removal of the placenta.

An abdominal examination may elicit pain from the uterus and parametria. A bimanual examination may elicit increased tenderness, if the abdominal examination is equivocal. Speculum examination may demonstrate foul smelling lochia, but this finding is neither sensitive nor specific (Lasley, Eblen, Yancey, & Duff, 1997).

LABORATORY AND IMAGING STUDIES

The diagnosis of postpartum endometritis is a clinical one. An elevated white blood count will support the diagnosis of infection. Blood cultures are typically negative and should not be obtained unless the patient appears septic. An ultrasound may identify if coexisting retained products of conception are present, for these must be evacuated to ensure successful antibiotic treatment. Endocervical and vaginal cultures are not recommended in the routine postpartum woman with fever and pain, since it is difficult to obtain a specimen uncontaminated by cervical or vaginal flora. If microbiology of the organism is necessary, consider an endometrial biopsy under sterile conditions. The specimen is submitted to microbiology in normal saline for gram stain, culture, and sensitivity. Results will be available later in the hospital course and can focus the choice of antibiotics.

TREATMENT

For moderate to severe infections, intravenous therapy with broad spectrum antibiotics is indicated. A commonly used regimen, with a reported 90% to 97% success rate, is clindamycin plus gentamicin. A meta-analysis comparing clindamycin plus an aminoglycoside with other regimens found that the treatment failure was higher with all other regimens. Daily dosing of gentamicin is as efficacious and safe as every 8-hour dosing of gentamicin (Livingston et al., 2003). Improvement is generally seen in 48 hours.

TABLE 28.1 Antibiotic Regimens for Postpartum Endometritis

PARENTERAL DRUG REGIMENS	DOSES	SAFETY IN BREAST-FEEDING (AMERICAN ACADEMY OF PEDIATRICS)
Gentamicin *plus*	4–7 mg/kg/d	Yes
Clindamycin *may add*	900 mg q 8 hr	Yes
Ampicillin	2 g q 6 hr	Yes
Ampicillin-sulbactam	3 g q 6 hrs	Yes
Ceftriaxone	2 g q 12 hr	Yes
Levofloxacin *plus*	500 mg q 24 hr	Unknown
Metronidazole	500 mg IV or po q 8 hr	Yes
Ticarcillin-clavulanate	3.1 mg q 6 hr	Yes

Source: Adapted from Cunningham et al. (2010) and AAP (2001).

Persistent fever or incomplete resolution of tenderness on examination, dictates the need for further radiologic imaging studies to assess for the presence of an abscess, infected hematoma, and septic pelvic thrombophlebitis. If an inadequate response is seen to clindamycin and gentamicin, then antibiotic coverage should be broadened with the addition of ampicillin or vancomycin in the penicillin allergic woman. Antibiotics are continued until the woman is afebrile for 24 to 48 hours. At that time, antibiotics can be discontinued. In the case of bacteremia, oral antibiotics should be administered for a total of 14 days and the choice of outpatient antibiotics is guided by sensitivity results. In cases when retained products of conception are identified as the nidus for infection, it is recommended to administer one dose of clindamycin and gentamicin before proceeding to dilation and curettage. Antibiotic regimens, the recommended doses and potential effects on breast-feeding, are noted in Table 28.1.

REFERENCES

Alexander, J., Thomas, P. W., & Sanghera, J. (2002). Inervention review: Treatments for secondary postpartum haemorrhage . *Cochrane Database of Systematic Reviews, (1)*, CD002867.

American Academy of Pediatrics (AAP) (2001). The transfer of drugs and other chemicals into human milk. *Pediatrics, 108*, 776–789.

Barbarinsa, I. A., Hayman, R. G., & Draycott, T. J. (2011). Secondary post-partum haemorrhage: Challenges in evidence- based causes and management. *European Journal of Obstetrics & Gynecology and Reproductive Biology, 159(203)*, 255–260.

Bitti, A., Mastroantonio, P., Spigaglia, P., Urru, G., Spano, A. I., Moretti, G., & Cherchi, G. B. (1997). A fatal postpartum *Clostridium sordelli* associated toxic shock syndrome. *Journal of Clinical Pathology, 50(3)*, 259–260.

Burrows, L. J., Meyn, L. A., & Weber, A. M. (2004). Maternal morbidity associated with vaginal versus cesarean delivery. *Obstetrics and Gynecology, 103*, 907–912.

Cunningham, F. G., Leveno, K. J., Bloom, S. L., Hauth, J. C., Rouse, D. D. J., & Spong, C. Y. (2010). *Williams obstetrics* (pp. 661–664). New York: McGraw Hill.

Hoyveda, F., & MacKenzie, I. Z. (2001). Secondary postpartum hemorrhage: Incidence, morbidity, and current management. *British Journal of Obstetrics and Gyneacology, 108*, 927–930.

Jorup-Ronstrom, C., Hofling, M., Lunberg, C., & Holm, S. (1996). Streptococcal toxic shock syndrome in a postpartum woman: Case report and review of the literature. *Infection*, 24,164–167.

Lasley, D. S., Eblen, A., Yancey, M. K., & Duff, P. (1997). The effect of manual removal of the placenta on postcesarean endometritis. *American Journal of Obstetrics and Gynecology, 176*, 1250–1254.

Livingston, J. C., Llata, E., Rinehart, E., Leidwanger, C., Mabie, B., Haddad, B., & Sibai, B. (2003). Gentamicin and clindamycin therapy in postpartum endometritis: The efficacy of daily dosing versus dosing every 8 hours. *American Journal of Obstetrics and Gynecology, 188*(1), 149–152.

Kovo, M., Behar, D. J., Friedman, V., & Mailinger, G. (2007). Pelvic arterial pseudoaneursym—A rare complication of cesarean section: Diagnosis and novel treatment. *Ultrasound in Obstetrics and Gynecology, 30*(5), 783–785.

Lu, M. C., Fridman, M., Korst, L. M., Gregory, K. D., Reyes, C., Hobel, C. J., & Chavez, G. F. (2005). Variations in the incidence of postpartum hemorrhage across hospitals in California. *Maternal and Child Health Journal, 9*(3), 297–306.

Multic-Lutvica, A., & Axelsson, P.(2006). Ultrasound finding of an echogenic mass in woman with secondary postpartum hemorrhage is associated with retained placental tissue. *Ultrasound in Obstetrics and Gynecology, 28*(3), 312–319.

Neil, A., & Thorton, S. (2002). Secondary postpartum haemorrhage. *British Journal of Obstetrics and Gynecology, 22*(2), 119–122.

Riggs, J. C., Zaghami, F., Najid, K., Haber, K., & Schreffler, S. M. (2010). Postpartum hemorrhage from ruptured Sertoli-Leydig cell tumor: A case report. *Journal of Reproductive Medicine, 55*(9–10), 433–436.

29

Psychiatric Complications in the Postpartum Period

Margaret Howard and Rebecca Christophersen

Women are most likely to develop a mood disorder during the childbearing years and the postpartum period, which represents a particularly high-risk time for new-onset of psychiatric illness as well as exacerbation or recurrence of preexisting psychiatric conditions (Munk-Olsen, Laursen, Pedersen, Mors, & Mortensen, 2006). Because of the frequency and regularity of obstetric (OB) visits during pregnancy and the impact of the delivery experience, most women seek consultation from their OB providers even when experiencing psychiatric symptoms. For women with no prior psychiatric history, mood disorder symptoms can be experienced as both unfamiliar and distressing. A clear description may be challenging in that women will often misattribute psychiatric symptoms to the labor and delivery experience, or simply, new motherhood.

Since psychiatric symptoms can emerge with relative suddenness in the postpartum period, it is not uncommon for these women to present to OB triage or emergency settings. However, due to multiple societal messages that motherhood is synonymous with fulfillment and joy, many women feel a sense of shame and guilt and may be reluctant to disclose their mood symptoms. For this reason, it is imperative that key personnel in the triage setting be familiar with psychiatric symptoms most likely to emerge during peripartum and be equipped to evaluate, call for more thorough psychiatric consultation, and/or administer immediate treatment with necessary follow-up. When severe postpartum psychiatric symptoms go unrecognized and untreated, the consequences for both mother and infant can be dire. OB providers, as primary medical caregivers for perinatal women, are uniquely positioned to intervene when psychiatric complications are detected. Like all medical conditions, early detection and intervention can vastly improve outcomes for both mothers and infants.

POSTPARTUM DEPRESSION

Postpartum Depression (PPD) is the most frequently occurring postpartum psychiatric complication. It is estimated that up to 19.2% of women will experience either a major or minor depression in the 3 months following childbirth (Gavin et al., 2005). According to the "*Diagnostic and statistical manual of mental disorders, Fourth edition*" (DSM IV, American Psychiatric Association, 2000), PPD is formally classified as a major depression, either recurrent or single episode with a range from mild to severe and the specifier "postpartum onset" is used when symptoms follow childbirth. When unrecognized and untreated, PPD causes profound suffering for the mother and, although rare, can result in suicide. PPD can compromise mother-infant interactions and care practices and the long-term deleterious impact of untreated maternal depression on infant/child development is well-documented (Field, 2010). PPD occurs in women of all socioeconomic, cultural, ethnic, and age groups. Risk factors that render a woman more vulnerable to PPD include prior history of postpartum or other lifetime depression, depression or anxiety disorder that emerges during pregnancy, adolescence, poverty, recent immigrant status, conflict with primary partner, and poor social support (Pearlstein, Howard, Salisbury, & Zlotnick, 2009).

PRESENTING SYMPTOMOTOLOGY

The diagnosis of PPD is challenging due to inherent changes in sleep, appetite, and energy during the early postpartum weeks. Similarly, fatigue, emotionality, irritability, and worry over the infant's well-being are common postpartum and typically referred to as the "baby" or "postpartum blues." While not a true disorder, postpartum blues responds well to support, reassurance, and adequate sleep and resolves by week 3 postpartum.

PPD, on the other hand, is a serious disabling condition and is characterized by sad, depressed mood and loss of interest or pleasure persistent for at least 2 weeks. Additional symptoms include sleep disturbance most typically insomnia (e.g., unable to sleep when the infant sleeps), lack of energy, feelings of worthlessness or guilt, often with the belief of being a "bad mother," difficulty thinking, concentrating, making decisions, and thoughts of suicide or "everyone would be better off without me." Other hallmark symptoms of PPD include anxiety, lack of attachment to the infant and intrusive, and unwanted thoughts of harm befalling the infant. Research substantiates clinical observation that there is no correlation between the presence of intrusive harming infant thoughts and acting on them (Barr & Beck, 2008). Rather, these thoughts are experienced as highly distressing to the mother, can result in avoidance of the infant and signal the severity of the depression.

SUICIDE

Suicide rates are lower during pregnancy and the postpartum period and perinatal women who complete suicide do so by more violent and lethal means than nonperinatal women (Lindahl, Pearson, & Colpe, 2005). Risk factors for suicide include comorbid psychiatric and substance abuse disorders and having a stillbirth or infant death within the first postpartum year. It is recommended that when assessing suicidality in the pregnant or postpartum woman, specific inquiry must be made about suicide risk factors such as prior suicide attempts, previous trauma, current domestic violence, substance abuse, and access to firearms.

HISTORY AND DATA COLLECTION

In the triage setting, a brief, easily administered and scored self-report screening measure is an optimal first step in detecting depression. The most widely used and well-studied depression screening tool for perinatal women is the 10-item Edinburgh Postnatal Depression Scale (EPDS; Cox, Holden, & Sagovsky, 1987), which has demonstrated validity, sensitivity, and specificity in screening for the presence of PPD. Scores equal to or above a 13 are generally indicative of depression (see Exhibit 29.1).

The nine-item Patient Health Questionnaire-9 (PHQ-9; Kroenke, Spitzer, & Williams, 2001) is a more general depression screen commonly used in adult primary care settings and may be more familiar to primary care providers. The PHQ-2 (Kroenke, Spitzer, & Williams, 2003) consists of just the first two

EXHIBIT 29.1

Edinburgh Postnatal Depression Scale (EPDS)

Name: ______________________ Address: ______________________

Your Date of Birth: ______________________ ______________________

Baby's Age: ______________________ Phone: ______________________

As you have recently had a baby, we would like to know how you feeling. Please check the answer that comes closest to how you have felt IN THE PAST 7 DAYS, not just how you feel today.

Here is an example, already completed.

I have felt happy:
- ☐ Yes, all the time
- ☒ Yes, most of the time
- ☐ No, not very often
- ☐ No, not at all

This would mean: "I have felt happy most of the time" during the past week. Please complete the other questions in the same way.

In the past 7 days:

1 I have been able to laugh and see the funny side of things
- ☐ As much as I always could
- ☐ Not quite so much now
- ☐ Definitely not so much now
- ☐ Not at all

2 I have looked forward with enjoyment to things
- ☐ As much as I ever did
- ☐ Rather less than I used to
- ☐ Definitely less than I used to
- ☐ Hardly at all

*3 I have blamed myself unnecessarily when things went wrong
- ☐ Yes, most of the time
- ☐ Yes, some of the time
- ☐ Not very often
- ☐ No, never

4 I have been anxious or worried for no good reason
- ☐ No, not at all
- ☐ Hardly ever
- ☐ Yes, sometimes
- ☐ Yes, very often

5 I have felt scared or panicky for no very good reason
- ☐ Yes, quite a lot
- ☐ Yes, sometimes
- ☐ No, not much
- ☐ No, not at all

*6 Things have been getting on top of me
- ☐ Yes, most of the time I haven't been able to cope at all
- ☐ Yes, sometimes I haven't been coping as well as usual
- ☐ No, most of the time I have copied quite well
- ☐ No, I have been coping as well as ever

*7 I have been so unhappy that I have difficulty sleeping
- ☐ Yes, most of the time
- ☐ Yes, sometimes
- ☐ Not very often
- ☐ No, not at all

*8 I have felt sad or miserable
- ☐ Yes, most of the time
- ☐ Yes, quite often
- ☐ Not very often
- ☐ No, not at all

*9 I have been so unhappy that I have been crying
- ☐ Yes, most of the time
- ☐ Yes, quite often
- ☐ Only occasionally
- ☐ No, never

*10 The thought of harming myself has occurred to me
- ☐ Yes, quite often
- ☐ Sometimes
- ☐ Hardly ever
- ☐ Never

Administered/Reviewed by ______________________ Date ______________________

Source: Reprinted, with permission, from Cox JL, Holden JM, Sagovsky R. 1987. Detection of postnatal depression: Development of the 10-item Edinburgh Postnatal Depression Scale. British Journal of Psychiatry 150:782-786. WWW.brightfutures.org

EXHIBIT 29.2

PHQ-2

Over the last two weeks, how often have you been bothered by any of the following problems:

1. During the past month, have you often been bothered by feeling down, depressed, or hopeless? Yes No
2. During the past month, have you often been bothered by little interest or pleasure in doing things? Yes No

If the response is "yes" to either question, consider administering the PHQ-9, the EPDS, or asking more questions about possible depression.

If the response to both questions is "no," the screen is negative.

Source: Kroenke et al. (2003).

questions of the PHQ-9 and may be particularly appealing in a busy OB triage setting (see Exhibit 29.2).

The EPDS, PHQ-9, and PHQ-2 perform similarly in screening for depression in postpartum women (Gjerdingen, Crow, McGovern, Miner, & Center, 2009; Flynn, Sexton, Ratliff, Porter, & Zivin, 2011). Positive screens can be followed by careful additional inquiry about mood state, sleep, appetite, concentration, anxiety, intrusive negative thoughts, hedonic capacity, degree of attachment to infant, and presence of suicidal thoughts. History of prior episodes of depression, anxiety or other mood disorders, substance use, and interpersonal or environmental stress must also be obtained. Symptom onset, intensity, and duration are critical as well as information regarding the woman's degree of functional impairment and whether or not adequate social support is present.

OTHER POSTPARTUM PSYCHIATRIC CONDITIONS

PPD is a term that is universally recognizable among OB providers yet other postpartum psychiatric conditions exist that, while not as common as depression, are equally debilitating and just as likely to be encountered in the triage setting. These include postpartum psychosis, and postpartum anxiety disorders, and their subtypes.

POSTPARTUM PSYCHOSIS

Postpartum psychosis, although not part of the formal psychiatric diagnostic nomenclature, is a widely used term to describe a severe, and relatively uncommon psychiatric condition that occurs in one to two per 1,000 live births (Munk-Olsen et al., 2006). It requires immediate attention, likely inpatient psychiatric hospitalization and has a rapid onset, with symptoms evident in the first 2 to 4 weeks after delivery. Women with postpartum psychosis may present to the OB triage unit exhibiting confusion, disordered thinking, mood lability, and delusions. Disorganized, bizarre behavior may be witnessed as well as flat or inappropriate affect.

Women with psychotic symptoms are frequently accompanied by family members who may additionally report paranoia, suspiciousness, grandiosity, and evidence of auditory or visual hallucinations. There are likely to be reports of poor judgment and impaired functioning. Sleeplessness and other hypomanic symptoms such as agitation and irritability are common prodromal states, emerging within 72 hours of childbirth. Unrecognized postpartum psychosis can have serious consequences including infanticide, suicide, and infant abuse/neglect. Women with postpartum psychosis may have command auditory hallucinations telling them to kill the infant or delusional beliefs that the infant or themselves are, for instance, possessed by demons and only be saved through death. Risk factors include a previous episode of postpartum psychosis, previous hospitalization for a manic or psychotic episode, current or past bipolar disorder diagnosis, family history of bipolar disorder, primiparity, and recent discontinuation of mood stabilizers (Doucet, Jones, Letourneau, Dennis, & Blackmore, 2011).

POSTPARTUM ANXIETY DISORDERS

Worry is common in new mothers and is often regarded as an adaptive and protective response in the early postpartum period. When anxious worrying becomes excessive, occurs in multiple settings/situations, does not respond to reassurance, inhibits normal functioning, or interferes with self-care or care of the infant, it has moved along the continuum from "normal" to "disordered." Subtypes of anxiety disorders include generalized anxiety disorder (GAD), obsessive compulsive disorder (OCD), and panic disorder and posttraumatic stress disorder (PTSD). Because anxiety disorders and major depression are highly comorbid in the postpartum period, it is essential to screen for both (Austin et al., 2010).

Panic Disorder

Panic disorder is characterized by unpredictable, discrete, episodes of intense anxiety and includes symptoms of fear, heart palpitations, shortness of breath, chest pain, dizziness, numbness or tingling, nausea, sweating, choking, fear of dying, or losing control. Postpartum women who experience an episode or more of panic will frequently present to the emergency room believing they are having a heart attack or other catastrophic medical crisis. There has been some evidence that weaning may precipitate or exacerbate panic symptoms (Ross & McLean, 2006).

Posttraumatic Stress Disorder

PTSD develops in response to a traumatic event, which is either witnessed or experienced and involves actual or threatened death, serious injury, or threat to physical integrity. The response to the traumatic event includes intense fear, helplessness, or horror. Women who have undergone traumatic deliveries and/or women with histories of prior trauma are susceptible to PTSD during the postpartum period. Symptoms include hypervigilence, fear, irritability, poor concentration, sleeplessness, heightened anxiety, intrusive recollections of the traumatic event, flashbacks or "re-living" of the experience, and psychological and physiological reactivity when exposed to stimuli associated with the traumatic event. Additional symptoms include emotional numbing, avoidance of stimuli reminiscent of the event or evocative of the feelings, or thoughts associated with the traumatic event. Women who have been victims of childhood or adult sexual assault may become "triggered" and experience PTSD symptoms during childbirth procedures, examinations, and delivery.

OBSESSIVE COMPULSIVE DISORDER

Intrusive, distressing, and short-lived thoughts of inflicting harm to the infant (e.g., dropping, smothering) are universal among new mothers (Fairbrother & Woody, 2008). OCD, however, is an extreme form of this and interferes with a woman's ability to care for herself and/or the infant. OCD is characterized by intrusive, unwanted images, thoughts or impulses either with or without accompanying compulsions. The most common obsessions experienced by postpartum women include contamination, intentionally or accidentally harming infant, need for order/symmetry, and catastrophic images. Compulsions are goal-directed, driven, and repetitive or ritualized behaviors whose engagement in, results in temporary reduction of anxiety associated with the obsessive thoughts or beliefs. Compulsions include cleaning, checking (often resulting in sleep deprivation due to incessant checking on infant), washing, praying, counting, repeating certain phrases, or other ritualized behaviors. The postpartum period represents a time of increased vulnerability to onset of OCD and a time of symptom exacerbation in women with preexisting OCD (Zambaldi et al., 2009).

PHYSICAL EXAMINATION

Typically, mental illnesses are not conceptualized as resulting in abnormal physical findings as one would expect in detecting illnesses such as high blood pressure or gestational diabetes mellitus. Aspects of brain dysfunction and its effect on the body as a whole continue to be a mystery despite decades of advancing research, especially for the postpartum period. However, symptoms of PPD, anxiety, and psychosis can result in physical abnormalities. Table 29.1 differentiates physical findings for depression, anxiety, and psychosis. It is important to conceptualize these disorders as interrelated resulting in symptom overlap.

DIFFERENTIAL DIAGNOSIS

Postpartum women will likely present to an emergency room or OB triage setting if they experience mental status changes. A family member or friend may be the first to notice or first to bring attention to these changes, as women may contribute these changes to expected postpartum experiences, have limited insight to describe the symptoms or may be too ashamed to verbalize what she is experiencing. There are multiple medical conditions that can either be mistaken for or result in psychiatric symptoms, therefore, ruling out differential diagnoses is imperative.

Depressive symptoms can result from anemia, vitamin deficiencies, alcohol abuse, gestational diabetes, and thyroid dysfunction. Hypertension, anemia, and thyroid dysfunction may result in symptoms of anxiety and

TABLE 29.1 Postpartum Physical Exam Findings

	BEHAVIORAL	AFFECTIVE	PHYSIOLOGICAL	SYMPATHETIC	PARASYMPATHETIC	COGNITIVE
Depression	Decreased energy Anhedonia Poor grooming Tearfulness	Flat Overwhelmed Irritability Hopelessness Uncertainty	Psychomotor retardation Change in appetite	Anorexia Weakness	Constipation Decreased blood pressure Decreased pulse	Guilt Worthlessness Thought blocking Decreased insight Poor judgment Thoughts of death
Anxiety	Fidgeting Glancing about Restlessness Repetitive actions Avoidance	Apprehensive Distressed Fearful Overexcited Worried	Facial tension Perspiration Muscle tension Shakiness Trembling	Cardiovascular excitation Diarrhea Dry mouth Facial flushing Increased reflexes Increased respiration Shortness of breath Vasoconstriction	Abdominal pain Faintness Nausea Tingling in extremities Urinary frequency, hesitancy, or urgency	Preoccupation Rumination Heightened awareness Intrusive thoughts Ego-dystonic thoughts of harming infant
Psychosis	Disorganized speech Mood swings Agitation Sleeplessness	Guarded Blank Bizarre	Hypomania			Delusions Hallucinations Paranoia Ego-dsyntonic thoughts of harming infant

Source: Adapted from Ackley & Ladwig (2011); Beck & Driscoll (2006).

panic. Use of illicit substances, thyroid disease, autoimmune disease, HIV, Sheehan's syndrome, tumors, and eclampsia must be ruled out given their association with mental status changes congruent with psychosis (Ebeid, Nassif, & Sinha, 2010).

LABORATORY FINDINGS

Evaluation of specific laboratory studies can assist in uncovering contributing factors of the etiology of symptom presentation. Thus, the recommended laboratory studies in Table 29.2 will provide evidence of possible differential diagnoses.

CLINICAL MANAGEMENT

Once diagnosis has been determined, the next step is to consider treatment options. Due to the fast pace and limited time to provide treatment to woman suffering from mental health symptoms in OB triage settings, pharmacotherapy is preferably the first-line treatment recommendation. Initiation of psychotropic medication, even at lower starting doses can be crucial in managing and preventing further exacerbation of symptoms. Alternative treatment options such as support groups and psychotherapy will require referral to a mental health provider. Psychiatric partial (or day) hospitalization in a specialized mother-baby unit is an optimal and effective form of treatment for postpartum women with severe symptoms. One such model is the Women & Infants Hospital PPD Day hospital in Providence, Rhode Island and consists of

TABLE 29.2 Postpartum Laboratory Tests

Thyroid function tests: TSH & Free thyroxine	• Hyperthyroidism, most common cause during pregnancy being Graves' disease, is associated with dysphoria, anxiety, restlessness, mania, depression, and impaired concentration. More severe symptoms include psychosis, delirium, and hallucinations • Hypothyroidism, most common cause for women of reproductive age being Hashimoto thyroiditis, is associated with psychomotor slowing, poor sleep, appetite changes, apathy, and poor concentration
Vitamin B12	• Deficiency associated with symptoms of depression, mood lability, and psychosis
Complete blood count	• Anemia is associated with depression, reduced cognitive function, fatigue, and emotional lability
Folate	• Utilized by the brain to synthesize of norepinephrine, serotonin, and dopamine • Deficiency can be associated with symptoms of depression
Electrolytes	• Imbalances resulting from inadequate nutritional intake • Imbalances may cause delirium
Vitamin D	• Deficiency associated with depressive symptoms
Drug toxicology	• Substances may induce symptoms of depression, anxiety, and psychosis

Source: Basraon & Costantine (2011) and Fischbach & Dunning (2008).

intensive 2 to 3 week daily (up to 6 hr/d) multidisciplinary/multimodal psychiatric intervention in a setting, which allows mother and infant to remain together for the duration of treatment (Howard, Battle, Pearlstein, & Rosene-Montella, 2006).

When initiating treatment in the postpartum period, it is necessary to weigh the difference of the risk of treatment versus the risk of untreated symptoms. The symptoms of depression, anxiety, and psychosis have been outlined earlier in this chapter and are critical to consider when presenting treatment options to women. Women typically have heard about medication risks to them and/or their breastfeeding infant, but unfortunately the source of their information is unlikely to be systematic and evidenced based. As OB providers, this is a unique opportunity to adequately inform women of the risks and benefits of treatment versus no treatment or undertreatment.

Although data are limited, evidenced-based research continues to gain momentum providing a broader base of knowledge and understanding of the risks and benefits of psychotropic treatment in the peripartum period. The following paragraphs discuss the most commonly chosen psychotropic medications for postpartum women.

Antidepressants

The first-line treatment for depression and anxiety symptoms currently are selective serotonin reuptake inhibitors (SSRIs) for their effectiveness and low side effect profile for women. If a woman has been on SSRIs during pregnancy, there are risks of neonatal side effects. These may include jitteriness, mild respiratory distress, decreased muscle tone, and irritability (Hale, 2004). Sertraline (Zoloft) and fluoxetine (Prozac) are the most well-studied SSRIs. Sertraline has not been associated with adverse infant response and has a relatively low amount that is actually transferred through breast milk (Hale, 2004). Fluoxetine, however, has a longer half-life and has been associated with adverse infant response including fussiness, drowsiness, and decreased weight gain. Of the two, sertraline is usually favored for breastfeeding mothers. Citalopram (Celexa) and escitalopram (Lexapro) have shown the highest percentage in breast milk. Table 29.3 summarizes relative infant dose (RID) of SSRI and other antidepressants used in the postpartum period.

TABLE 29.3 Maternal Transfer to Breast Milk

ANTIDEPRESSANT	AVERAGE RID (%)
Sertraline	2.2
Fluoxetine	6.8
Citalopram/escitalopram	3.6
Paroxetine	2.1
Bupropion	0.7
Venlafaxine	6.4
Mirtazapine	1.9
Trazodone	0.7

Source: Hale (2004).

Benzodiazepines

When initiating treatment, benzodiazepines are effective in acute treatment of anxiety disorders. The relative risk for breastfeeding infants is low; however, caution should be taken to watch for sedation and withdrawal effects in infants (Hale, 2004).

Hypnotics

There is no available systematic data regarding sleep aids. However, since insomnia is a significant precursor to worsening depression, anxiety, and psychosis, the risk of unknown data may be warranted when weighing against symptomatology.

Mood Stabilizers

Mood instability can occur postpartum. In fact, the postpartum period may be the first hypomanic/manic episode for women and is closely linked to the risk of psychosis. There may be several depressive episodes prior to a bipolar spectrum disorder emerging. Lithium requires systematic monitoring and transfers to breast milk at high percentages (Hale, 2004). Lamotrigine (Lamictal) is an effective mood stabilizer as well, but also has a high transfer through breast milk. It may be difficult to distinguish between benign infant rashes and severe life-threatening lamotrigine rash. With this being said, neither lithium nor lamotrigine are completely contraindicated during breastfeeding, therefore, close monitoring of the infant is prudent.

Antipsychotics

The second-generation antipsychotics (SGAs) are not only a preferred choice for psychotic symptoms, but there is clinical evidence to support that SGAs are useful as alternative options for treatment of anxiety and insomnia. Little data exist on antipsychotics during breastfeeding. The main symptom to watch for is sedation in both mother and infant (Hale, 2004). Due to the risk of sedation, starting at unconventionally low doses may assist in compliance and adherence.

Considerations for Psychotropic Use

Questions to consider when prescribing include the following: Will mom be breastfeeding? Will mom be too sedated from medication choice to tend to baby or parent? Will mom be more troubled by risk of weight gain, coupled with exiting pregnancy weight? Will sexual side effects be more problematic since postpartum women already have a low sexual drive?

When assessing the risks and benefits of medication choice, choosing a treatment that has been effective in the past may outweigh the risks of trying a new, better-studied medication. Remitting symptoms in the postpartum period is time sensitive in order not to prevent decline of a women's ability to care for self and infant.

Finally, noting the limitations of the Food and Drug Administration (FDA) pregnancy risk categories is imperative. No psychotropic medications

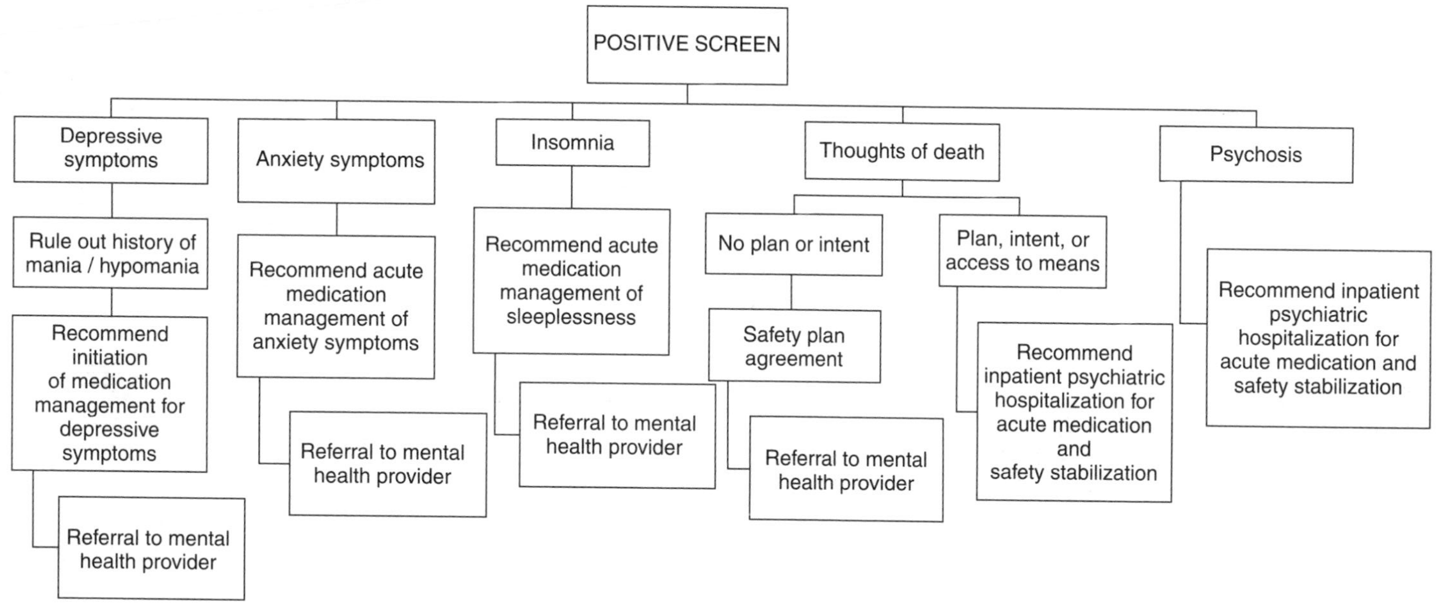

FIGURE 29.1 Guide for management of postpartum mood symptoms

are yet FDA approved for use during pregnancy. Psychotropic medications all cross the placenta so are never "no risk." Adverse medication effects do not generalize from one species to another and drugs can get "demoted" the more they are studied in humans. The most reliable data are systematic, prospective, controlled studies.

FOLLOW-UP

The most ideal approach to treatment and follow-up with postpartum women is multidisciplinary utilizing physicians, nurses, social workers, and community resources within medicine and psychiatry. Unfortunately, this approach may not be available in all settings. The algorithm in Figure 29.1 assists as a guide for decision making.

Postpartum mood changes significantly impact not only mother but children and family as well. Early detection and treatment initiation by providers that come in contact with postpartum women will reduce the detrimental effects of symptoms promoting healthier mothers, infants, and families.

REFERENCES

Ackley, B. J., & Ladwig, G. B. (2011). *Nursing diagnosis handbook: An evidenced-based guide to planning care* (9th ed.) St. Louis, MO: Mosby Elsevier.

American Psychiatric Association. (2000). *Diagnostic and statistical manual of mental disorders, fourth edition, text revision*. Washington DC: American Psychiatric Association.

Austin, M-P. V., Hadzi-Pavlovic, D., Priest, S. R., Reilly, N., Wilhelm, K., Saint, K., Parker, G. (2010). Depressive and anxiety disorders in the postpartum period: How prevalent are they and can we improve their detection? *Archives of Women's Mental Health, 13*(5), 395–401.

Barr, J. A, & Beck, C. T. (2008). Infanticide secrets: Qualitative study on postpartum depression. *Canadian Family Physician, 54*(12), 1716–1717.e-5.

Basraon, S., & Constantine, M. M. (2011). Mood disorders in pregnant women with thyroid dysfunction. *Clinical Obstetrics and Gynecology, 54*(3), 506–514.

Beck, C.T. & Driscoll, J.W. (2006). *Postpartum mood and anxiety disorders: A clinician's guide*. Boston, MA: Jones & Bartlett.

Cox, J. L., Holden, J. M., & Sagovsky, R. (1987). Detection of postnatal depression. Development of the 10-item Edinburgh postnatal depression scale. *British Journal of Psychiatry, 150*, 782–786.

Doucet, S., Jones, I., Letourneau, N., Dennis, C. L., & Blackmore, E. R. (2011). Interventions for the prevention and treatment of postpartum psychosis: A systematic review. *Archives of Women's Mental Health, 14*(2), 89–98.

Ebeid, E., Nassif, N., & Sinha, P. (2010). Prenatal depression leading to postpartum psychosis. *Journal of Obstetrics and Gynaecology, 30*(5), 435–438.

Field, T. (2010). Postpartum depression effects on early interactions, parenting, and safety practices: A review. *Infant Behavior & Development, 33*(1), 1–6.

Flynn, H. A., Sexton, M., Ratliff, S., Porter, K., & Zivin, K. (2011). Comparative performance of the Edinburgh postnatal depression scale and the patient health questionnaire-9 in pregnant and postpartum women seeking psychiatric services. *Psychiatry Research, 187*, 130–134.

Fairbrother, N., & Woody, S. R. (2008). New mothers' thoughts of harm related to the newborn. *Archives of Women's Mental Health, 11*(3), 221–229.

Fischbach, F., & Dunning, M. B. (2008). *A manual of laboratory and diagnostic tests* (8th ed.). Philadelphia, PA: Lippincott Williams & Wilkins.

Gavin, N. I., Gaynes, B. N., Lohr, K. N., Meltzer-Brody, S., Gartlehner, G., & Swinson, T. (2005). Perinatal depression: A systematic review of prevalence and incidence. *Obstetrics and Gynecology, 106*, 1071–1083.

Gjerdingen, D., Crow, S., McGovern, P., Miner, M., & Center, B. (2009). Postpartum depression screening at well-child visits: Validity of a 2-question screen and the PHQ-9. *Annals of Family Medicine, 7*, 63–70.

Hale, T. W. (2004). Maternal medications during breastfeeding. *Clinical Obstetrics and Gynecology, 47(3)*, 697–711.

Howard, M., Battle, C. L., Pearlstein, T., & Rosene-Montella, K. (2006) A psychiatric mother-baby unit for pregnant and postpartum women. *Archives of Women's Mental Health, 9*, 213–218.

Kroenke, K., Spitzer, R. L., & Williams, J. B. W. (2001). The PHQ-9: Validity of a brief depression severity measure. *Journal of General Internal Medicine, 16*, 606–613.

Kroenke, K., Spitzer, R. L., & Williams, J. B. (2003). The patient health questionnaire-2: Validity of a two-item depression screener. *Medical Care, 41*, 1284–1292.

Lindahl, V., Pearson, J. L., & Colpe, L. (2005). Prevalence of suicidality during pregnancy and the postpartum. *Archives of Women's Mental Health, 8*, 77–87.

Munk-Olsen, T., Laursen, T. M., Pedersen, C. B., Mors, O., & Mortensen, P. B. (2006). New parents and mental disorders: A population-based register study, *Journal of American Medical Association, 296*, 2582–2589.

Pearlstein, T., Howard, M., Salisbury, A., & Zlotnick, C. (2009). Postpartum depression. *American Journal of Obstetrics and Gynecology,* 200, 357–364.

Ross, L. E., & McLean, L. M. (2006). Anxiety disorders during pregnancy and the postpartum period: A systematic review. *Journal of Clinical Psychiatry, 67*, (*8*), 1285–1298.

Vesga-Lopez, O., Blanco, C., Keyes, K., Olfson, M., Grant, B. F., & Hasin, D. S. (2008). Psychiatric disorders in pregnant and postpartum women in the United States. *Archives of General Psychiatry, 65(7)*, 805–815.

Zambaldi, C. F., Cantilino, A., Montenegro, A. C., Paes, J. A., de Albuquerque, T. L. C., & Sougey, E. B. (2009). Postpartum obsessive-compulsive disorder: Prevalence and clinical characteristics. *Comprehensive Psychiatry, 50(6)*, 503–509.

Critical Postpartum Medical Complications

30

Courtney Clark Bilodeau and Srilakshmi Mitta

The postpartum woman who presents to triage can be a clinical challenge. Common postpartum complaints can result from benign causes in the postpartum course or from a serious, potentially life-threatening complication. For example, a postpartum woman complaining of fatigue and dyspnea may be mildly anemic and sleep deprived or could be symptomatic from a pulmonary embolism or congestive heart failure. Triage clinicians must be thorough in their history taking and physical examination, and quickly determine the appropriate clinical management. Three of the most critical conditions in postpartum that a triage clinician may face are cardiomyopathy, deep vein thrombosis, and pulmonary embolism.

PERIPARTUM CARDIOMYOPATHY

Maternal hemodynamics rapidly change post delivery. Cardiac output temporarily increases immediately following birth secondary to a decompression of the vena cava from the gravid uterus and auto transfusion of utero-placental blood to the intravascular space. Over several days, the cardiac output and maternal heart rate decrease to prepregnancy levels. Postpartum diuresis peaks by the fifth postpartum day and lasts for several weeks (Davies & Herbert, 2007). A postpartum woman without underlying cardiac disease can typically handle these cardiovascular changes without difficulty. In cases of a more complicated course, such as with preeclampsia and diastolic dysfunction, symptomatic pulmonary edema can occur. Postpartum heart failure can also be caused by the rare idiopathic condition of peripartum cardiomyopathy (PPCM). PPCM is defined as a dilated cardiomyopathy causing heart failure in the last month of pregnancy or within 5 months postpartum. The diagnosis requires no other identifiable cause of heart failure or recognizable heart disease prior to the last month of pregnancy. Diagnostic criteria include echocardiographic findings of left ventricular (LV) systolic dysfunction with an LV ejection fraction (EF) less than 45% (Pearson et al., 2000). In 2005, data from an epidemiologic study described women diagnosed with cardiomyopathy earlier in pregnancy (pregnancy-associated cardiomyopathy) and had similar presentations and outcomes as traditional PPCM patients. The authors suggested that the two forms of idiopathic cardiomyopathy may be within a spectrum of the same disease (Elkayam et al., 2005). A more recent definition proposed by the Heart Failure Association of the European Society of Cardiology Working Group excludes women who develop cardiomyopathy earlier in pregnancy. The group also suggested that LV dilation may not always be found on echocardiograph (Sliwa et al., 2010).

The etiology of PPCM is unknown and multiple factors may contribute to its pathogenesis. Some proposed hypotheses include apoptosis (Sliwa et al., 2006), oxidative stress (Hilfiker-Kleiner, Sliwak, & Drexler, 2007), and maternal immune response to fetal antigens (Nelson, 1998; Pearson et al., 2000). Genetic factors may also play a part in PPCM development (Morales et al., 2010; van Spaendonck-Zwarts, 2010). Risk factors for the development of PPCM are listed in Exhibit 30.1.

PRESENTING SYMPTOMATOLOGY

The clinical presentation of PPCM is highly variable. Symptoms can often be confused with benign peripartum complaints. The most common presenting symptoms of PPCM are noted in Exhibit 30.2.

HISTORY AND DATA COLLECTION

The woman suspected of having PPCM warrants a thorough history taking regarding the pregnancy as well as the labor and delivery. The woman's family medical history is important, especially regarding cardiac diseases including dilated cardiomyopathy and sudden cardiac death. Social history includes activity level prior to and during pregnancy to contrast with current exercise capacity. Questions regarding illicit drug and alcohol use are also imperative. It is recommended that the time course for the woman's complaints is clearly recorded.

PHYSICAL EXAMINATION

There is a wide range of objective findings that can help to diagnosis PPCM. Increased heart rate and respiratory rate and a decreased pulse oximetry may be found. Blood pressure can vary, including postural hypotension (Sliwa et al., 2010). The jugular venous pressure may be increased. Cardiac auscultation findings include systolic ejection murmurs and a prominent pulmonic valve component of the second heart sound and a third heart sound. If there

EXHIBIT 30.1

Risk Factors for the Development of PPCM

- Advanced maternal age
- Multiparity
- Multifetal pregnancy
- African descent
- Preeclampsia and eclampsia
- Prolonged tocolytic therapy with beta-agonists

Source: Elkayam et al. (2005), Gentry et al. (2010), and Lampert et al. (1993).

is cardiomegaly, the point of maximal impulse (PMI)/apical impulse can be displaced. Pulmonary auscultation may reveal wheezes and rales. Peripheral edema, ascites, and hepatomegaly may also be found. Preeclamptic women are commonly hyperreflexive.

LABORATORY AND IMAGING STUDIES

Electrocardiograms (ECGs) are frequently obtained in suspected cases of PPCM. Exhibit 30.3 lists potential findings on ECG.

Laboratory values of brain natriuretic peptide (BNP) and troponin-I may be elevated in PPCM. Preeclampsia is both a risk factor for the development of cardiomyopathy and can cause non-PPCM symptomatic pulmonary edema. It is critical to exclude the diagnosis of preeclampsia when determining if a woman has PPCM. In addition to history and physical examination, laboratory studies used to diagnose preeclampsia include creatinine, hemoglobin, platelets, liver enzymes, urine protein, and uric acid.

EXHIBIT 30.2

Common Symptoms of PPCM

- Dyspnea
- Decreased exercise tolerance
- Pedal edema
- Orthopnea
- Paroxysmal nocturnal dyspnea
- Dizziness
- Chest pain
- Palpitations
- Cough
- Hemoptysis
- Fatigue
- Abdominal pain

Source: Sliwa et al. (2010)

EXHIBIT 30.3

Potential ECG Findings in PPCM

- Normal (no abnormalities)
- Tachycardia
- Atrial Fibrillation
- Low Voltage
- Anterior precordium Q waves
- PR and QRS interval prolongation
- Voltage criteria consistent with LV hypertrophy
- ST-T wave abnormalities

Source: Sliwa et al. (2010).

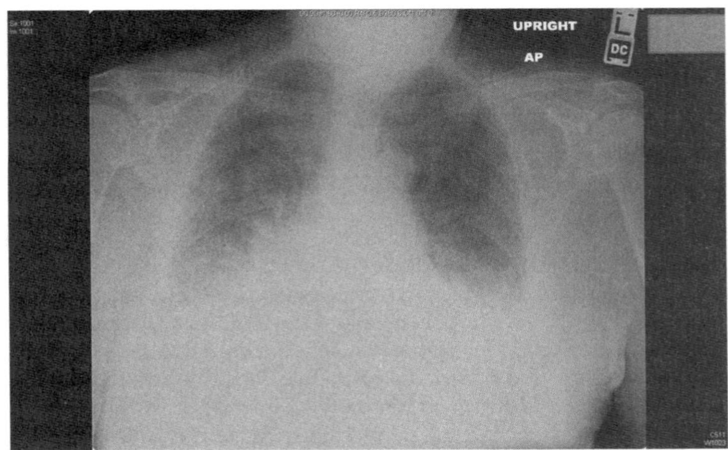

FIGURE 30.1 Chest radiograph: Cardiomegaly and pulmonary congestion.

Source: Courtesy of the Department of Radiology, Women & Infants Hospital, Providence, RI.

Chest radiography in women with PPCM may show enlarged cardiac silhouette, patchy lower lung infiltrates, vascular cephalization, and pleural effusions. Figure 30.1 shows cardiomegaly, and pulmonary congestion.

An echocardiograph is recommended for all peripartum women suspected of having PPCM. An immediate ("bedside") echocardiograph can be useful to rapidly diagnose and evaluate the severity of cardiac dysfunction. The echocardiography findings may include reduction in contractility, LV enlargement, reduction in LVEF, regional abnormalities in systolic wall thickening, pericardial effusion, left atrial enlargement, and mitral and tricuspid valve regurgitation (Elkayam et al., 2005; Modi et al., 2009; Sliwa et al., 2010).

Incidence of venous thromboembolism (VTE) is increased in women with PPCM. If indicated, evaluation for embolic phenomena is performed (see deep venous thrombosis [DVT]/Pulmonary embolism [PE] below).

DIFFERENTIAL DIAGNOSIS

The differential diagnoses for PPCM include preexisting cardiomyopathy, hypertensive heart disease, congenital heart disease, myocardial infarction, and pulmonary embolism. Noncardiogenic pulmonary edema, most commonly secondary to preeclampsia, tocolytics, or sepsis must be ruled out as an alternative diagnosis (Sliwa et al., 2010).

CLINICAL MANAGEMENT AND FOLLOW-UP

The initial management goals for postpartum PPCM are to stabilize the woman's cardiovascular status and provide symptomatic relief. The woman is placed on continuous cardiac and pulse oximetry monitoring and supplemental oxygen is administered. Intravenous access is obtained and a urinary catheter is placed to monitor urine output. Consultation with specialists may include an obstetric internist (internist with special training in the care of medical illness in pregnancy), pulmonary critical care specialist, cardiologist, and maternal fetal medicine specialist.

Pharmacologic therapy in postpartum PPCM is similar to nonobstetric congestive heart failure treatment plans (Dickstein et al. 2008; Sliwa et al., 2010). In suspected preeclamptic women, who are frequently intravascularly depleted and have decreased renal function, the medication dose and frequency of administration may need to be adjusted. Morphine can be cautiously administered for anxiety and pain control. Diuresis with loop diuretics (furosemide with a starting dose of 10 mg) is a first-line treatment. Angiotensin-converting enzyme inhibitors (ACEI) are used for afterload reduction and are preferred over the vasodilators, such as hydralazine, which are typically used instead of ACEIs during pregnancy. Beta-blockers help to improve systolic function in the long-term and are typically given after the acute decompensation of heart failure has resolved, and the patient is euvolemic. Digoxin and inotropes may be used in select cases for acute heart failure management. Thromboprophylaxis is frequently considered due to the high risk for thrombus formation, especially in the postpartum state. Once stabilized, the postpartum woman with PPCM is transferred to the appropriate inpatient service for further management.

POSTPARTUM DVT AND PULMONARY EMBOLISM

Pregnancy and the puerperium (the 6–8week postpartum period between childbirth and the return of the uterus to its normal size) are times of increased risk for VTE secondary to fulfilling Virchow's Triad of hypercoagulability, venous stasis, and vascular injury (Bagot & Arya, 2008). While VTE is relatively rare in otherwise healthy young women, it can be up to 10 times more common in pregnant women of similar age. In fact VTE has been recognized for many years as a leading cause of maternal morbidity and mortality worldwide, especially among developed and developing nations (Andersen, Steffensen, Sorensen, Nielsen, & Olsen 1998; CMACE, 2011).

Population-based studies have shown an increasing incidence of VTE in pregnancy, which may be due in part to increasing vigilance on the part of clinicians as well as improved diagnostic techniques and standards (Andersen et al., 1998; Heit et al., 2005). In addition to this, the postpartum period has been identified as a time of even greater risk, with one study showing that the annual incidence was 5 times higher among postpartum women than pregnant women (Heit et al., 2005). Additional risk factors for postpartum VTE are essential determinants for diagnoses, treatment, and outcomes and can be found in Exhibit 30.4.

PRESENTING SYMPTOMATOLOGY

DVT can cause various symptoms including lower extremity swelling, pain, erythema, warmth, or induration. It is critical to remember that DVT during pregnancy and the postpartum period may develop in uncommon locations such as pelvic or abdominal veins. Therefore, women may present with atypical complaints such as abdominal, groin, thigh, buttock, or flank pain.

PE can present with nonspecific symptoms making the diagnosis in both pregnant and nonpregnant patients difficult. PE should be considered if the presenting complaint includes chest pain or heaviness, shortness of breath, dyspnea (at rest and on exertion), hemoptysis, palpitations, or syncope. Most

EXHIBIT 30.4

Risk Factors for Postpartum VTE

- Past history of VTE
- Family history of VTE
- Thrombophilia
- Obesity
- Age > 35 years
- Tobacco use
- Cesarean section
- Preeclampsia
- Prolonged bed rest or immobility

Source: RCOG (2009).

of these symptoms are common in normal pregnancy and some are present postpartum, making the diagnosis even more challenging.

DIFFERENTIAL DIAGNOSIS

Differential diagnosis for DVT includes cellulitis, superficial thrombophlebitis, lymphedema, musculoskeletal strain, ruptured baker's cyst, or trauma. PE has a wider differential and can include any other cardiopulmonary processes such as pulmonary edema (both cardiogenic and noncardiogenic), pneumothorax, pneumonia, pleurisy, myocardial infarction, and pericarditis.

HISTORY AND DATA COLLECTION

The diagnosis of VTE starts with a detailed history, which will then guide the clinician with further options for future workup and management. Thorough information about the woman's presenting complaints and pregnancy course is critical. Personal history of a past VTE, superficial thrombophlebitis, pregnancy loss, or any inherited or acquired thrombophilias can further narrow the differential. Finally, it is imperative to ask about a family history concerning thromboses and social history regarding smoking and daily activities.

PHYSICAL EXAMINATION

DVT can present with lower extremity edema (pitting and nonpitting), erythema, warmth, and palpation of a cord or induration. Physical examination findings such as Homan's sign (pain with forced dorsiflexion of the ankle) has traditionally been recommended, however, this maneuver has been shown to have low specificity and sensitivity when diagnosing DVT.

As opposed to DVT, PE can present with a variety of symptoms including fever, tachypnea, tachycardia, hypoxia (at rest and exertion), pleuritic chest pain, rales, loud second heart sound, cough, arrhythmia, syncope, or cardiopulmonary collapse.

DVTs are largely diagnosed with a combination of history, examination, and a confirmatory imaging study. The gold standard for the diagnosis is venography; however, because of ready availability, lack of radiation and high specificity, compression ultrasound (CUS) has become the initial test of choice. CUS is useful in detecting femoral and popliteal venous thrombi. However, if clinical suspicion for DVT is high or if a more proximal vessel is suspected, further imaging is warranted (Cogo et al., 1998). Serial ultrasounds (over a 2-week period) to identify a clot as it progresses or pelvic/abdominal imaging may be necessary to detect a possible thrombus.

D-Dimer, a fibrin degradation product, can be elevated in the setting of an acute clot. It is, however, also elevated in many situations including trauma, postsurgery, malignancy, pregnancy, and the puerperium. D-Dimer testing, using an enzyme-linked immunosorbent assay (ELISA) is highly sensitive with a good negative predictive value, which, in conjunction with a low clinical suspicion for PE, can help rule out PE in nonpregnant patients. D-Dimer use in pregnancy and the puerperium has not been sufficiently studied and can be misleading since elevation is not indicative of acute thrombosis.

When PE is suspected, it is crucial to accurately make the diagnosis, but also exclude other potential etiologies for the woman's complaint. Initial workup includes an arterial blood gas, ECG, and chest x-ray, although none of these tests should be used to definitively rule in or rule out a PE (Rodger et al., 2000). In nonpregnant patients, the incidence of sinus tachycardia and evidence of right heart strain (i.e., right bundle branch block [RBBB]) was found to be slightly increased in patients with PE. Chest x-rays are not helpful in diagnosing a PE but rather can be used to help exclude other possible diagnoses such as pneumothorax, pulmonary edema, or pneumonia.

The biggest challenge for a clinician when trying to diagnose a pregnant woman with PE is determining what imaging test will be most useful and also minimize fetal radiation exposure. The scope of this chapter will focus on postpartum diagnosis of VTE; therefore, fetal exposure other than via breast milk is not an issue.

Both ventilation perfusion (V/Q) scan and computed tomography pulmonary angiogram (CTPA) are acceptable options for use in the postpartum period, and the decision to use one over the other can vary based on institution. CTPA, however, is being used more frequently due to ease of testing and a higher sensitivity and specificity over V/Q scans (Rathbun, Raskob, & Whitsett, 2000). Figures 30.2 depicts filling defects in segmental branches of the pulmonary arteries, consistent with the diagnosis of PE.

Another advantage of CTPA is its ability to detect other possible cardiopulmonary diagnoses such as pulmonary edema or even aortic dissection. In spite of all its benefits, CTPA does confer an increased amount of radiation to lactating breast tissue and is relatively contraindicated in the setting of renal failure, at which point V/Q scan may be a more suitable alternative.

Finally, it is critical to ask whether the woman is breast-feeding or not, as this can be of great concern to a new mother. Small amounts of iodinated or gadolinium based contrast agents reach breast milk. The American College of Obstetrics and Gynecology and the American Association of

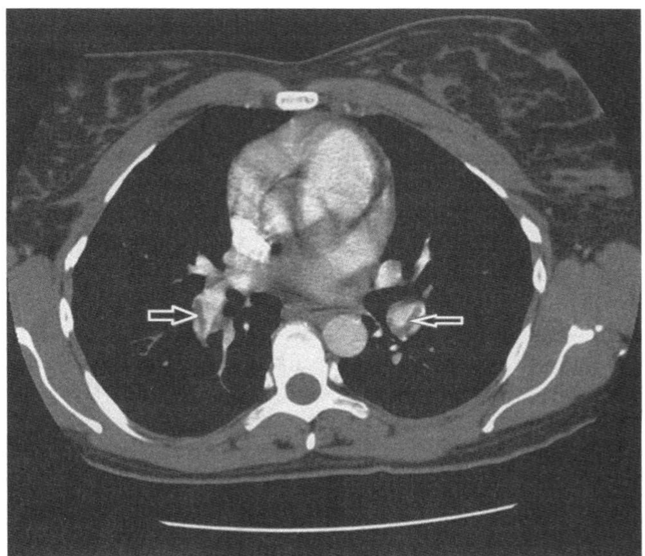

FIGURE 30.2 CTPA of PE.

Source: Courtesy of the Department of Radiology, Women & Infants Hospital, Providence, RI.

Family Physicians both support continued breast-feeding without interruption in lactating women who receive iodinated contrast or gadolinium. If a mother feels uncomfortable, an alternative option is to discard pumped milk for 24 hours postprocedure (Ito, 2000; Webb, Thomsen, Morcos, & Members of Contrast Media Safety Committee of European Society of Urogenital Radiology (ESUR) 2005).

CLINICAL MANAGEMENT AND FOLLOW-UP

Once a diagnosis of VTE has been established, initial care can be initiated in either an inpatient or outpatient setting and is mostly dependent on a patient's clinical stability. For many postpartum women, being away from their newborn can cause much distress and anxiety, therefore whenever clinically possible, outpatient care is considered.

Therapeutic anticoagulation can last for 3 to 6 months and the most commonly used treatment options include low-molecular-weight heparin (LMWH) and warfarin. Unfractionated heparin (UH) is rarely used in the postpartum period, unless the woman is deemed at high risk of bleeding, and therefore, the potential rapidity of reversal of UH may be an advantage. LMWH is a more convenient and safe option. Due to the ease of administration, pharmacokinetic predictability and decreased risk of heparin-induced thrombocytopenia (HIT) and osteopenia, LMWH is an ideal choice for initial outpatient therapy of postpartum VTE (Greer & Nelson-Piercy, 2005). LMWH can be continued for the complete duration of therapy; however, transition to warfarin for the long-term is another option.

At baseline, lab work includes a complete blood count (CBC) and coagulation studies including prothrombin time (PT) and activated partial thromboplastin time (aPTT). Close outpatient follow-up with a hematologist or the patient's primary care doctor is essential to ensure proper monitoring of anticoagulation levels and for potential complications such as bleeding or HIT. Thrombophilia workup is debatable and not all tests are useful in the setting of recent pregnancy and/or recent thrombus, thereby warranting good follow-up with a specialist in the field. Postpartum VTE can be a difficult diagnosis to make; however, better care for new mothers can be given with increased education and awareness by providers as well as improving laboratory and imaging studies.

REFERENCES

Andersen, B. S., Steffensen, F. H., Sorensen, H. T., Nielsen, G. L., & Olsen, J. (1998). The cumulative incidence of venous thromboembolism during pregnancy and puerperium—An 11 year Danish population based study of 63,300 pregnancies. *Acta Obstetricia et Gynecologica Scandinavica, 77*, 170–173.

Bagot, C. N. & Arya, R. (2008). Virchow and his triad: A question of attribution. *British Journal of Haematology, 143*, 180–190

Centre for Maternal and Child Enquiries (CMACE). (2011). Saving Mothers' Lives: Reviewing maternal deaths to make motherhood safer: 2006–08. The Eighth Report on Confidential Enquiries into Maternal Deaths in the United Kingdom. *British Journal of Obstetrics and Gyneacology, 118*, 1–203.

Cogo, A., Lensing, A. W., Koopman, M. M., Piovella, F., Siragusa, S., Wells, P. S.... Prandoni, P. (1998) Compression ultrasonography for diagnostic management of patients with clinically suspected deep vein thrombosis: Prospective cohort study. *British Medical Journal, 316(7124)*, 17–20.

Davies, G., & Herbert, W. (2007). Assessment and management of cardiac disease in pregnancy. *Journal of Obstetrics and Gynaecology Canada, 29*(4), 331–336.

Dickstein, K., Cohen-Solal, A., Filippatos, G., McMurray, J. J., Ponikowski, P., Poole-Wilson, P. A.... ESC Committee for Practice Guidelines (CPG). (2008). ESC guidelines for the diagnosis and treatment of acute and chronic heart failure 2008: The Task Force for the diagnosis and treatment of acute and chronic heart failure 2008 of the European Society of Cardiology. Developed in collaboration with the Heart Failure Association of the ESC (HFA) and endorsed by the European Society of Intensive Care Medicine (ESICM). *European Journal of Heart Failure, 10*, 933–989.

Elkayam, U., Akhter, M. W., Singh, H., Khan, S., Bitar, F., Hameed, A., & Shotan, A. (2005). Pregnancy-associated cardiomyopathy: clinical characteristics and a comparison between early and late presentation. *Circulation, 111(16)*, 2050–2055.

Gentry, M. B., Dias, J. K., Luis, A., Patel, R., Thornton, J., & Reed, G. L. (2010). African-American women have a higher risk for developing peripartum cardiomyopathy. *Journal of American College of Cardiology, 55*(7), 654–659.

Greer, I. A., & Nelson-Piercy, C. (2005). Low-molecular-weight heparins for thromboprophylaxis and treatment of venous thromboembolism in pregnancy: A systematic review of safety and efficacy. *Blood, 106*(2), 401–407.

Heit, J. A., Kobbervig, C. E., James, A. H., Petterson, T. M., Bailey, K. R., & Melton, L. J. 3rd. (2005). Trends in the incidence of venous thromboembolism during pregnancy or postpartum: A 30-year population-based study. *Annals of Internal Medicine, 143(10)*, 697–706.

Hilfiker-Kleiner, D., Sliwak, K., & Drexler, H. (2008). Peripartum cardiomyopathy recent insights in its pathophysiology. *Trends in Cardiovascular Medicine, 18*,173–179.

Ito, S. (2000). Drug therapy: Drug therapy for breast-feeding women. *New England Journal of Medicine, 343*, 118–126.

Modi, K. A., Illum, S., Jariatul, K., et al. (2009). Poor outcome of indigent patients with peripartum cardiomyopathy in the United States. *American Journal of Obstetrics and Gynecology, 201*, 171.e1–171.e5.

Morales, A., Painter, T., Li, R., Siegfried, J. D., Li, D., Norton, N., & Hershberger, R. E. (2010). Rare variant mutations in pregnancy-associated or peripartum cardiomyopathy. *Circulation, 121(20)*, 2176–2182.

Nelson, J. L. (1998). Pregnancy, persistent microchimerism, and autoimmune disease. *Journal of the American Medicine and Women's Association, 53*,31.

Pearson, G. D., Veille, J. C., Rahimtoola, S., Hsia, J., Oakley, C. M., Hosenpud, J. D.,... Baughman, K. L. (2000) Peripartum cardiomyopathy: National heart, lung, and blood institute and office of rare diseases (national institutes of health) workshop recommendations and review. *Journal of American Medical Association, 283*, 1183–1188.

Rathbun, S. W., Raskob, G. E., & Whitsett, T. L. (2000). Sensitivity and specificity of helical computed tomography in the diagnosis of pulmonary embolism: a systematic review. *Annals of Internal Medicine, 132(3)*, 227–232.

Rodger, M., Makropoulos, D., Turek, M., Quevillon, J., Raymond, F., Rasuli, P., & Wells, P. S. (2000). Diagnostic value of the electrocardiogram in suspected pulmonary embolism. *American Journal of Cardiology, 86(7)*, 807–809, A10.

Royal College of Obstetricians & Gynaecologists (RCOG). (2009). *Reducing the risk of thromboembolism during pregnancy, birth and the puerperium. Guideline no. 37.* London: *RCOG*.

Sliwa, K., Forster, O., Libhaber, E., Fett, J. D., Sundstrom, J. B., Hilfiker-Kleiner, D., & Ansari, A. A. (2006). Peripartum cardiomyopathy: Inflammatory markers as predictors of outcome in 100 prospectively studied patients. *European Heart Journal, 27*, 441–446.

Sliwa, K., Hilfiker-Kleiner, D., Petrie, M. C., Mebazaa, A., Pieske, B., Buchmann, E.... Heart Failure Association of the European Society of Cardiology Working Group on Peripartum Cardiomyopathy. (2010). Current state of knowledge on aetiology, diagnosis, management, and therapy of peripartum cardiomyopathy: A position statement from the Heart Failure Association of the European Society of Cardiology Working Group on peripartum cardiomyopathy. *European Journal of Heart Failure, 12(8)*,767–778.

van Spaendonck-Zwarts, K. Y., van Tintelen, J. P., van Veldhuisen, D. J., van der Werf, R., Jongbloed, J. D., Paulus, W. J.,... van den Berg, M. P. (2010) Peripartum cardiomyopathy as a part of familial dilated cardiomyopathy. *Circulation, 121(20)*, 2169–2175.

Webb, J. A., Thomsen, H. S., Morcos, S. K., & Members of Contrast Media Safety Committee of European Society of Urogenital Radiology (ESUR). (2005). The use of iodinated and gadolinium contrast media during pregnancy and lactation. *European Radiology, 15*, 1234–1240.

Index